ANTI/VAX

A VOLUME IN THE SERIES

The Culture and Politics of Health Care Work

Edited by Suzanne Gordon and Sioban Nelson

For a list of books in the series, visit our website at cornellpress.cornell.edu.

ANTI/VAX

Reframing the Vaccination Controversy

BERNICE L. HAUSMAN

ILR PRESS

AN IMPRINT OF

CORNELL UNIVERSITY PRESS

ITHACA AND LONDON

First published 2019 by Cornell University Press

Printed in the United States of America

Library of Congress Cataloging-in-Publication Data

Names: Hausman, Bernice L., author.
Title: Anti/vax : reframing the vaccine controversy /
    Bernice L. Hausman.
Description: Ithaca, New York : ILR Press, an imprint of Cornell
    University Press, 2019. | Series: The culture and politics of health
    care work | Includes bibliographical references and index.
Identifiers: LCCN 2018052013 (print) | LCCN 2018052991 (ebook) |
    ISBN 9781501735639 (pdf) | ISBN 9781501735646 (ret) |
    ISBN 9781501735622 | ISBN 9781501735622 (cloth ; alk. paper)
Subjects: LCSH: Anti-vaccination movement—United States. |
    Vaccination—Social aspects—United States. | Vaccination of
    children—Social aspects—United States.
Classification: LCC RA638 (ebook) | LCC RA638 .H38 2019 (print) |
    DDC 614.4/7083—dc23
LC record available at https://lccn.loc.gov/2018052013

In memory of Rose Gomez Hausman

CONTENTS

PREFACE AND ACKNOWLEDGMENTS

While I was working on this book, one of my brothers took ill. We were together for a family vacation on Long Island during Labor Day weekend. He had been hiking in California a few weeks earlier, had a low fever and rash, and seemed to recover. Once on the East Coast, he became very sick: lethargic, nauseated, and feverish. He had the chills and shook violently at times. By the time we took him to the emergency room at a local hospital, he was dehydrated and quite wobbly.

We have little experience with serious illness in my family. My brother's illness—undiagnosed initially despite a full tick panel and tests for other infectious diseases—was a startling and illuminating experience for someone writing about vaccination controversy. My brother thought for sure he had West Nile virus disease (and later tests proved him right), as he had encountered unusually large numbers of mosquitoes during his camping trip, but the infectious disease doctors at the hospital didn't think so. Were they just oriented toward ticks because the problem on Long Island is Lyme disease? At dinner one night while he was still in the hospital, the rest of us talked about Lyme disease on the island and the difficulty of diagnosing and treating it. "If I get a tick bite," my other brother announced, "I am just going to demand doxycycline, right away."

My brother's illness was scary. It is the quintessential experience of infectious disease that vaccines are meant to guard against. Pain, fear, and uncertainty characterized the immediate experience of illness for my brother, who endured strange symptoms that he had trouble describing, and fear and uncertainty definitely dominated the experience for the rest of us. I resisted the impulse to google his symptoms and try to figure out what was going on, after the one night I spent reading about tick-borne diseases on the CDC's website. Figuring out what was going on was the job of the doctors at the hospital, and surely they knew more than I did about infectious disease in the United States and elsewhere (clearly they did, as one of the docs told us his theory of how Lyme infection was carried to Iceland by puffin birds). But the impulse was there, and I was aware that I should stifle it. (Fortunately, I had other work to do during long boring hours at the hospital.) And yet, in the end, those smart doctors were wrong; not respecting my brother's explanation for what was wrong with him, they didn't do the easy test that would have acknowledged his account. He had to go back to Los Angeles and his own doctor to get the right diagnosis, and even then he had to fight to get tested for West Nile.

Vaccines, in general, are meant to end this kind of experience by preventing infectious diseases and the disruptions they cause in people's lives (including ending many of those lives). Having gone through the scary part of that experience, and being now on the other side, as my brother is well, I see the attractiveness of vaccination for West Nile, Lyme, or other insect-borne infectious diseases. He keeps saying that he might never go camping again, which is hard for me to believe, since it is something he has enjoyed for decades and now he is immune to West Nile virus. After having gone through this experience, though, who would want to risk something like it again? If a vaccine could make such activities safer, who wouldn't want it?

Four months after my brother's illness, just as I was starting the final revisions to this manuscript, my mother went to the hospital with a gastrointestinal bleed. I took the train from Roanoke to Philadelphia to help my father and spend time with her in the hospital. A biopsy of a lesion in her stomach came back with a diagnosis of large B-cell lymphoma.

A subsequent PET scan of her abdomen showed widely disseminated cancer. On a second trip north, I finished revisions to the conclusion when the train to Philadelphia got stopped in Washington because of a March snowstorm. My mother had decided that she wanted hospice care; then she stopped eating and drinking. Two weeks later, she passed away in her sleep.

There was nothing redeeming or valuable about her final illness, except that it was what she died of. My father kept talking about the fact that the cancer was discovered after it had spread, presumably as a way of understanding why my mother was in such discomfort, why she didn't want to undergo chemotherapy, why it was incurable. I think of it as his way of managing the situation and trying to control it: scientific medicine works if you can use it at the right time. Most of my mother's illness was very physical and very uncomfortable: her legs were swollen; she couldn't eat; she was nauseated, had diarrhea or constipation; and she was exhausted all the time. Mercifully, because she decided to take control of the situation, her suffering was limited. She initially entered the hospital on January 12, 2018. She passed away in hospice early in the morning of March 12, 2018, two weeks after deciding to die.

It was awful, and it was completely normal. My mother was eighty-nine years old. What did we think was going to happen? At some point, the body gives up, makes abnormal cells, calls it quits.

Illness is one of the fundamental dramas of human life. It is a reminder of our own mortality and a basic, humbling reminder of embodiment. When I think of the phrase *burden of disease*, this is what I think of—how much it hurts, how tired we are, how confusing it is to be so out of control, so weak, so uncaring about others. How being sick is burdensome—heavy, slow, and hard. The physicality of it is unrelenting.

My own feelings after these two experiences are unresolved. My brother's illness made me realize that we are vulnerable in ways I had known intellectually but not actually experienced. I learned that very healthy people can be struck by serious illness in unexpected ways. I entered that zone of fear and uncertainty that serious illness creates. These are emotions that modern technological advances protect us against, or at least aim to protect us against, with (fantasies of) control and regulation.

My mother's final illness I was more prepared for but still shocked by. Even though we know it will come, our mortality never ceases to startle us. Perhaps that is why the other illnesses along the way are so important—they prepare us, albeit incompletely, for the final one. They teach us what it is to be dependent, needy. They give us hope that we can pull through, even though, eventually, there will always be one time when we do not.

This book is dedicated to the memory of my mother, Rose Gomez Hausman, who faced her death squarely and fearlessly, indomitable to the end.

I had plenty of help writing this book, although the sentiments expressed in it are entirely my own. I started the Vaccination Research Group (VRG) in spring 2010, with the support of the Center for the Study of Rhetoric in Society in the English Department at Virginia Tech, then directed by Kelly Belanger. Karen Roberto, director of the Institute for Society, Culture, and the Environment at Virginia Tech, provided key funds to support my research. Heidi Lawrence was my first graduate assistant to work on this project, and her insights have been and will always be crucial to the way I understand vaccination controversy. Phil Hayek and Lenny Grant also assisted the VRG and propelled the research forward in significant ways. Tarryn Abrahams is an inspiration and the current emerging scholar who leads me to deeper understandings of vaccine skepticism than I would be capable of by myself. Other graduate students involved in the project include Amy Reed, Libby Anthony, Shelby Turner, Kari Putterman Campeau, Michelle Seref, and Lauren Fortenberry. Colleagues Clare Dannenberg, Susan West Marmagas, François Elvinger, and Molly O'Dell also contributed to this research. Rachel Wurster formatted the first draft and cleaned up the bibliography and notes for the initial submission to the press.

The following undergraduate students have been the primary researchers of the VRG, and all have influenced my understanding of vaccine skepticism: Erica Frempong, Jonathan Chapman, Lauren Cobert, Carly Smith, Andria Wallen, Megan Casady, Jessica Fuller, Leanne Shelley, Josh Trebach, Kelsey Soppet, Aubrey Sozer, Rachel Dinkins, Karen Spears, Olivia Kasik, Darya Nesterova, Sarah Brown, Erin Mack, Mecal Ghebremichael, Aimee Sutherland, Jonathan Lutton, Elena Patel, Varsh Peddireddy, James Foley, Kelsey Patel, Maggie Cashion, Nick Lucchesi, Jonathan Roberts, Erica Palladino, Kathryn Buss, Travertine Orndorff, Lakshya Ramani,

Prerna Das, Neil Feste, Margaret Eddleton. These students read original research articles; wrote annotations; created posters, information sheets, media analysis reports, and flowcharts; suggested novel analytical models; assisted in grant writing; created and maintained websites; conducted and analyzed surveys; and interviewed research participants. They were and are true collaborators, and working with them has been one of my greatest joys as a professor.

I have presented papers and posters on vaccination controversy to the American Society for Bioethics and Humanities, the International Conference Immunity and Modernity in Leuven, Belgium, the International Society for the Study of Narrative, the Virginia Humanities Conference, the National Immunization Conferences in Atlanta, the Centers for Disease Control and Prevention, Emory University, the Ohio State University, University of California-Riverside, and Georgia Tech. Colleagues at Virginia Tech—especially Kelly Pender, to whom I owe a huge debt of gratitude for listening to me think through various parts of this book—helped me through the arduous stages of planning and writing a book manuscript. Peter Potter, director of VT Publishing Strategies, gave me sage advice about pitching the book and led me to Cornell University Press. Sioban Nelson has been especially helpful as series editor, along with Suzanne Gordon, and Fran Benson was particularly supportive in how to craft the final arguments. Elena Conis, Melinda Wharton, Carol Colatrella, Jim Phelan, Chikako Takeshita, Lisa Keranen, Rebecca Garden, and many others provided opportunities for me to share my ideas as I worked out the arguments of this book.

I was fortunate to have research leave for a semester to muscle out a first draft of the book before I became chair of the Department of English at Virginia Tech. The Edward S. Diggs Professorship in the Humanities at Virginia Tech provided funds for research assistance and travel to conferences; my utmost gratitude goes to Hattie Diggs, who endowed the professorship in her husband's name, and to the faculty committee that conferred on me the honor of the position while I was writing this book.

My father looks forward to reading *Anti/Vax*, and I thank him for being patient with me while I bend his ear about modern medicine and its problems. I am sure that, as a retired physician, he bites his tongue often while in conversation with me. My brothers, sisters-in-law, cousins, spouse, and children all had to hear me talk about vaccines and vaccine skepticism for years; I thank them for their forbearance. Since most of them are vaccine supporters, these conversations helped me model arguments about vaccine skepticism for this audience.

The administrative staff in the Department of English at Virginia Tech—Patty Morse, Sandra Ross, Judy Grady, Sarah Helwig, Laura Ferguson, Bridget Szerszynski, Sally Shupe, and Kristen Cox—have all facilitated my work on this book, even if they didn't know it, by helping me be an effective administrator and supporting my work as chair.

Clair James lives with me and therefore with my books in all stages of development, providing editing advice, proofreading, and, in the case of this book, formatting the final manuscript and fixing the notes and bibliography. Thank you isn't enough for that kind of detailed attention to someone else's ideas and writing. My children, Rachel and Sam, became adults while I worked on *Anti/Vax*. I thank them for their patience with me and my academic obsessions.

Finally, I want to thank the many people who have agreed to talk to my research team about their beliefs and practices with respect to vaccination. These research participants provide the evidentiary basis for my arguments in chapter 10. Reading their interview transcripts, I have come to learn things about how people's ideas about health, illness, the body, and medicine are interwoven with personal experience and philosophical perspectives about life on planet Earth. I have learned things about myself and how I characterize the meaning of health and illness in my own life, and I have come to understand, at least a little bit, how to think generously about the beliefs of those whose practices are different from mine. I thank them for the courage to speak to us in a highly charged, inflammatory context in which some of the choices that some of them make are vilified. They have made the labor of writing *Anti/Vax* worthwhile.

ANTI/VAX

Introduction

Vaccination Stories and Why I Wrote This Book

The first definition of the word *safe* is "harmless." This definition
would imply that any negative consequence of a vaccine would make
the vaccine unsafe. Using this definition, no vaccine is 100 percent
safe. Almost all vaccines can cause pain, redness or tenderness at the
site of injection. And some vaccines cause more severe side effects. For
example, the original pertussis (whooping cough) vaccine could cause
persistent, inconsolable crying, high fever or seizures associated with
fever. Although none of these severe symptoms resulted in permanent
damage, they could be quite frightening to parents.

But, in truth, few things meet the definition of "harmless." Even
everyday activities contain hidden dangers. For example, every year
in the United States, 350 people are killed in bath- or shower-related
accidents, 200 people are killed when food lodges in their windpipe,
and 100 people are struck and killed by lightning. However, few of
us consider eating solid food, taking a bath, or walking outside on a
rainy day as unsafe activities. We just figure that the benefits of the
activity clearly outweigh the risks.

VACCINE EDUCATION CENTER, CHILDREN'S HOSPITAL OF
PHILADELPHIA, "VACCINE SAFETY: ARE VACCINES SAFE?"

In 2013, a physician committee at the Institute of Medicine reported
that there were fewer than 40 studies examining the safety of the
government's vaccine schedule for children under age six.

Only 40 studies.

Vaccine safety science has so many knowledge gaps that the Institute
of Medicine could not determine whether the timing and numbers

of vaccinations given to babies and young children is or is not responsible for the development of learning disabilities—asthma—autoimmunity—autism—developmental and behavior disorders—seizures—and other kinds of brain and immune system problems.

NATIONAL VACCINE INFORMATION CENTER,
"IS THE CHILDHOOD VACCINE SCHEDULE SAFE?"

This book explores the particular vaccination controversies that surround us today. *Anti/Vax* tries to answer questions that are not currently being asked and, in so doing, to reorient a stalemated public debate. Such a reorientation is necessary in order to move beyond the inflammatory impasse in which we find ourselves—speaking past one another, blaming, and settling into our entrenched positions. In writing this book, I do not proclaim which side is right, but investigate the controversy itself—why this debate, why so charged, and why now? I bring to the foreground ideas and values that are not fully understood or accounted for in media reporting and medical research. As a result, my discussion moves away from predictable arguments about scientific literacy and toward questions about people's worldviews and how they understand the role of health and illness in their lives. To have a meaningful public discussion about vaccination, its value, and its potential adverse consequences (both biological and social), we must do more to understand the minority positions that are so frequently vilified.

I study medical controversies in the public sphere as social controversies. This approach has bearing on what we think such controversies are about and how to remediate them. In rhetoric, an *exigence* is something that presents as a problem that can be addressed by communication or some form of discourse.[1] A problem that can be addressed nondiscursively does not present a rhetorical exigence. By analogy, a social controversy is something that must be addressed by social means—by social interaction, by community decision-making, by democratic deliberation and lawmaking, for example. It cannot be addressed by scientific or biomedical data dumped into the public sphere—it represents a problem *in society* that requires a social solution.

In eight years of research on vaccination controversy, I have found that it is energized by contrasting visions of human life on earth and the vulnerability of human bodies. In my view, vaccine skepticism is not a problem of misunderstanding evidence or thinking the wrong things. Vaccine resisters approach problems of the body in ways that can be at odds with mainstream scientific approaches. Their protest demands a *social* response because the problems they point toward are problems of social and political disagreement. After all, vaccination would not engender a controversy if there were not laws mandating certain vaccines for children's school entry or requiring vaccination for certain jobs. Vaccination controversy is ultimately a controversy about what it is to be a modern human, including questions about the responsibility one has to oneself, one's family and community, and the human community overall, as well as to the earth and its sustainability. That is, vaccination controversy, investigated deeply and with attention to the foundational concerns that animate it, concerns fundamental questions of human existence and flourishing. To describe it and also to suggest remedies to a stymied social debate, we have to think differently about what kind of problem it is, who is at fault for creating and/or sustaining the problem, and what should be done in order to make the problem go away.

I begin with my own vaccination story. Vaccination stories are stories of our relationships to both our health care providers and the state, our compliance or noncompliance with the law, our experiences and understanding of health and illness, and the way in which important medical events are recorded (or not) by our parents, health care providers, and selves. I had my children just as the current set of vaccination concerns was percolating, but, as I show in this book, vaccination concerns have been around as long as vaccinations have. It was my research into vaccination controversy that made me think about my own vaccination story and those of my children, not the other way around. Indeed, my research has complicated my feelings about vaccination, making me less likely to simply accept the idea that the answer to each and every infectious disease is vaccination, and more inquisitive about vaccines that are recommended to me as a patient.

My Vaccination Story

I was born early in 1962. The 1960s were a golden age for vaccine development, riding on the wave of successful polio vaccines in 1955 and 1961, and as vaccines were developed for measles, mumps, and rubella,

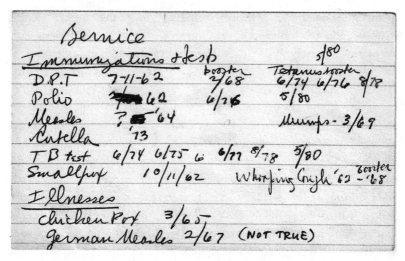

Fig. 1. Bernice Hausman handwritten vaccination record

vaccination became a routine aspect of pediatric care. In the 1970s, which I spent in elementary, middle, and high school, almost every state instituted mandatory vaccination against the routine illnesses of childhood.

My childhood vaccination record is an old 3 x 5 card in my mother's almost illegible handwriting. The card, given to me by my mother when my parents sold their big house to move to an apartment, complicates, rather than clarifies, my vaccine history:

Immunizations & tests

DPT 7–11–62 booster 2/68 Tetanus booster 6/74 6/76 8/78 5/80
Polio 62 booster 6/76 5/80
Measles ? '64
Mumps 3/69
Rubella '73
TB test 6/74 6/75 6 6/77 8/78 5/80
Smallpox 10/11/62
Whooping Cough '62 booster '68

Illnesses

Chicken Pox 3/65
German Measles 2/67 (NOT TRUE)*
*I wrote "(NOT TRUE)" next to German Measles record.

Why there is a rubella vaccination when there is also a date for when I had German measles is unclear to me: these are two names for the same disease. When I was a child, rubella vaccines were given at school; I remember being pulled out of line because my parents thought I'd had the illness. So why there is a record of vaccination in 1973 is a mystery. My parents don't remember. It may be that the vaccination became mandatory for school entry that year. Over a decade later I needed proof that I had been vaccinated against or had the measles to attend graduate school. Since I did not show antibodies to measles, I was vaccinated again, but that vaccination is not on my 3 x 5 card, nor in any other record that I can find.

I also have a smallpox "successful vaccination" certificate. The date on my mother's handwritten card is for October 11, 1962, while the certificate has October 12 as the date. Probably this distinction doesn't matter, but it does suggest a certain level of inaccuracy in my records.

Since childhood, I have had many more vaccinations, especially because I have traveled to Africa twice. These later vaccines (including yellow fever, required for a visa to visit Uganda, typhoid, hepatitis A and B, and meningococcal) now show up on my electronic medical record.

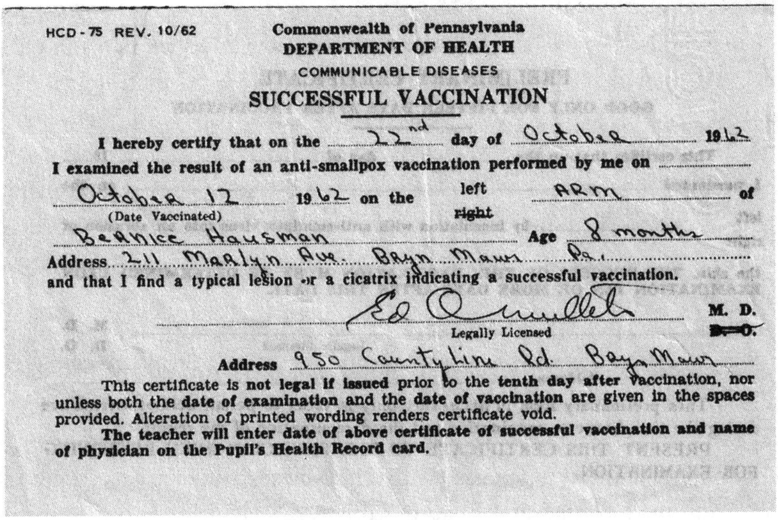

Fig. 2. Bernice Hausman smallpox "Successful Vaccination" certificate

I have another vaccination story about decisions I made about my children. Or, as the case may be, decisions I did not make. I learned to think of these as nondecisions when, about a decade after my kids were born, I realized that new parents were making actual decisions about the vaccinations their children received—refusing or delaying some.

My kids were born in the mid-1990s. At that time, some mainstream parents were concerned about vaccination, but these apprehensions were not widespread in my social circles. I was very conscious about decisions I made during my two pregnancies—decisions against technological intervention if I didn't think it was necessary and somewhat careful choices about what I ate while pregnant. While pregnant with my daughter during 1993 and 1994 in Chicago, I chose hospital-based midwives to supervise the pregnancy and birth and avoided as many screening tests as I could out of a desire to allow the pregnancy to proceed as naturally as possible. I didn't have any pain relief while in labor or during delivery, although, since I tested positive for Group B strep, I did have an antibiotic drip when I arrived at the hospital. Yet my daughter received the hepatitis B vaccine the day she was born—indeed, I really didn't think twice about it. When my son was born two years later in southwestern Virginia, I proceeded pretty much as I had with the first baby. In the local hospital, which I reached about twenty minutes before he was born, there was no time for the antibiotic drip. He got his Hep B vaccination on his second day of life.

My children's vaccination records are more orderly than mine, in part because their first vaccinations were recorded by a hospital nurse. My daughter's is written in a small booklet that also has her height and weight, tracked over her first year, as well as other subsequent vaccinations given her in the pediatric clinic of the University of Chicago hospital. Of course, both children also now have electronic medical records of their vaccinations reaching back into their infancy, although the electronic format has not always led to greater accuracy.

I didn't question their vaccinations, not when they were born nor during their childhoods. My son became ill and was hospitalized five days after he was born, with a fever of unknown origin, but we never suspected an adverse reaction to the hepatitis B vaccine. I was pleased that both my children got chicken pox, even though my son's experience was so miserable, and my husband and I had to take turns staying at home with the kids while they were sick. I took pictures of them in the bath to prove that they'd actually had it, as the varicella vaccine was new in the 1990s and beginning to be required for day care and school entry. My children are members of one of the last birth cohorts of American kids to get sick with chicken pox.

It was only when I realized that colleagues of mine with younger children, those born in the early 2000s, were concerned about vaccination, delaying their children's shots or simply worried each time their children had a vaccination, that I came to see that I had missed this particular concern even though I had been hypervigilant about other medical interventions that might have predisposed me to be concerned about vaccines. The signal event for me was hosting a baby shower for a friend and having a colleague give her two books about vaccine risks and alternative schedules. Yet knowing others were concerned didn't affect my own attitude a whole lot. The HPV vaccine Gardasil became available when my daughter was twelve, and my husband and I had a quick conversation about whether there was enough safety data before we signed her up.

I think that my own vaccination story is probably typical of Americans my age. Lots of late baby boomers, I imagine, have an index card with their vaccination record scrawled on it by their mother. We were vaccinated for smallpox, one of the last American cohorts to undergo that ordeal. Our more recent vaccination records are probably more orderly and stored electronically, yet we are often lax about adult vaccinations. Many television commercials for pertussis vaccinations are aimed at us. An adverse event makes us wary of particular vaccines, or perhaps vaccines in general. And we had chicken pox as children.

My vaccination stories date me, historically situating my experience but also distinguishing it from alternatives that might have been. As I show later in the book, the 1960s and 1970s were not void of vaccine skeptics, like Robert Mendelsohn, MD. If my parents had married earlier than 1955, I might have contracted measles or polio. If I had been born after 1971, I would not have been vaccinated for smallpox, and I might have been in that cohort of parents increasingly concerned about vaccines when I had my own kids in the early 2000s. And my parents might have joined Dissatisfied Parents Together, in 1982, over concerns about the DPT shot.

Except that my specific parents wouldn't have. As a pathologist and full believer in scientific medicine, my physician father is a staunch supporter of vaccines and always has been. Both my parents, born in the 1920s, had some of the diseases I was vaccinated against, and fear of polio certainly dominated my father's childhood. My father told me that whooping cough was the worst illness he can remember because it hurt so much. (He contracted the mumps as an adult, however, when my older brother, born too early for the vaccine, came down with it as a toddler.) Both my parents strongly support mainstream medicine, to the point that when I was pregnant with my first child, my father consistently referred to the certified nurse midwives who were my primary caregivers as the "ladies in the hospital" and worried every time I went to a chiropractor to help with my lower back pain.

My attitude toward vaccines as a new mother in the middle 1990s is somewhat less typical, however, as this was a time of increasing vaccination concern, and my dedication to breastfeeding and unmedicated childbirth put me in the kinds of social circles that, for some parents, facilitated forms of vaccine hesitancy. For whatever reason, these concerns did not surface in my experience. I came to vaccination controversy out of an intellectual interest in medical controversies in the public sphere, not from any personal experience of vaccine concern. Initially, I wanted to know why some people refused vaccination for their children. Eventually, I wanted to understand why the social context provided such a fertile ground for vaccine skepticism to flourish.

Understanding Vaccination Controversy

When I began my research into vaccination controversy in spring 2010 with an avid group of undergraduate students, I called us the Vaccine Refusal Research Group. It took a semester to realize that such a title was inappropriate for research that seeks to understand a public controversy. Sometime during the following year, we renamed it the Vaccination Research Group (VRG). In the time since, as the public discussion concerning vaccination in the United States has become more heated and media reporting increasingly inflammatory, it has become clear that a neutral approach to the topic is necessary in order to understand it. In the context of a research group filled with undergraduates who plan to go to medical school, this neutral stance has sometimes been a hard sell.

But as we developed several interview studies that invited nonvaccinating parents to tell their stories to us, the neutral research stance was crucial to convincing them to enroll in the studies and speak forthrightly about their experiences and beliefs. The inflammatory reporting context of vaccination controversy also became a focus of our research efforts, as we came to understand it as actively shaping the social context we seek to explain.

We have learned many things together. One is that vaccination concerns are as old as vaccination itself. Whether you date vaccination first to variolation, a centuries-old practice in which matter from active smallpox pustules was scraped into the skin of someone uninfected, or to Edward Jenner's experiments with cowpox in the 1790s, there have been people who objected to vaccination or worried about its consequences.[2] Since the nineteenth century, vaccination concerns have coalesced around two primary issues: (1) compulsory vaccination, and (2) adverse medical consequences. The first concern can be expressed in a number of ways; in the United States, it can be grounded in arguments about individual freedom, religious belief, or bodily autonomy. It might also be expressed as a concern about governmental overreach, or a conspiracy between the government and medical authorities or practitioners or between the government and the pharmaceutical industry. Consistent within this theme is a concern that families (not bureaucrats) should make decisions about the health care of their members, and that the government should not reach into domestic life to upset the authority of parents. In *Jacobson v. Massachusetts*, a United States Supreme Court decision in 1905, the court decided that government had the right to mandate vaccination to protect the public's health, but that the individual had the right to be exempted if vaccination posed a risk to his or her health as an individual.

Vaccine mandates were initially established in the nineteenth century to stop outbreaks of smallpox once they had started. After the advent of polio, measles, mumps, and rubella vaccines in the 1950s and 1960s, vaccine mandates were enacted across the United States in the 1970s and enforced through school-entry mandates in order to establish herd immunity against particular diseases and hasten the eradication of some, like measles.[3] Recently, mandates have come to the fore of public debate and legislative action because liberal exemption laws are perceived to allow parents to inappropriately opt out of vaccinating their children, thereby threatening herd immunity in particular localities. Getting rid of personal belief, philosophical, or religious exemptions is seen as getting tough on vaccination compliance and not allowing people's misinformed views to interfere with public health goals. In a particularly dramatic move in 2015, California ended its personal belief exemption for vaccination after an outbreak of measles originated at Disneyland the preceding December. This change of law has led to a political campaign to recall the bill's proponents in the legislature and rescind the law itself.

Current public discussion about mandates is dominated by arguments about adverse medical consequences. For parents concerned about vaccine injury, vaccine mandates enforce acceptance of potentially dangerous medical treatments. For the most strident supporters of vaccination, such concerns are the result of scientific illiteracy and lack of understanding that the benefits of vaccination far outweigh the risks. These vaccine advocates believe that the success of vaccines in lessening rates of infectious disease has resulted in a medical paradox in which the lack of disease incidence makes the vaccines seem riskier than the illnesses they prevent. To counteract this perceived ignorance, vaccine promoters try to convey clear risk/benefit scenarios for vaccination, hoping to persuade parents and others skeptical of vaccination that vaccination is not only a public good but a personal one as well.

The Vaccine Education Center (VEC) at the Children's Hospital of Philadelphia (CHOP) is a good example of this strategy, as the first epigraph to this chapter demonstrates. The brainchild of vaccine advocate and inventor Paul Offit, MD, the VEC defines vaccine safety in terms of its risk/benefit ratio, arguing that when a vaccine's benefits to a population outweigh its risks, the vaccine is safe. The question of whether a vaccine can cause a serious adverse event is always interpreted through this calculus. Thus, for example, rotavirus vaccines are understood to be safe even though they cause a small number of cases of intussusception (a rare form of bowel blockage), because rotavirus disease itself causes a small number of cases of intussusception. The VEC puts the matter this way, in two parts of its entry on rotavirus vaccine:

> Because both current rotavirus vaccines prevent rotavirus—and therefore prevent a rare form of intestinal blockage—the question became which was

rarer, intestinal blockage caused by the vaccine or by natural infection. The question can be answered by looking at what happened to the rate of intestinal blockage once vaccination started to replace natural infection. Most recent evidence shows that the incidence of intestinal blockage of infants in the United States has not increased because of rotavirus vaccines.

Without a rotavirus vaccine, approximately 55,000 to 70,000 children born in the United States would be hospitalized with rotavirus each year. Since the vaccine has been in use, this number has decreased by about 80 percent. There are no severe side effects from rotavirus vaccine. Therefore, the benefits of the rotavirus vaccine clearly outweigh the risks.[4]

However, vaccine-skeptical parents might see the issue differently.

For example, this standard framework of risk versus benefit will always suggest that choosing against vaccination is choosing irrationally because to be approved vaccines must show that adverse reactions to them are less dangerous, across the population, than the diseases they protect against. Such evidence is a requirement of FDA licensure. And the solution to fears of vaccine risk within this framework is to educate about scientific approaches to risk. If the number of cases of intussusception has not increased with the widespread use of the vaccine, and the vaccine prevents serious rotavirus disease in the vast majority of those vaccinated, one could say, in agreement with the VEC information, that the vaccine is safer than being sick with rotavirus.

Yet some cases of intussusception *are* being caused by the rotavirus vaccine; that fact is implicit in the presentation of evidence. The claim made by the VEC that "there are no serious side effects from rotavirus vaccine" is thus not true. Some children experience intussusception from the vaccine. For parents, there may be a difference between a side effect from vaccination and one from an illness: the meaning of an adverse event may be perceived differently if the precipitating action is a chance occurrence of illness in comparison to a medical intervention like vaccination. In other words, if my child gets intussusception from being sick with rotavirus I may feel differently than if my child gets intussusception because I had her vaccinated.

On the other hand, if I don't know how serious rotavirus is and I forgo vaccination because of the uncertainty of its effects, and then my child becomes very ill or dies, I may feel that I have been ill served by the information that I used to make my decision not to vaccinate.

Interestingly, both vaccine-promoting and vaccine-skeptical popular books use a similar narrative to either support or question the safety profile of vaccines, through a typical "injured child story." Popular books questioning vaccination often use the injured child story to stage an argument about false medical advice supporting vaccination that led to a catastrophic injury. Here the authors argue that the risks of vaccination were downplayed and the child suffered (or died). The obverse story concerns a parent who didn't understand the risk of not vaccinating and the child who suffered severe illness, injury, or death. Popular books promoting vaccination often use this kind of story to demonstrate the risks of vaccine refusal.

In the interview studies of the Vaccination Research Group, we see alternative approaches to illnesses and a high valuation of the biological experience of illness in families that don't vaccinate. While our sample sizes are quite small, these findings deserve further investigation, as they suggest a wholly different approach to the idea of infectious disease risk. Many of our informants embrace the experience of illness and believe the body must be properly supported while ill in order to regain health. The risk/benefit scenarios that are propounded by the VEC would be unpersuasive to these families, as the safety of a particular vaccine would not be expressed as a population-based ratio of the prevalence of adverse events compared to the disease-preventing benefits, nor could it be understood as a comparison to the same adverse event experienced as a result of vaccination or disease. This is not to say that these families would never vaccinate, although that is probably true for some. Rather, it is to suggest that reasons to vaccinate might be persuasive only if they took account of other kinds of concerns, such as how vaccination itself changes disease experience, occurrence, and treatment, and thus overall human health, or took account of other values and beliefs, such as the experience of illness and the value of supportive care. In a context characterized by uncertainty, these families trust domestic practices to enhance health and support those who are ill, rather than medicines and treatments that they see as potentially damaging and interventionist.

In any event it is difficult to accept the typical public health approach that vaccine skeptics lack scientific literacy or a proper sense of community responsibility (another common argument). Both of these characterizations exemplify what scholars call the *deficit approach to scientific knowledge*, which is shorthand for how scientists and bureaucrats see members of the public as ignorant when they disagree with mainstream scientific positions. Thoughtful exploration of the views of vaccine skeptics reveals some people with extremely unorthodox views of science and medicine, as well as many folks who are well versed in a variety of scientific discourses and who disagree with mainstream assessments of vaccine safety and efficacy, who believe that adverse reactions to vaccinations are underreported and improperly studied, and who hold diverse views on the true threat of infectious disease on human populations. I am not saying that I agree with vaccine skeptics on any of these issues. In any event, my expertise and my research do not allow me to make scholarly claims about vaccine safety or the reality of vaccine injury. What I can say is that studying vaccination controversy—and studying it not as a problem of "those people" who won't accept vaccination for the miracle that it is but as a public controversy with various constituents—has led me to understand it as a complex problem that is as much social as it is scientific.

Are some people who refuse vaccination ignorant of the scientific arguments made on behalf of vaccination? Absolutely. Are some people who accept vaccination equally ignorant of those arguments? Sure. The point here is not to ferret out the beliefs of those who don't vaccinate in order to change their minds or demonstrate how they are wrong. The point of this book is to show that vaccine skepticism is linked to various beliefs and practices that are actually not that unusual in American society, and that such skepticism is sustained by popular suspicions of the government, sponsored scientific research, and pharmaceutical companies. Many Americans join vaccine skeptics in their deep concerns about the profit motive in drug development and research. The increase in vaccines on the recommended infant and child schedules has been a catalyst for parents who wonder if there is a limit to a child's tolerance for what some perceive to be an aggressive immunization regime.

In addition, negative views of so-called antivaxxers are established and upheld in public debate. The public controversy over vaccination depends upon a particularly damaging kind of group character assassination, much to the detriment of ongoing democratic dialogue. Both vaccine promoters and vaccine skeptics are guilty of pernicious forms of argument, but in this book I explore how the image of the gullible, misinformed parent circulates in provaccine portrayals. This kind of representation allows the news media and others to avoid the varied cultural influences on vaccine skepticism. Indeed, it allows everyone to avoid confronting the complex social contexts in which vaccine skepticism makes sense.

Anti/Vax shows how vaccination controversy animates the US imagination, suggesting why the controversy festers in a context in which most parents vaccinate their children and in which outbreaks of infectious disease are contained handily. As I show throughout the book, the vaccination debate gathers up and consolidates a number of concerns and fears about contemporary medicine and the future of humankind in the context of medical experimentation. As a result, it is unlikely to be ameliorated by attempts to educate parents in scientific literacy. Indeed, in this scenario such education only feeds concerns with vaccination as it empowers individuals to access scientific studies themselves and make their own assessments of vaccine efficacy and safety, not all of which are likely to coincide with professionals' perspectives.[5]

Readers might wonder why I spend so much time discussing other people's arguments, usually through analysis of published books or scholarly articles. One reason is that I have been trained to do just that—to establish my own arguments through the close reading of others' claims. This form of argumentation is a staple in the humanities. But another, and more pertinent, reason is that this method reveals that there are *already* arguments that can explain voluntary nonvaccination within public debates about science, medicine, and the meaning of illness. That is, there already exist ideas that allow us to understand vaccine skepticism, and plenty of scholars and popular writers are talking about them. Yet somehow no one has pulled together these ideas to situate vaccine skepticism within current cultural preoccupations with medicine and its limits. I use this argument strategy—working through texts that circulate around and through vaccination controversy both publicly and in published scholarship—to show how vaccine skepticism makes sense, instead of treating it as a fundamental irrationality.

The book ranges widely, considering news reporting on vaccines, viruses, and bioterrorism; popular book-length treatments of vaccination controversy; Holocaust and science denial; how we know the truth and what a fact is; medicalization and the antimedicine movement; zombie apocalypse fiction; and research findings from interviews with vaccine skeptics.

Initially, when I thought of the book as "making sense of vaccine skepticism," I thought of it as explaining vaccine skeptics to everyone else. But as I revised the manuscript, it became clear to me that *Anti/Vax* is really about medicine and modernity, and how vaccine skepticism reveals pervasive cultural worries about how the things that save us also just might kill us. While writing this book, I went down the rabbit holes of inquiry as far as I could go, and I thought through the big questions and issues that emerged from these journeys. The result is a book that argues that vaccination controversies are examples of decidedly modern questions about human community and understanding—how we live together, what knowledge binds us, how we come to believe things, and what we require of one another.

Vaccine proponents argue, somewhat uniformly, that with respect to infectious disease these questions can be answered by scientific inquiry and findings. I show that for many people, however, science is not a simple matter, and human motivations and history complicate trust in others, especially trust in the scientific establishment and government. Really understanding vaccination controversy means acknowledging that reliance on the abstract systems, expert knowledges, and bureaucratic management that are characteristic of modernity really bothers many modern people. Vaccine skeptics' concerns, rendered this way, reflect many preoccupations of contemporary culture. Everyone would do well to take vaccination controversy seriously—not necessarily as evidence of vaccine skeptics' claims, but as evidence of deeper and widespread disgruntlement with cultural assumptions about technoscientific advancement, triumph over infectious disease, and other myriad accomplishments of biomedicine.

Only when we do so will we be able to discuss national public health goals, the role of vaccine mandates, the politics of vaccination exemptions, and the role of illness and infectious disease in our lives in ways that represent the democratic aspirations of our nation and honor public health efforts as collective, rather than punitive, exercises in national character.

1

So What Bothers You
about Vaccines?

There never was a golden age of vaccine acceptance. Immunization has never been universally accepted in any population as a method of disease prevention. The British gastroenterologist Andrew Wakefield's 1998 *Lancet* article did not transform American parents' perceptions of vaccines, although that article later became emblematic of vaccine skeptics in troubling ways.[1] Vaccination has always had its detractors and its resistors, even as vaccinology in the twentieth century has been accepted wholeheartedly by mainstream medicine, public health, and most American parents as a primary method to prevent infectious disease.[2]

Historians have been clear on this issue in their analysis of vaccination in the United States and elsewhere. For example, James Colgrove shows that persuasive measures were necessary in the 1920s to convince wary American parents to vaccinate against diphtheria, which was a feared disease, although vaccine acceptance increased steadily through the 1930s.[3] David Oshinsky writes in *Polio: An American Story* that frustration with parents not vaccinating their children for polio emerged quickly after the first few years that the Salk vaccine was available, suggesting that as soon as mass vaccination became federal policy, public health concerns about vaccine-wary parents emerged as well.[4] For all the talk about "polio pioneers," hundreds of thousands of parents did not volunteer their children for the experimental shots when they could have. Elena Conis's *Vaccine Nation: America's Changing Relationship with Immunization* demonstrates the rhetorical efforts of scientists and public health officials alike to get parents (and physicians!) to accept vaccines for the so-called mild diseases of childhood (measles, mumps, and rubella) in the 1960s and 1970s.[5] Concerns about the pertussis vaccine were expressed beginning with its initial use in the 1930s, and came to prominence in the 1970s just as vaccine mandates for school entry swept the states and a British study suggested that the vaccine could cause neurological disorders. And in 1982, an NBC affiliate in Washington, DC, aired a documentary about vaccine dangers called *DPT: Vaccine Roulette*.[6] This program is often credited with starting the contemporary antivaccination movement.[7] Whether it did or not is up for debate.

This chapter describes the broad array of concerns about vaccination and viral and bacterial illnesses that have animated the public from the 1980s through the first decade and a half of the twenty-first century. The purpose here is to better understand what, precisely, the current perceived vaccination crisis is about, given existing data on vaccination attainment among children. This chapter and the next use news reporting as a way of gauging public concern, but also provide the opportunity to examine how reporting shapes public views. Ultimately, we can see how reporting has focused on certain positions about the nature of vaccine hesitancy and skepticism, and how the public has been deflected from its own complex expressed worries about vaccination.

Federal Vaccination Provision and Vaccination Attainment

Elena Conis and James Colgrove have written the two most authoritative histories of vaccination in twentieth-century and early twenty-first-century America, *Vaccine Nation* and *State of Immunity* (respectively). Readers interested in fuller historical treatments of vaccination in the United States should consult these sources. *State of Immunity* begins in the Progressive Era (early twentieth century) and focuses on the periodic oscillation between persuasion and compulsion in public health efforts to expand vaccination. *Vaccine Nation* focuses on the postpolio period, explaining how the expansion of vaccination in the last forty years of the twentieth century occurred in tandem with vaccine skepticism and outright refusal. Conis pays special attention to the social contexts and effects of federal action to broaden vaccine uptake, from John F. Kennedy's Vaccination Assistance Act (1962) through Jimmy Carter's Childhood Immunization Initiative (1977) and Bill Clinton's Vaccines for Children program (part of the Omnibus Budget Reconciliation Act of 1993). Both of these sources offer insights into how past federal action on vaccination provides a context for the current vaccination controversy.

The polio vaccine was the first to be provided nationally through a coordinated federal effort. When vaccine proponents worked to ensure better immunization rates against poliomyelitis in the 1960s, they confronted an old challenge—middle-class citizens were more likely to line up themselves and their children for shots than were poor people. In the early 1960s, Kennedy's Vaccination Assistance Act thus targeted poor children, those older than five years of age, and provided the four vaccines that were then available: polio, diphtheria, pertussis, and tetanus. That act was renewed during the Johnson administration, but the funding mechanism changed under President Nixon to a set of block grants to states, some of which chose to put the funds to other public health uses. In the 1970s, Jimmy Carter's plan, which included shots for seven vaccine-preventable diseases (diphtheria, pertussis, tetanus, polio, measles, rubella, and mumps—the latter three having been developed since 1963), also focused on poor children. Carter's Childhood Immunization Initiative relied more on volunteers and attempted to keep the federal footprint subordinated to state oversight. Conis points out that the Carter initiative involved significant moralized messaging that identified parental ignorance, misunderstanding, and lack of attention to the importance of vaccines as reasons parents didn't immunize their children. Thus, the 1990s were not the first period in which parental belief or disposition was understood to be a problem in achieving optimal vaccination levels nationally.

After leveled or diminished funds for childhood vaccination during the Reagan administration, and a measles epidemic from 1989 through 1991, reporting on US vaccination policies often compared them (rather

TABLE 1. National vaccination rates at 35 months

Vaccine acronym	Disease(s)	Number of doses up to 35 months	Children vaccinated 2015 (%)	Children vaccinated 1995 (%)	Notes
DTaP	Diphtheria, tetanus, and pertussis	3+	95.0	94.5 (DTP)	Acellular pertussis vaccine introduced in 1996
IPV	Poliovirus	3+	93.7	87.8 (both IPV and OPV)	Inactivated poliovirus vaccine (IPV); until 2000, both IPV and OPV (oral poliovirus vaccine) were used in the United States
MMR	Measles, mumps, and rubella	1+	91.9	89.8	Booster at 4–6 years
HepA	Hepatitis A	1+	85.8	n/a	1+ dose; 2 doses by 2 years for all children recommended since 2005
HepB	Hepatitis B	3+	92.6	67.9	Introduced as routine vaccine in 1990s
Hib	Bacterial meningitis caused by Haemophilus influenzae type b	3+	94.3	91.2	Primary series: receipt of greater than 2 or 3 doses depending on product type received
RV	Rotavirus	2+ or 3+	73.2	n/a	Rotarix® (RV1; 2+ doses; approved for use in 2008) and Rota Teq® (RV5; 3+ doses; approved for use in 2006)
VAR	Varicella or chicken pox	1+	91.8	25.8 (1997)	First available 1995
PCV	Pneumococcal disease	3+	93.3	73.2 (2004)	Pneumococcal conjugate vaccine, started 2000

Sources: National Immunization Survey (NIS)—Children (19–35 months), Centers for Disease Control and Prevention, CDC.gov, https://www.cdc.gov/vaccines/imz-managers/coverage/nis/child/index.html; Holly A. Hill et al., "Vaccination Coverage among Children Aged 19–35 Months—United States, 2015," *MMWR* 65, no. 39 (October 7, 2016): 1065–71.

negatively) to those of poor countries. Bill Clinton's plan, like his over-
haul of welfare a few years later, relied on what was termed *personal
responsibility*, even though it was clear at the time that vaccination rates
were related to socioeconomic status. Regardless of the semantics, the
program has been successful in diminishing nonvaccination among the
poor and improving rates overall. A comparison of vaccination rates from
the mid-1990s to today demonstrates that over a twenty-year period that
began in 1995, significant gains were made in improving rates of MMR
and polio vaccination for infants up to thirty-five months, and that most
other childhood vaccination rates have improved marginally over time. In
2015, only 0.8 percent of US children under the age of three years received
no vaccinations at all.[8]

The data in table 1 demonstrate that, contrary to popular belief, this
country is not currently experiencing a national crisis in vaccination attainment. This is not to say that clusters of unvaccinated children and
adults do not pose a public health risk, as public health officials are quick
to point out, or that there is not room for improvement in these immunization rates (at least from the perspective of public health). The data shown
in the table do not include the final boosters in some series, and these are
often the very shots that are most difficult to attain, as toddlers and young
children go to the doctor less frequently than infants, and other logistical
obstacles present themselves. In addition, the table does not include some
vaccines that target adolescents, like the HPV or meningococcal vaccines.
Nevertheless, the data presented here suggest that hyperbolic claims of increasing rates of unvaccinated children across the nation are not based on
data collected by the Centers for Disease Control and Prevention (CDC).

A Short History of Vaccine Concerns since 1980

In 1980 seven vaccines were given routinely to children in the United States
to prevent the following illnesses: diphtheria, tetanus, pertussis, measles,
mumps, rubella, and polio. At the time these were usually administered in
two shots and a liquid dose: DTP, MMR, and oral polio.[9] There were also
boosters. By the end of this period, however, the recommended vaccination schedule for US infants and children had ballooned significantly to
shots against a total of sixteen diseases. (It is difficult to quantify exactly

the number of shots, given the variety of multiple-vaccine formulations that children can receive and that the number of doses recommended varies according to the age of the child.) The historian Mark Largent argues that the sheer number of vaccines given to infants and children is a primary, legitimate concern.[10] Understanding how and why vaccinations have increased in number is helpful in getting a handle on a generalized heightened anxiety about infant and childhood vaccines.

Historically, legislation has set the context for steadily increasing recommendations and mandates for infant and childhood vaccination. In the early 1990s, the Clinton initiative made it likely that vaccine manufacturers would seek recommended status by the CDC's Advisory Committee on Immunization Practices (ACIP) and try to be on the list of vaccines mandated for school entry. The Obama administration's Affordable Care Act of 2010 expanded on Clinton's program, requiring that insurance plans cover ACIP-recommended vaccines for children without cost to them or their families. What this means is that getting a new vaccine onto ACIP's recommended list is a priority for vaccine manufacturers, because it ensures a reliable stream of vaccine-eligible children or adults whose immunizations are covered by insurance. (Better yet is getting onto the list of vaccines mandated for school entry, which is often a consequence of being put on the list of recommended vaccines.) This feature of federal legislation, while clearly making vaccinations affordable and thus accessible for children and adults from lower socioeconomic strata, also created the context for parental resistance to childhood vaccines, simply because there were so many added to the schedule and many are often administered at the same office visit. Immunization overload thus became a focus of parental concern in the early twenty-first century.[11]

But while increased immunizations for infants and children is an important part of this story, it is not the only, or necessarily the most important, part. In what follows I trace a history of vaccination and infectious disease concern that tacks back and forth between fears of vaccine shortage in the context of disease outbreak and nervous attention to vaccine risk. It is important to understand that these tendencies occur together, suggesting ambivalence about medicalized approaches to health at the same time that illness is feared. The high vaccination attainment demonstrated in table 1 came about in the context of growing concerns about vaccination and the emergence of what we think of today as a highly charged vaccination controversy in the public sphere. What we have, then, is something of an enigma—high attainment in the context of growing concern. What we normally don't think about, however, is the range of concerns about vaccines that have been raised historically and how those relate to what sometimes seems a narrow focus on childhood vaccines and, in particular, the possibility of a connection between childhood vaccines and autism. This section of the chapter traces concerns about vaccines that were documented in news reporting from the early 1980s through 2015.

The acceleration of vaccine approval and insertion into the recommended schedule during the 1980s and 1990s coincided with the emergence of the AIDS epidemic and the changes it wrought on drug development regulations and activist medical culture at large. Because developments concerning HIV/AIDS were so prevalent in news reporting during this period, I have not included them in this discussion, but they do provide a context for vaccination controversy as it emerged. It also bears noting that in 1976, during a time when there were significant concerns about the whole-cell pertussis vaccine causing neurological damage, a vaccine against a strain of swine flu was thought to have caused increased incidence of Guillain-Barre syndrome (GBS), a temporary form of paralysis. A huge rollout of swine flu vaccinations during Gerald Ford's presidency was halted when GBS was thought to be caused by that vaccine.

What should be clear by this point is that concerns about vaccines did not arise de novo in the 1980s or 1990s but have persisted since the rollout of federally supported vaccination programs in the 1950s. Indeed, many historians have traced long-standing concerns back to the 1790s, when Edward Jenner invented the smallpox vaccine. But the thirty-five-year period from 1980 to 2015 is long enough to demonstrate significant and diverse worries about vaccines in the United States, as well as the triumphant development of many vaccines that have lowered infant morbidity and mortality.

The early to mid-1980s saw increased concerns about vaccines in the media as well as the development and approval of two important vaccines for children. In 1982 an NBC affiliate in Washington, DC, aired *DPT: Vaccine Roulette*, a documentary about vaccines and their dangers. Excerpts were also shown on the *Today Show*. The documentary followed concerns about the whole-cell pertussis vaccine from the 1970s, when British researchers claimed that it caused neurological damage. A vaccine safety group, Dissatisfied Parents Together (with the same acronym, DPT), established itself at this time. (This group later became the National Vaccine Information Center, one of the country's largest and most vocal vaccine safety organizations, with an expansive website.) A few years later, in 1985, a vaccine against Haemophilus influenzae type b (Hib, a bacterial disease) was released. Before the vaccine, Hib was a major cause of meningitis in infants. Updated in 1987, the vaccine allowed physicians to rule out meningitis when infants presented at emergency rooms with high fevers. And in 1986, a recombinant vaccine for hepatitis B (Hep B) was developed as an improvement over the older vaccine, released in 1981, which was made from human blood products.

From 1989 to 1991, tens of thousands of Americans were sickened by a measles outbreak that spread across the United States. The outbreak was thought to be the result of low vaccination rates that were themselves the outcome of more than a decade of lagging attention to childhood vaccination attainment. The outbreak motivated Bill Clinton, once he was president, to initiate the Vaccines for Children program in 1993, which aimed to reduce socioeconomic and racial disparities in vaccine availability and receipt by lowering logistical barriers to vaccination for poor children. In the public imagination, however, the outbreak was partly overshadowed by the Gulf War, also known as Operation Desert Shield and Operation Desert Storm. The war was a response to Iraq's invasion of Kuwait and involved a coalition of forces led by the United States. Gulf War Syndrome, a controversial diagnosis involving numerous complaints (including fatigue, diarrhea, rashes, cognitive difficulties, and other symptoms), was linked by some to the anthrax vaccines given to soldiers deployed to the Persian Gulf. Thus, just as in the early to mid-1980s vaccine development occurred in tandem with vaccination concerns, so too at the beginning of the 1990s worries about epidemic-level infectious disease emerged at the same time that new illnesses were being blamed on vaccination receipt.

The pattern would continue throughout the decade, as new vaccines were released and included in the recommended schedule for infants and children. In 1991 ACIP recommended a change in the schedule for hepatitis B vaccination, with a goal of total disease elimination in the United States. Trying to vaccinate adults and those at risk of hepatitis B had not worked to lessen transmission in the United States in line with CDC goals. As a result, ACIP recommended universal childhood vaccination against

Hep B that would begin, optimally, on the day of their birth. In 1995 a vaccine against chicken pox (varicella) was added to the recommended immunization schedule for children, although most states would not include it as a mandatory vaccine for school entry for a few more years. In 1996 an acellular version of the pertussis vaccine replaced the whole-cell version, partly in response to concerns about neurological injury presented in *DPT: Vaccine Roulette*.

Thus, one new vaccine, one redesigned vaccine, and a new schedule for yet another preceded the emergence of significant new concerns about childhood vaccination in the mid- to late 1990s. In 1997, the Food and Drug Administration (FDA) Modernization Act led to studies concerning mercury in FDA-regulated compounds, including vaccines. Mercury, in the form of ethylmercury, is a component of thimerosal, a vaccine preservative. Research would indicate that children might be getting too much mercury across all of the infant and early childhood vaccines, especially as these were increasing in number. In the end, the FDA found that infants receiving all recommended vaccines could, by six months of age, be injected with 187.5 micrograms of mercury. With the American Academy of Pediatrics (AAP), in 1999 the FDA urged vaccine makers to reduce thimerosal, albeit controversially by allowing manufacturers to use up existing stocks. While the FDA stated that there was no evidence of harm from thimerosal in children's vaccines, it made its recommendation on the basis of the precautionary principle.

The thimerosal controversy would continue into the new century, however. The FDA request to remove thimerosal from vaccines was the beginning of an effort to determine if there were any adverse consequences of ethylmercury in vaccines, especially for children. In June 2000 the CDC invited scientists to a meeting to consider possible adverse reactions to thimerosal in vaccines. Held at the Simpsonwood Conference Center in Norcross, Georgia, the conference now bears that name in common parlance (the official title of the conference was "Scientific Review of Vaccine Safety Datalink Information"). At the closed-door meeting, CDC-invited scientists examined data from the Vaccine Safety Datalink Project, a network of HMOs across the country that gathers electronic health information related to vaccinations to monitor potential adverse reactions to vaccines. Robert F. Kennedy Jr., in a famous article titled "Deadly Immunity" that was published in *Rolling Stone* magazine and on Salon.com in 2005 (and discussed at greater length in chapter 2), later pointed to the Simpsonwood conference as evidence of a government cover-up of the dangers of mercury in vaccines.[12] At the time, the scientists in attendance concurred that further research was needed to confirm or repudiate claims of neurological damage due to thimerosal in vaccines. The Institute of Medicine (IOM) study released in 2004, which found no link between thimerosal and autism, would be one result of this decision.

In the meantime, technological innovations and the introduction of new vaccines through the 1990s and early 2000s occurred simultaneously with growing concerns. It should be no surprise that a British gastroenterologist who had been working with families of autistic children on a potential connection between gut disorders and autism published a paper in *The Lancet* in 1998 titled "Ileal-Lymphoid-Nodular Hyperplasia, Nonspecific Colitis, and Pervasive Developmental Disorder in Children."[13] The study suggested a possible link between the MMR (measles, mumps, and rubella) vaccine and a condition called *autistic enterocolitis*. Diagnoses of autism were accelerating in the period, and Andrew Wakefield, the gastroenterologist in question, was engaged in long-term research on these possible connections, as well as related research on measles and gut problems.[14] The same year that Wakefield's *Lancet* article was originally published, the first rotavirus vaccine, Rotashield, was introduced. Rotavirus is a gastrointestinal disease that affects very young infants, causing diarrhea and vomiting. The following year the vaccine was withdrawn after cases of intussusception, a condition in which the bowel telescopes into itself, increased marginally postvaccination. The withdrawal of the vaccine was controversial among vaccine advocates, who argued that even with the possibility of elevated cases of intussusception, many millions of children would be protected against potentially severe disease.

In 1999 a different set of concerns about vaccines surfaced in the public imagination: the journalist Edward Hooper published *The River*, a lengthy and detailed argument that HIV/AIDS was caused by the use of kidneys from monkeys infected with simian immunodeficiency virus (SIV) to grow polio vaccine.[15] The vaccine researcher Hilary Koprowski had run trials for an attenuated live-virus polio vaccine in the Congo in the late 1950s. He was competing against Albert Sabin for the development of a live-virus polio vaccine; Koprowski's vaccine was not approved. Hooper argued that SIV present in diseased monkeys could have been transmitted to humans with the vaccine and then mutated to become HIV. His contention rests, in part, on the knowledge that another simian virus, SV40, was discovered to have contaminated polio vaccines in the late 1950s and early 1960s. To this day there are arguments that SV40, which was present in both injected and oral polio vaccines until about 1963 in the United States and perhaps later in some other countries, is a cause of cancer in humans.[16]

Hooper's argument is controversial and has been debunked by mainstream AIDS researchers, who generally agree that vaccination aided the spread of HIV in Africa but not that vaccines caused SIV mutation. Rather, the generally accepted theory is that SIV mutated as a result of mixing chimpanzee or other primate blood contaminated with SIV with human blood during butchering. This theory is known as the "bushmeat hypothesis" or "cut hunter hypothesis." Initially the virus remained isolated in rural communities, but political and social upheaval in early to mid-twentieth-century Africa—accompanying decolonization and independence—led to its introduction in larger population centers. Mass vaccination campaigns carried out in the second half of the twentieth century accelerated the spread of HIV due to inadequate needle sterilization or needle reuse without sterilization, as there was widespread use of injectable penicillin and other medications across the African continent in the 1950s and after.[17] But Hooper maintains the plausibility of his claims on a website (aidsorigins.com), and he has many adherents who are sympathetic to the notion that contamination of vaccines with animal products is both a primary cause of HIV and, more generally, a widespread danger of contemporary vaccination regimes.

In the following year, 2000, Patrick Tierney published *Darkness in El Dorado: How Scientists and Journalists Devastated the Amazon*, which was preceded by an article in the *New Yorker*, "The Fierce Anthropologist."[18] Both of these publications claimed that the anthropologist Napoleon Chagnon, along with the physician James Neel, purposefully infected Amazonian Yanomami Indians with measles in a kind of eugenics experiment in 1968. Chagnon and Neel were accused of injecting the Yanomami with a poorly attenuated live-virus measles vaccine to see who would survive, instead of vaccinating them to protect them from an ongoing epidemic, as they claimed. Tierney's claims set off a firestorm of controversy within academic anthropology concerning the ethics of research on vulnerable populations and the potential harms of human experimentation to prove dubious scientific hypotheses. In the context of vaccination skepticism, both Tierney's and Hooper's books raised the specter of scientists run amok in the forests of Africa and South America, seeding infections among the world's poorest and most vulnerable people.[19] They also expressed grave concerns about vaccines that actually caused diseases rather than preventing them, as a result of either technical problems (using monkey kidney cells to grow virus) or purposeful malevolent experimentation (testing isolated populations to prove questionable sociobiological theories). These kinds of concerns—that the techniques to make vaccines are vulnerable to accident and contamination, that the public cannot trust physicians or researchers—are prevalent in the long history of vaccination concern.[20] It is telling that they continue even in an era of seemingly stringent regulation and oversight.

The year 2000 also saw three significant developments in vaccination policy in the United States. Yet another vaccine was recommended for infants—the pneumococcal conjugate vaccine, or PCV—bringing the total number of recommended vaccines for infants and children to eleven (diphtheria, pertussis, tetanus, hepatitis B, measles, mumps, rubella, varicella, polio, Haemophilus influenzae type b, pneumococcal disease). Oral poliovirus vaccine was discontinued in the United States, as a result of the continued, albeit rare, incidence of illness caused by reversion of the attenuated live virus in the vaccine to wild type (a possibility disputed by Albert Sabin, the creator of the approved live-virus oral polio vaccine, throughout his entire life). The injected polio vaccine, which used a killed virus, again became the standard, although oral polio vaccine continued to be used around the world because of its ease of administration and low cost, and because it is better at protecting communities where vaccination rates may be low. In addition, measles was declared eliminated in the United States, which meant that there was no longer any endemic circulation of measles in the country. This declaration continues to confuse people to this day, who often think that it means that there is no more measles at all in the United States. For public health authorities, it is a technical term that means all infections are understood to come from beyond the US border; it also means that any measles infection is considered an outbreak.

The new millennium would escalate concerns about illnesses as well as vaccines, exacerbating existing worries about both potential epidemics and the medicines meant to prevent them. The September 2001 attacks on the World Trade Center and Pentagon, and the subsequent anthrax letters sent through the US Postal Service, renewed concerns about bioterrorism. The federal government used existing smallpox vaccine stores as an exigence to create more vaccine for American citizens and instituted a program to vaccinate frontline health care workers and military personnel. Many of those targeted for smallpox vaccination resisted because of known adverse reactions to the vaccine. In 2003 severe acute respiratory syndrome (SARS) emerged in China and quickly spread to Toronto and elsewhere through air travel. From 2003 through 2008, a series of court cases was initiated to fight the compulsory administration of anthrax vaccine to military troops. And in 2004, a flu vaccine shortage, due to a decrease in manufacturing capacity, caused a flurry of concern about availability and rationing, both in the immediate context and in terms of future possible pandemic events.

That same year, the IOM published a review of the science concerning autism and MMR, as well as autism and thimerosal, discounting any link holding vaccines responsible for rising rates of autism. The report was derided by vaccine skeptics but lauded by the government and physicians as putting an end to public concerns about autism and childhood vaccines. As if to put an exclamation point on the report, in 2004 ten out of thirteen coauthors of the 1998 Wakefield study published in *The Lancet* formally retracted the study.

All the while, new vaccines were being developed and recommended for infants, children, and adolescents. In 2005 the hepatitis A vaccine was recommended for all infants, and the first conjugate meningococcal vaccine, MCV4 (Menactra), was licensed. In 2006 two new vaccines were rolled out—RotaTeq, against rotavirus, and Gardasil, against HPV. RotaTeq was later joined, in 2008, by Rotarix, both vaccines replacing the disgraced Rotashield, which had been pulled in 1998 because of increased incidence of intussusception. But any lingering controversy around the rotavirus vaccines was overshadowed by the immediate public debates occasioned by the first vaccine marketed to protect against cancer: Gardasil.

Created by Merck, which was still suffering from the Vioxx debacle, at the time Gardasil protected against four strains of the human papillomavirus (HPV), which can cause cervical cancer in women and genital warts and anal and oral-pharyngeal cancers in both sexes.[21] ACIP recommended

Gardasil for girls eleven to sixteen years of age, primarily because the vaccine was understood to be most effective before girls became sexually active. Some states wanted to add the vaccine to those required for middle-school entry, and Merck mounted a significant lobbying campaign to that effect. But conservative families objected to a vaccine that they thought might encourage young girls to be sexually promiscuous. When concerns about side effects of Gardasil emerged on social media in 2008, these linked up with existing resistance to a vaccine for an infection spread by sexual, rather than casual, contact. The CDC authorized a study to examine its safety, but even when that was published in 2009, confirming the safety profile of Gardasil, a robust network of websites and organizations continued to question its necessity and safety. Many of these websites contain video narratives of girls who had been injured by the HPV vaccine, which is administered in three rather expensive doses a prescribed number of months apart.

Against this backdrop, influenza emerged as a new focus of concern. In 2006, a highly pathogenic strain of avian flu (H5N1) began to spread because of wild bird migrations and the inadequacy of containment of domesticated fowl. Prior to this period, the virus was largely confined to small poultry holdings in Southeast Asia, although it had occasionally caused more widespread culling of contaminated flocks. But in 2006 the potential spread of H5N1 led to increasing speculation about how it might mutate and spread between humans. Concerns about pandemic influenza energized existing worries about flu vaccine uptake in ordinary contexts, and in 2008 ACIP recommended annual vaccination against influenza for children six months to eighteen years of age. This change was backed up by evidence that children were responsible for spreading flu to their elders, especially more vulnerable grandparents. Then, in 2009, there actually was a global outbreak of influenza, the swine flu (H1N1) pandemic. The disease was mild for most of those infected, but it spread rapidly across the globe. Fears of a repetition of the 1918 Spanish flu pandemic led to quick development of a vaccine and then shortages through fall 2009 when rollout of the vaccine was slow. From the end of 2007 through 2009 there was also a shortage of Hib vaccine because of bacterial contamination at a Merck manufacturing site. As a result of the Hib shortage, rates of Hib vaccination fell sharply as public health authorities rationed the vaccine for vulnerable infants. In 2010, ACIP finally recommended an annual flu vaccine for all US citizens over six months of age, with some exceptions for medical contraindications. That decision to expand recommendations for influenza vaccination was made, in part, to ensure adequate supply and manufacturing capacity in the event of a pandemic occurrence.

The end of the first decade of the twenty-first century witnessed more action on the vaccines and autism connection, even though the IOM's 2004 report was supposed to have put that controversy to rest. In 2009 and 2010, the Omnibus Autism Proceeding declared that there was no evidence that thimerosal or MMR causes autism.[22] The Omnibus Autism Proceeding was an action taken by the federal vaccine court (established in the 1980s to adjudicate cases of vaccine injury) to consolidate the thousands of claims being made that thimerosal and/or the MMR vaccine caused autism. In 2010, *The Lancet* formally retracted the 1998 Wakefield study, and the Affordable Care Act (ACA; also known as Obamacare) was signed into law. The ACA included enhanced provisions for vaccination, mandating that vaccines be covered under all health plans. It also required, upon implementation, that hospitals report flu vaccination rates of their employees; lower rates of vaccination meant lower reimbursements.

The following year, ACIP recommended that boys ages eleven to twelve be vaccinated against HPV. But the stories coming out of the second decade of the twenty-first century, at least its first five years, were more about diseases and outbreaks than vaccines. In 2012, Middle East respiratory syndrome (MERS) emerged in Saudi Arabia. MERS is a coronavirus, like SARS. Like SARS, it caused significant concern about spread through travel, especially because of the yearly hajj, the annual Islamic pilgrimage to Mecca. In 2014 in the United States, cases of measles spiked upward of 600 as a result of a very large outbreak in a largely unvaccinated Amish community in Ohio. The disease was thought to have been brought in by returning missionaries who had been in the Philippines. The same year, Ebola virus outbreaks in West Africa caused the deaths of tens of thousands, and one death of a traveler to the United States, as well as a few cases among medical personnel treating Ebola patients in the United States.

And at the end of 2014, a measles outbreak began at Disneyland, in California. In 2015, over 100 cases across the country were linked to this outbreak, which caused a flurry of inflammatory reporting and attacks on nonvaccinating parents.[23] The total number of measles cases in 2015 was 189, however, matching almost exactly the number in 2013 (187). Yet as a direct effect of the outbreak, California ended its personal belief and religious exemptions for vaccination, which were historically quite flexible, with a law signed in June 2015 to take effect the following year. Finally, in 2016 dramatic increases in rates of microcephaly in infants in Brazil and other South American countries suggested that Zika virus infection in pregnant women was dangerous to developing fetuses. The only existing public health efforts to be marginally effective in preventing Zika infection were standard antimosquito actions (use insect repellant, stay inside during peak mosquito hours, wear protective clothing). Predictably, developing a Zika vaccine quickly became a focus of public health activity in the United States, as did killing mosquito populations with insecticides.

Reporting and the Problem of Parental Belief

While stories of infectious disease dominated the news in 2010–2015, vaccination controversy itself became an inflammatory focus of reporting, as documented in the next chapter. One of the things that accompanied inflammatory reporting on vaccination was an increasing focus on voluntary nonvaccination. That is, reporting tended to focus on the vaccine debate itself, and when outbreaks of infectious viral disease occurred, voluntary nonvaccinators tended to be mentioned as a primary cause. Thus, as the twenty-first century unfolded, outbreaks of infectious disease—SARS, H5N1 influenza, H1N1 influenza, MERS, Ebola virus, measles, and Zika—caused significant concern, as did voluntary nonvaccination. The juxtaposition of these trends—the increasing emergence of infectious disease and some people's beliefs that vaccines are dangerous—underlines the double nature of public concern throughout this whole period, in which vaccinology advanced significantly and vaccines were developed, approved, and recommended at a swift pace, while concerns about vaccination also increased. In a context in which there is a heightened concern about emerging infectious diseases and the dangers of a globalized world in spreading them, the fact that some people repudiate vaccines becomes a significant focus of public health concern.

In this way, belief, and parental belief in particular, seemed to be the cause of infectious disease spread, and the supposed vaccination crisis became a crisis of belief rather than, for example, a problem of logistical barriers or financial barriers (although it continues to be both for some families). While the overall rate of complete nonvaccination of children remains extremely low (less than 1 percent of the population), there is a perception that nonvaccination is a significant and widespread threat.[24] Because there were so many professional attestations to the safety of vaccines—the 2004 IOM report on autism, thimerosal, and MMR; the retraction of the 1998 *Lancet* article by Wakefield and colleagues; the findings of the 2009 Omnibus Autism Proceeding, for example—beliefs against vaccination were easily presented as irrational and the result of the improper public influence of celebrities, fake science, experts who were really charlatans, or just the Internet. Thus, despite the fact that concerns about vaccines and their potential dangers have dogged vaccinology for over a century, the persistence of such concerns today contributes to the sense of a new crisis, especially as reporting on emerging infectious disease unsettles peoples' equanimity in a globalized world.

In *Vaccine Nation*, Elena Conis discusses the role of the media in shaping public perception of vaccination in the 1990s and 2000s. She focuses on the primacy of the MMR-autism connection in media stories about vaccination after 2000, showing that, over the course of a decade or more, the media simplified a complex vaccination controversy into a single and simple story: "the misinformed, irrational, vaccine-fearing parent."[25] Across multiple domains—in medical research, in news reporting, on Facebook, in popular nonfiction—the same *imago* of the fearful and irrational vaccine-refusing parent was held up as the main challenge to national immunity. Indeed, the "misinformed, irrational, vaccine-fearing parent" is a topos in the classic rhetorical sense, a place or topic from which one can make an argument. The argument that tends to be made from this topos is that the primary problem with vaccine skepticism is *belief*.

The idea that *belief* is the primary problem has significant consequences. If the problem with low vaccination rates or clusters of children exempted from mandatory vaccination is belief, specifically *wrong beliefs*, then the solution is to change those beliefs through education. Yet studies have shown that this kind of public health intervention—the attempt to change the views of firm vaccine refusers, especially through correction with scientifically approved information—is not successful.[26] There are a number of theories as to why this is the case, although many of these seem to further entrench the idea that vaccine skeptics are irrational (such as the idea that they cling to psychologically self-reinforcing ideas that bolster their identities, as if other folk, like scientists, do not do the same thing). As I will show later in the book, vaccination resistance is often labeled *denialist* and likened to climate change skepticism or refutations of the fact that HIV causes AIDS. That argument portrays vaccine skeptics as people who purposefully ignore or repudiate good scientific evidence for no evident reason other than ignorance, prejudice, or self-interest. Indeed, some have argued that vaccine skeptics seem immune to convincing scientific arguments about the value of vaccination.

To make the argument that vaccine skepticism is a problem of belief and not, for instance, a problem of public health policy and practice, concerns about government overreach, fears about corruption in medical research and the development of pharmaceuticals, or the result of actual bad experiences with vaccination, these other possible ways of framing vaccination concerns have to be discounted or obscured. News reporting is one context in which the public's views are framed and interpreted; thus, it is a primary venue for the assessment of what a particular trend means, what its basis is, and how it should be understood broadly. In addition, representations of vaccination controversy affect the way we think about it and shape our responses to disease outbreaks. As published debates about vaccination became more and more focused on the problem of the nonvaccinating parent and the threat of the unvaccinated child, they left behind other concerns that preoccupied parents and others in previous decades. This newer media focus reveals how the beliefs of nonvaccinating parents were targeted as a primary problem of national health. In the process, the reporting contributed to the controversy rather than ameliorating or really explaining it. Because of these trends, reporting on vaccination has done and continues to do a disservice to the American public.

I have presented this history in order to show the complex context in which vaccine skepticism has emerged as a forceful public controversy in the United States. Rather than demonstrating a historical narrowing of public interest in the vaccine-autism controversy, this overview demonstrates the numerous vaccine- or virus-related events that focused national and international attention on disparities in vaccination availability, risks of emerging infectious diseases, public health readiness, possible adverse health consequences of vaccines for soldiers and others, biosecurity concerns, and emerging infectious diseases, among other issues. It is a story of varying and potentially clashing concerns about diseases and methods of preventing them. It is also a story that enfolds increasing reliance on vaccination as a primary public health strategy—made evident in the development of new vaccines and their recommendation by federal advisory boards and agencies—with concerns about vaccination that continue to be voiced and coalesce around particular vaccines and their perceived dangers.[27]

The changes that occurred across more than three decades of reporting on vaccination suggest that the problem of parental belief emerged only when other concerns about vaccination were stripped of their authority or believability, or simply stopped being reported on. News reporting on vaccination has not always portrayed nonvaccinating parents as dangerous to their children, and reporters took up various topics concerning vaccination before the current focus on vaccine skepticism itself. When misinformed parents became the target of vaccine promoters, representations of parental concerns were narrowed significantly. The typical vaccine-skeptical parent was described as white, middle class, and educated. Other kinds of parents who might have concerns that do not register publicly because they lack the resources to maneuver through the exemption mechanism in their state, or because they are afraid that any parental behavior outside of public health norms might alert child protective services, were not represented. Indeed, while current stereotypes and most reporting imply that wealthy educated parents are most likely to voluntarily forgo vaccination for their children, a 2015 Pew study shows that parents with college degrees are *more* likely to see the MMR vaccine as safe (92 percent) than parents with only a high school degree or less education (77 percent).[28] Data like this suggest that there is inadequate reporting on parental concerns about vaccines. Concerns about vaccinations required by the military, which continue to this day, challenge the view of vaccine opponents as comprised almost entirely of misinformed parents. And the Internet, heralded in other contexts as an advance that democratizes knowledge and makes specialty expertise broadly available, comes under criticism for directing gullible parents to misinformation and deceptive science about vaccination.

The next chapter takes this history and interprets news reporting about it. While conducting this research, it became apparent to my undergraduate researchers that in order to keep track of the news reporting and its increasingly inflammatory tone we needed a better fix on the sequence of events and concerns—thus, we created the timeline on which this chapter is based. But turning the timeline into a narrative has taught me something that I hadn't considered before—that the juxtaposition of concerns reveals an oscillation that is, in some ways, the significant story. Worries about vaccine risks and the continual increase in acceptance of vaccines occurred in tandem; advances in vaccinology are evident at the same time that people are skeptical about rapidly developed vaccines or attempts by pharmaceutical companies to have their products mandated by state governments. Heightened concerns about emerging infectious diseases were reported on at the same time that nonvaccinating parents became a focus of attention. Because of the simultaneity of concerns and medical developments, the perceived acceleration of worries that fuel vaccination controversy is really a kind of slow boil of existing and developing trends. What has made vaccine skepticism jump to the forefront of public consciousness, however, is the way it is reported on in both old and new media, and the increasingly inflammatory tone in which concerns about vaccination are addressed. The next chapter comments on how and when the reporting became more highly charged, and speculates about specific instances in the history just presented that allowed that to happen.

2

Immune to Reason

Earlier this month, a bill surfaced in the New York State Legislature
proposing that parents be permitted to reject vaccinations for their
children simply because they opposed them philosophically, as one
might oppose Oreos or the Disney Channel. The bill had emerged
before and gone nowhere; in the unlikely event that it was enacted, it
would give parents even greater leeway to reject science for children
who were ostensibly in school to gain an understanding of it.

On this occasion, the timing was especially bizarre, given the recent
measles outbreak tied to Disneyland and the renewed fury it has
brought to vaccine resistance. It was as if a plane had again crash-
landed in the Hudson River and lawmakers seized the moment to
spare airlines the expense of inflatable rafts.

New York Times, February 13, 2015

With these two paragraphs, the "Big City" columnist Ginia Bellafante begins an article about vaccination skepticism and legal attempts
to broaden exemption laws in New York State.[1] I read this piece as my
research team and I were covering the Disney measles outbreak that began
in late December 2014. We had been tracking the outbreak, as well as the
reporting on vaccine exemptions in the Los Angeles school district during
fall 2014. This article struck me as unusual for the New York Times, in
that it seemed highly inflammatory. After all, it's not every day that, in
the space of two paragraphs, a journalist likens philosophical commitments to an opposition to cookies or television, makes a snide comment

about the irony of parental rejection of science, and uses the example of an airplane crash-landing in the Hudson to bring home the notion that vaccine resistant parents are kooks who would prefer evident danger to proven precautionary measures. This article made me wonder: when had such reporting started? And what were the precipitating causes, if there were any? I asked two undergraduate students working with me that semester to explore the tone of reporting on vaccination controversy from the 1980s to the present day.

My students, Kate Buss and Travertine Orndorff, found a subtle but decided increase in highly charged reporting on vaccination since 2000, and especially since 2005. Before then, there was little reporting in mainstream venues that blamed parents for not vaccinating their children or sought to disparage those who did not vaccinate. There was very little that used the belittling language or florid examples evident in the excerpt above. There was reporting on parent vaccine watchdog groups that was respectful about parental concerns about vaccination risks, and reporting on vaccines covered a variety of topics: reporting in general was not confined to disparaging parental beliefs or the idea that vaccines caused autism. Indeed, Travertine found that, in *Mother Jones*, reporting on vaccination in the 1990s tended to be very sympathetic to parental concerns about contaminants. It was only around the middle of the first decade of the twenty-first century that reporting shifted in that magazine, as well as others, to be predominantly against vaccine skepticism and to be decidedly inflammatory in its tone.

By 2014 and 2015, inflammatory reporting about vaccine skepticism was common. The *Los Angeles Times* and the *Hollywood Reporter* published a series of articles in September 2014 claiming that the rates of personal belief exemption from vaccination in some Los Angeles schools were similar to rates of nonvaccination in poor countries like Chad and South Sudan.[2] The implication, of course, is that wealthy white Angelenos should know better than to act like impoverished black Africans. The stories were picked up in *Slate* and the *Atlantic*.[3] Such reporting primed readers to respond with alarm to the measles outbreak that began in late December 2014 in Disneyland. Stories in the *Los Angeles Times* were particularly charged, even though national numbers for measles for the entirety of 2015 were similar to those in 2013, meaning that the Disney outbreak was part of a relatively typical year for measles cases in the United States.

This chapter addresses reporting and public commentary on vaccination and vaccine skeptics, examining how a particular view of so-called antivaxxers is created, one that implies their irrationality, lack of scientific literacy, and unwillingness to act as responsible citizens. Popular books written by vaccine proponents frame vaccination skepticism as fear-based and self-centered. Vaccine proponents also often target the media as increasing coverage of and legitimating vaccine skeptics' views, casting the media as a primary cause of vaccination concern itself. Our research shows that news media, at least since around 2005, has increasingly focused on vaccination controversy, specifically parental concerns about autism and vaccines, and that its reporting has become increasingly hyperbolic and inflammatory. But it wasn't always this way—since the 1980s, various concerns about vaccination have surfaced across national media, and it appears that only recently has there been a consensus about the irrationality of vaccine fears. In examining how these views are created and sustained in news reporting, we can understand how certain ideas—for example, that vaccine skeptics are scientifically illiterate—become truisms, and, in the current climate, memes that are shared across social media platforms without comment or thoughtful reflection.

How Reporting Became Inflammatory

Studying the news is an academic field unto itself, and the discussion here does not constitute an exhaustive analysis. I use a selective investigation of a few mainstream and progressive publications to explore how the topics covered and tone of news reporting on vaccination and vaccination controversy changed from the 1980s to the present. Most of the primary analysis discussed here was developed by undergraduate researchers Kate Buss and Travertine Orndorff in the Vaccination Research Group during spring 2015.[4] To amplify their work on *Time* magazine, the *New York Times*, and *Mother Jones*, I searched past articles from *Slate* and *Salon*, two Internet-only magazines. Obviously, neither of these latter sources provided content from the 1980s, when the Internet did not exist. Both *Slate* and *Salon* published broadly on vaccination issues and controversy, becoming progressively more assertive against vaccine skepticism after 2005.[5]

Chapter 1 offered a narrative chronology of events and issues concerning vaccination and infectious disease during this period. That narrative was created by examining news reporting as well as consulting other sources. As I showed there, reporting revealed a rich mixture of triumphant scientific discovery, ongoing concerns about safety, pandemic or emerging disease preparedness, parental fears and convictions, bioterrorist threats (both real and imagined), legal claims about injury, narratives about vaccine dangers, ethically questionable vaccine trials or infectious disease experiments, and lengthy considerations of the meaning of scientific evidence. Until recently, the tone of most reporting was neutral, although more emotional and politically charged language did surface at key moments. Since 2005 and especially after 2010, the tone of online publications in particular became notably inflammatory, although the *New York Times* article with which I started this chapter shows that even traditional news outlets display hyperbolic prose in reporting on vaccination controversy.

Reporting in *Time* and the *New York Times* in the 1980s focused primarily on low vaccination rates, measles outbreaks, and extending recommendations for physicians to get the flu vaccine. Especially in New York City, efforts to ensure that schoolchildren were vaccinated for the measles dominated coverage. Late in the decade a series of measles outbreaks dominated news on vaccination, but earlier reporting on Dissatisfied Parents Together, the group that formed after the airing of *DPT: Vaccine Roulette* in 1982, portrayed parents as well-meaning advocates of vaccine safety. The measles outbreaks of 1989–1991 were widespread, and President George H. W. Bush was attacked for not prioritizing public health (immunization programs of the 1970s had lapsed during the Reagan/Bush years). President Clinton's Vaccines for Children program was, in large part, a response to low vaccination rates that were thought to have caused the 1989–1991 measles outbreaks. Parent blaming emerged in reporting after the passage of this program in 1993, although much of that reporting also suggests that many parents faced multiple difficulties getting their children vaccinated, so the blame was tempered by sympathy. As immunization rates rose through the 1990s, though, the mildly inflammatory reporting associated with the topic's overt politicization diminished.

Vaccine reporting in the mid-1990s focused, in part, on the mysterious illness dubbed "Gulf War Syndrome," a perfect vehicle for the circulation of concerns on the newly emergent Internet. In one of its first issues, *Slate* included an article by Atul Gwande on Gulf War Syndrome.[6] Among the possible culprits for the debilitating symptoms ("Common complaints are fatigue, joint pain, headache, difficulty sleeping, diarrhea, or nausea") were the required immunizations received by the troops, including vaccines for anthrax and botulinum toxin. Later in the decade *Slate* published an article about brewing rebellion in the military against required immunizations against anthrax, suggesting that one contributor to the resistance to the anthrax vaccine was "the availability to soldiers of vaccine misinformation on the Internet."[7] These concerns about required vaccines for troops—usually anthrax and smallpox—became more common after the terrorist attacks of 2001, when a slew of articles in *Slate* and a few in *Salon* reported on them, and continued sporadically through 2004.[8] Other coverage in the late 1990s continued to consider possible negative reactions to vaccines.[9]

In the late 1990s and early 2000s other kinds of conspiratorial stories about viruses and vaccines circulated. Critical reviews of Patrick Tierney's book *Darkness in El Dorado: How Scientists and Journalists Devastated the Amazon*, published in 2000, appeared in *Slate* that same year. A number of articles were published in fall 2000 about Tierney's argument that anthropologist Napoleon Chagnon, along with physician James Neel, purposefully infected Yanomami Indians in the Amazon with measles.[10] This coverage, along with news about Edward Hooper's 1999 polemic *The River*, which argued that a 1950s polio vaccine trial in the Congo was the origin of AIDS, expressed concerns about inadequate virus attenuation in live-virus vaccines, contamination of vaccines with other species' DNA, and scientific and pharmaceutical misconduct in general.[11]

Tierney's and Hooper's books, both of which feature stories about prominent vaccines that made people ill rather than protecting health, emerged the year before the September 11 attacks in 2001. In the immediate aftermath of 9/11, bioterrorism claimed a lot of media attention. Concerns about vaccine availability in the event of an attack and possible adverse events associated with vaccination show up simultaneously, perhaps feeding worries that scientists were not really in control of the infectious agents used in vaccines or the process of testing their safety. But the primary importance of the September 11 attacks to a changed tone in reporting on vaccination has to do with a heightened tone in news reporting in general. The fact that vaccinations were one response to concerns about bioterrorism made resistance to those vaccinations seem unpatriotic and ill informed, leading to hyperbolic language: "Today the case for mandatory vaccination is even stronger. This is war. We need to respond as in war. . . . And the government's highest calling is to protect society—a calling even higher than protecting individuals."[12]

The first decade in the new century brought a variety of concerns about emerging infectious diseases and vaccine availability. In 2003, along with continuing controversy about requiring American troops to be vaccinated against anthrax (coinciding with the war in Iraq, Operation Desert Freedom), severe acute respiratory syndrome, or SARS, caused a spike in concern about vaccine development and availability in the context of emerging infectious diseases. SARS also demonstrated how quickly an infectious disease can hop from country to country by air travel, as an outbreak occurred in Toronto because of a sick air passenger, even though SARS emerged first in China and most cases were located there. During that year and the next, *Slate* also reported on flu vaccine shortages. Mid-decade there were a number of articles about avian flu and the prospect of a vaccine. There was a perceived threat of a global pandemic if H5N1, the avian flu virus that previously spread only from fowl to humans and not very successfully, mutated so that it could pass between humans and, especially, in airborne droplets. Also, at mid-decade an article in *Slate* ("A Shot in the Dark," a very popular title for articles about vaccinations, particularly critical ones[13]) criticized the 1996 varicella (chicken pox) vaccine for being unnecessary and expensive in a society with limited funds for children's health.

Thus, coverage of vaccination in *Slate*, *Time*, and the *New York Times*—and the controversies it elicited—was varied at mid-decade, although it was during this period that the tone and focus of the coverage began to shift, albeit unevenly across the publication venues I am considering here.[14] Concerns about vaccines (chicken pox, anthrax) were reported on at the same time that concerns about shortages of other vaccines (flu) received attention, and emerging infectious diseases were highlighted.[15] In 2005 the science writer Arthur Allen began reporting on vaccination for *Slate*—a prominent promoter of vaccination, he later published a book, *Vaccine: The Controversial Story of Medicine's Greatest Lifesaver* (2007)—and played a significant role in *Slate*'s developing trend of arguing *against* vaccine skeptics and *for* the value of vaccination. Indeed, gradually, from around 2004 through to the present, most reporting on vaccination in these publications coalesced around vaccination controversy itself, including the claim that science had answered questions about vaccine risks. In this way, vaccination controversy became the problem of voluntary nonvaccination. In tandem with this trend, reporting became significantly more inflammatory. Jenny McCarthy, often referred to as "the former Playboy model," although she was also an actress, comedian, and talk show host, emerged as a prominent vaccine safety advocate and promulgater of the theory that vaccines can cause autism. She became a common, if not frequent, target.[16]

Thimerosal and possible links between the MMR vaccine and autism were slow to become predominant themes in news reporting in the 2000s. Reporting on thimerosal's possible dangers was initially taken quite seriously. Most reporting venues treated concerns about thimerosal in the late 1990s as if they had merit, probably because the FDA initiated a study on levels of mercury in vaccines. Additionally, the FDA's subsequent decision to remove thimerosal from single-vial vaccines in the United States by 2002 seemed both to address and to validate concerns about the ethylmercury preservative. Arthur Allen's first article for *Slate* in 2005 concerned thimerosal, and while he attacked both Robert F. Kennedy Jr. and David Kirby (the author of *Evidence of Harm*, a 2005 book that claims thimerosal in vaccines may cause autism), Allen also wrote positively about SafeMinds, a group that later came under withering criticism for its continued support for the thimerosal-autism connection.[17] After thimerosal's proposed ties to autism were discredited in 2004 (IOM report) and again in 2009 (Omnibus Autism Proceeding), claims about heavy metal contaminants in vaccines drew increasingly charged rhetoric in news reporting. Similarly, the Wakefield article published in *The Lancet* in 1998 did not seem to affect reporting much until after 2004 and the release of the IOM report that discredited links between MMR and autism. After 2005, reporting focused increasingly on the problems with Wakefield's article. Its eventual retraction in 2010 made the news seemingly everywhere.[18]

In *Slate* after 2007, all of the reporting is vehemently opposed to vaccine skepticism; *Mother Jones* followed a similar trajectory. In 2002 *Mother Jones* published an article skeptical of the need for required anthrax and smallpox vaccinations for the military in the post-9/11 era, and in 2004 published an article sympathetic to concerns about thimerosal in vaccines.[19] After 2007, however, all *Mother Jones*'s articles on vaccination focused on vaccine controversy itself and promulgated inflammatory arguments against vaccine skeptics. *Salon* had a similar conversion, but it occurred later in the decade. It published two prominent vaccine-skeptical articles in 2005: Kennedy's "Deadly Immunity," about the dangers of thimerosal, which was published concurrently in print in *Rolling Stone*, and "The World Just Fell Out from Under Me," by a mother whose child had Asperger's syndrome, which she blamed on thimerosal in vaccines.[20] Not until later did *Salon* shift consistently to reporting that criticized vaccine skepticism.

Kennedy's "Deadly Immunity" is an interesting piece in the context of increasingly charged rhetoric about vaccination concerns. In it, he makes a series of damning allegations against the CDC and the physicians, scientists, and pharmaceutical company employees who attended the Simpsonwood conference in 2000, largely for covering up known concerns about thimerosal and its neurotoxic effects on developing brains. He repeatedly uses terms like "laced" to describe the thimerosal in vaccines. Written as an exposé, the article claims that the government and the scientists at the meeting tried to bury clear evidence that thimerosal "appeared to be responsible for a dramatic increase in autism and a host of other neurological disorders among children."[21] He also accuses the writers of the 2004 IOM report of doing the government's bidding by determining that there was no evident link between vaccines or thimerosal and autism. Kennedy's article, in other words, is a full-on assault against government science and the drug industry.

The science writer Seth Mnookin, among others, disputes Kennedy's claims, arguing in *The Panic Virus* that Kennedy both distorts the existing public record and misunderstands what can be proved with scientific research. But what is important to my discussion here is how Kennedy's article serves as an example of an increasingly inflammatory debate. Using his experience as an environmental activist and lawyer, Kennedy accuses top public health officials in the United States and the world of trying to hide evidence of harm. As a result, his article becomes an emblem of vaccine skeptics' refusal to accommodate the facts as they are understood by vaccine supporters. It is this kind of article that people like Seth Mnookin and Paul Offit are referring to when they claim that "the media" have inflamed vaccination controversy.[22] (More on this in chapter 3.) But *Salon*'s later shift to reporting *against* vaccine skepticism, and its eventual removal of the article from its website, attest to the changing headwinds of the debate. "Deadly Immunity" expresses a core set of beliefs characteristic of some radical vaccine skeptics—that the government is hiding data that demonstrate the dangers of metals used as preservatives or adjuvants in vaccines, that pharmaceutical companies and the government are too cozy with one another to ensure vaccine safety, and that seemingly independent scientific organizations cannot be trusted to conduct ethically valid research. It also provides an easy target for criticism from the other side, with its seemingly slipshod use of selective quotation and its consistent use of correlative statistics to strongly (and, from the perspective of scientists, wrongly) imply cause and effect. For many people, the inflammatory elements in the debate are exemplified by articles like "Deadly Immunity," rather than in the more routine castigation of vaccine skeptics that became more and more common after its publication.

In retrospect, and despite the importance of "Deadly Immunity," three other events that occurred between 2004 and 2009 appear to have motivated inflammatory reporting focused increasingly on vaccination controversy itself: the 2004 IOM report, the 2006 rollout of Gardasil (the HPV vaccine), and the 2009 Omnibus Autism Proceeding judgment finding no connection between thimerosal and autism or between MMR vaccine and autism.[23] Once the Immunization Safety Committee of the IOM had published its report (2004), the culture wars concerning the HPV vaccine began (2006), and the vaccine court rendered its verdict (2009), the focus of articles on vaccination invariably concerned, at some level, vaccination controversy and the problem of vaccine refusal. It was no longer possible to represent voluntary nonvaccination as a rational behavior, at least in the context of reporting in *Slate* and *Salon*, as well as in *Mother Jones*. Even mainstream reporting venues like *Time* and the *New York Times* were using highly charged language and portraying voluntary nonvaccinators as ridiculous, as the quotation that began this chapter demonstrates. Thus, reporting on vaccination became reporting on vaccine refusers and the dangers that they pose to the nation as a whole.[24]

Why were these events so important to changes in reporting tone? When the Immunization Safety Committee of the IOM published its review of the science concerning autism and MMR, as well as autism and thimerosal, discounting any link that would hold vaccines responsible for rising rates of autism, it seems to have fueled a change in sympathy for those who continued to claim that vaccines cause autism. It was as if "science had spoken," even if activists like Robert F. Kennedy Jr. didn't believe it. Then, in 2009, the vaccine court confirmed the IOM report in its verdict. The year following the Omnibus Autism Proceeding, 2010, Britain's General Medical Council found Andrew Wakefield to have engaged in unprofessional conduct, and a month later *The Lancet* retracted the 1998 article. He subsequently lost his license to practice medicine in the United Kingdom.[25]

In between, in 2006, the HPV vaccine Gardasil was approved for use by the FDA. Two of the strains that the vaccine protected against cause 70 percent of cervical cancers in women. The strains also cause cancers of the anus and throat as well as genital warts in both sexes. Nevertheless, the vaccine was initially and rather aggressively marketed solely as a vaccine for women against cervical cancer. The CDC's Advisory Committee on Immunization Practices (ACIP) recommended Gardasil for girls ages eleven to sixteen. Both *Slate* and *Salon* published extensively on the Gardasil rollout and the subsequent cultural controversy that positioned vaccine advocates against those members of the religious right who believed that it would promote promiscuity. *Mother Jones* published three articles on this topic alone in 2007.[26] The *New York Times* and *Time* magazine also covered the Gardasil rollout and the controversy that ensued. In the *New York Times*, articles both for and against the vaccine appeared, with physicians lining up on both sides of the debate. Concerns ranged from cost to uncertainty about the vaccine's safety and effectiveness to the all-important question of whether a vaccine against a sexually transmitted disease would encourage girls to be sexually active. In state legislatures, there were extensive discussions about making Gardasil part of the list of vaccines required for school entry, a measure that would have reduced costs to families (because then the vaccine would have been included in the Vaccines for Children program) but that also enraged social conservatives.

Because the HPV vaccine debate became entangled in culture wars concerning girls' sexual behavior, reporting language became increasingly inflammatory, although for the most part the *New York Times* remained neutral in its coverage. But criticism of vaccine skeptics became more common and more florid across the other publication sites, especially after the 2009 judgment in the Omnibus Autism Proceeding against the alleged connection between thimerosal and/or MMR vaccine and autism. That ruling came in the middle of a serious set of concerns about Gardasil safety, which had motivated the CDC to conduct a study confirming that the vaccine was not causing adverse events beyond mild discomfort and a rash of fainting by preteen and teenage girls.[27] That study was published in August 2009, in the middle of the most recent swine flu outbreak, which became another focus of vaccine concerns.

In spring 2009 H1N1 (swine) flu emerged in the southwestern United States and Mexico and quickly became pandemic, although the illness itself was generally mild (with some notable exceptions, such as in pregnant women). The development of a vaccine and its quick dissemination in early fall raised concerns about safety and efficacy, and then, predictably, there was a shortage of the vaccine, which caused its own kind of panic. The H1N1 pandemic came a year after the broadening of recommendations for seasonal flu vaccines to all children, and a year before the further enlargement of that recommendation to all citizens over the age of six months. At this point, increasingly inflammatory language and attitudes became common in articles about vaccine skeptics in both *Slate* and *Salon*, especially in *Salon* during the 2015 Disney measles outbreak. In *Slate*, vaccine skepticism was linked to anti-GMO activism in a 2015 article, presenting both to be antiscience and evidence of widespread science denial.[28] At this point, all instances of vaccination concern seem to be perceived as opportunities to comment on voluntary nonvaccinators and their troublesome decisions.

Vaccination controversy initially developed in a context that was not simply focused on fears about autism, although that is how the discussion is often framed now. My analysis confirms Elena Conis's conclusion that concerns other than autism have simply been left aside in the way that vaccination is treated in the media now. She reports that the vaccine-autism story became increasingly frequent in the media as the twenty-first century progressed: "U.S. newspapers mentioned the link four hundred times in 2001 and more than three thousand times in 2009. And there were five times the number of evening news stories on the link in 2010 than there had been in 2001."[29] Most important in my view is the significant earlier reporting trend that challenged scientists about their ethics, reliability, and results, a reporting trend that simply dropped out of the publishing mix at a certain point. The concerns about shortages, soldiers, and various side effects also fell away, so that parental concerns about childhood autism appear to dominate the public sphere and are targeted as the primary reasons why vaccine skeptics don't vaccinate their children, as well as the primary problem with respect to vaccination in the country as a whole.

There is some evidence that the rise of social media on the Internet has affected reporting styles, as venerable news sources like the *New York Times* rely on website visitors to stay relevant. The advent of Twitter and Facebook as news sources influences the way that news is reported elsewhere. Most significant for my argument, however, are three of the issues that are evident even in the mainstream, and more neutral, news reporting venues—coverage of bioterrorism and measures to combat it, the debunking of proposed links between the MMR vaccine and autism and between thimerosal and autism, and the rollout of an HPV vaccine. These trends emphatically linked mandatory vaccination to national security, vilifying those who challenged that claim or expressed worry about side effects or adverse events. They also characterized anyone concerned about vaccine safety and unknown vaccine risks as scientifically illiterate and provided a context in which conservative opponents of a so-called cancer vaccine could be ridiculed publicly, even though most attempts to mandate the HPV vaccine for school entry failed. Taken together, these were game-changing trends in reporting on vaccination skepticism.

Changes in news reporting create as well as reflect changes in public perception. When parents express concerns about the ingredients in vaccines or worry about how many vaccines their children receive at single well-child visits to the doctor, authorities often respond that "science" has rendered their concerns moot. The analysis provided in this chapter suggests that the narrowing of vaccination concern to the issue of autism causation does not necessarily reflect the range of vaccination worries in the United States. Some of the most contentious issues that emerged in the HPV vaccine debate concerned whether the government should mandate a vaccine for a disease that is sexually transmitted. That is, if an illness is not communicable through casual contact, and thus not likely to be spread easily in a school, is it appropriate to require the vaccine against it as a criterion for school entry? The classic reason that vaccines have been required for school entry is that the school itself threatens children because of the required close physical proximity, and, consequently, they need to be protected from each other. But if a specific and intimate behavior—like sex—is necessary to spread the disease, is it appropriate to require the vaccine for everyone? The hepatitis B vaccine rehearsed this question in the 1990s, and vaccine promoters won that battle.[30] But with Gardasil, the situation ended differently, with only Virginia, Rhode Island, and the District of Columbia requiring the vaccine for middle-school girls.[31] Because the vaccine was labeled the cancer vaccine, though, and because the objection to the vaccine came largely from the religious right, reporting portrayed these issues as typical culture war problems that conservatives have with teenage sexuality, not concerns about the reach of the government on the bodies of citizens.

3

WHOM DO YOU TRUST?

This chapter and the next look at nonfiction books on vaccination skepticism that are written for the general public. The authors of these books consistently portray vaccine-hesitant parents as easily manipulated, although the books differ in their arguments about how and why antivaccinationists gain influence over them. In all, the question of whom to trust and how to trust are paramount, demonstrating that vaccination controversy funnels more widespread concerns about citizen faith in modern governments and medical science. I start with two provaccine jeremiads, Dr. Paul Offit's *Deadly Choices: How the Anti-vaccine Movement Threatens Us All* and Seth Mnookin's *The Panic Virus: A True Story of Medicine, Science, and Fear*, the first released right at the end of 2010 and the other early in 2011. Published to significant media attention, they both fed on and contributed to shifts in tone in vaccination reporting that were examined in chapter 2.

Reading these books, one would think that media reporting on vaccination controversy was tipped in favor of vaccine skeptics and that, as a consequence, the media were poisoning the minds of mainstream American parents with misinformation about the dangers of vaccines. Yet seven years past their publication dates, it is clear that much has changed about reporting on vaccination controversy. For example, in the wake of the Disney measles outbreak in late December 2014, the media have been engaged in a persistent argument *against* nonvaccinating parents. Almost all news reporting on the Disney outbreak emphasized the need to vaccinate and blamed voluntary nonvaccination for causing lowered herd immunity in areas beset by the outbreak. Opinion pieces, such as Frank Bruni's op-ed article in the *New York Times* entitled "The Vaccine Lunacy: Disneyland, Measles, and Madness" and other articles like the one by Ginia Bellafante quoted at the start of the previous chapter, have been particularly charged.[1] My local paper, the *Roanoke Times*, ran an article speaking specifically to concerns raised during the Disney outbreak, in which mothers defended their right not to vaccinate their children and complained about their portrayals in mainstream media: "Critics question their intelligence, their parenting, even their sanity. Some have been called criminals for foregoing shots for their children that are overwhelmingly shown to be safe and effective."[2]

The reporting on vaccine hesitancy that Offit and Mnookin target has changed since the publication of their books in 2011. Indeed, their books helped to change it, finding fault with nonvaccinating parents for believing wrong information and endangering others and blaming the media for promoting these views to others. Offit and Mnookin are not the only vaccination proponents who make arguments about the gullibility of vaccine-skeptical parents and the reasons why they are swayed by antivaccine sentiments, but they are perhaps the most prominent. Their books provide a glimpse into the frustrations of mainstream vaccine promoters.

Already in 2011, reviewers expressed surprise that the public needed more information about why vaccines are important. Abigail Zuger, MD, asked, in the first sentence of her *New York Times* review of *The Panic Virus*, "Does the reading public really need yet one more rundown of the repeatedly debunked claims linking childhood vaccinations and autism?" Her answer, after reading the complete book, is a resounding yes. Mnookin, she writes,

> really hits his stride when he turns to the social history of autism advocacy; his section on the actress Jenny McCarthy is a tour de force. To promote her

2007 book describing the purported vaccine-induced autism of her young son and his subsequent cure, Ms. McCarthy staged a media blitz, a medical tent show writ large. Blond and charismatic, she waved away science, energized the people who wanted to believe her message . . . and managed to do quite nicely for herself as well, netting a deal with Oprah Winfrey's production company.[3]

Of course, both Mnookin and Offit also profited from their books' popularity. Publication of these books transformed Mnookin's career from more general investigative reporting to a focus on science writing—*The Panic Virus* was named one of the five best books on health and medicine in 2011 by the *Wall Street Journal*, and he is now a professor and the director of the program in science writing at MIT. Offit, who published previously on vaccination controversy—most notably in *The Cutter Incident*, about inadequately inactivated polio vaccines that caused thousands of cases of polio just after licensure in the mid-1950s—also saw his cultural capital increase as a result of the timely publication of *Deadly Choices*. Both Mnookin and Offit were featured, among other notable scholars, physicians, and writers, at a 2014 symposium on vaccination at the NYU medical school to honor Jonas Salk on what would have been his 100th birthday, where Offit spoke about his then forthcoming book, *Bad Faith: When Religious Belief Undermines Modern Medicine*.

In the period directly after the Omnibus Autism Proceeding's finding (in 2009) that neither MMR nor thimerosal contributed to autism, railing on vaccine skeptics became predictable in media messaging about the perils of nonvaccination. Indeed, when Stephen Colbert interviewed Paul Offit on the *Colbert Report* on January 31, 2011, he did the interview relatively straight, without his alter ego's trademark double dealing.[4] I remember that I was actually up late enough to see the show and was looking forward to watching Offit squirm. Instead, Colbert soft-pedaled questions to him that were easily answered in favor of the official public health line on vaccination—indeed, his questions, delivered in Colbert's familiar tone, were clearly meant to enable Offit to highlight his primary arguments, rather than challenge them.

Quite soon after publication, these two prominent, popular books came to exemplify the tone of public debate, and they are heralded within the provaccine community as explaining vaccine refusal to the public.

Since one purpose of *Anti/Vax* is to explore how vaccination controversy is portrayed and understood by various constituents of the debate, in this chapter I examine how a prominent doctor (Offit) and a reporter-turned-science writer (Mnookin) see vaccine skepticism emerging from and being sustained by the cultural context. In the next chapter, I explore some of the same issues with books written by a historian, a sociologist, and an essayist. All of these authors understand vaccination controversy through the narrow lens characteristic of news reporting after 2005—concerns articulated by parents about the dangers that vaccines pose to their children. By following the lead of news reporting, these authors can be accused of augmenting the very problem that they seek to explicate and correct. They assert that vaccine skepticism is a problem of parental belief rather than an articulation of broader public concerns about science, medicine, and government intrusion on the bodies of citizens, and in so doing they cement that idea in the public sphere and make it seem true.

Deadly Choices

With his usual bravado, in *Deadly Choices: How the Anti-vaccine Movement Threatens Us All* Dr. Paul A. Offit blames lawyers, media reporting, opportunistic parents, and ignorant, disreputable doctors with fueling current vaccination controversy. His book begins with an account of the 1982 NBC documentary *DPT: Vaccine Roulette*, which, in his view and that of many others, started contemporary vaccination skepticism by claiming that the DTP vaccine caused neurological damage in children. At the time, the pertussis element of the combination vaccine was a killed whole-cell vaccine, with more proteins than any other current vaccine being used. In the late 1970s, a study in Britain had indicated one in 100,000 children would suffer permanent brain damage from the DTP vaccine. That study, Offit avers, was never replicated, and by the late 1980s most researchers and public health officials decided that the vaccine did not cause the harms identified in the 1970s. After his criticism of *DPT: Vaccine Roulette*, Offit discusses Barbara Loe Fisher and the National Vaccine Information Center (one of the most established vaccine-skeptical organizations, which began as Dissatisfied Parents Together in 1982), controversies about several vaccines in the 1990s and 2000s (hepatitis B, Hib, rotavirus, chicken pox, HPV), the MMR-autism connection and its fate in the Omnibus Autism Proceeding of 2009, historical and contemporary challenges to vaccine mandates, Jenny McCarthy and concerns about thimerosal and other metals in vaccines, Dr. Bob Sears and his alternative vaccine schedule, and, in a final chapter, the need to trust experts, vaccine proponents, and government public health officials, despite prominent examples, like former NIH head Bernadine Healy, who raised questions about vaccine safety. *Deadly Choices* offers a comprehensive argument against the most visible elements of vaccine skepticism in the public domain, ending with an appeal to shared humanity through herd immunity.

It is important to mention that Offit covers a number of historical vaccine injuries due to production error—a 1940s yellow fever debacle, in which soldiers receiving the vaccine were infected with hepatitis B; a 1929 tuberculosis vaccine (BCG) error in which ten-day old infants in France were injected with live human TB; and the Cutter incident, which occurred directly after the licensing of the Salk polio vaccine for national use in 1955 and during which thousands of Americans were injected with improperly prepared vaccine that contained live polio virus. Recounting these incidents allows Offit to make his primary argument: "The yellow fever, Cutter, and BCG vaccine disasters didn't spur significant anti-vaccine activity. . . . In America, people still trusted vaccines; and they trusted those who made and recommended them. It would take fear of pertussis vaccine to turn the tide; ironic, given that the pertussis vaccine tragedy was imagined."[5] That is, he is arguing, when *real* tragedies happen, no one distrusts vaccines; the incidents are recognized as mistakes of oversight or implementation, not science. The argument that follows is clear: the current antivaccination movement is based on *imaginary injuries*. The bulk of the text is taken up with demonstrating how fear of vaccines themselves emerged and continues to drive the public controversy.[6]

The book is filled with the usual suspects—television reporters who distort the truth, doctors who speak outside their areas of specialization, lawyers who can smell a retainer from a long way off, celebrities who are both manipulative and gullible, and parents who are easily swayed when confronted with confusing information or who seek immediate answers to unsolved medical conditions like autism. Along the way Offit never minces words—suggesting what Barbara Loe Fisher *should* have been doing if she had *really* been a vaccine safety advocate (like John Salamone, whose son was injured by the oral polio vaccine but who advocated for vaccine safety rather than becoming a vaccine skeptic), telling the doctors and lawyers who testified in the Omnibus Autism Proceeding what they *should* have done if they had *really* wanted to help children with autism—but it is at times difficult to determine what Offit's standards are for acceptable reasoning and the truth. He claims to base all of his positions on good science and reputable expertise (in one long section, criticizing evidence presented at the Omnibus Autism Proceeding by an unqualified doctor and presenting his own preferred expert).

Yet Offit uses both inflammatory discourse and misleading statistics to promote some of his views.[7] For example, the prologue to *Deadly Choices* starts this way:

> *There is a war going on out there*—a quiet, deadly war.
>
> On one side are parents. Every week they're bombarded with stories about the dangers of vaccines. . . . Understandably, some parents are backing away from vaccines; one in ten are choosing not to give one or more vaccines. Some aren't giving any vaccines at all; *since 1991 the percentage of unvaccinated children has more than doubled.*
>
> On the other side are doctors. Weary of parents who insist on individualized schedules, scared to send children out of their offices unvaccinated, and concerned that their waiting rooms, *packed with unvaccinated children*, are becoming a dangerous place, they're taking a stand. (ix; emphasis added)

References to war and the notion that doctors' waiting rooms are *packed* with children who aren't vaccinated are somewhat exaggerated, although one could argue that such language is not out of line in a book trying to capture the interest of readers to flip the page. But the statement that "since 1991 the percentage of unvaccinated children has more than doubled" is simply wrong (xv). The CDC's own statistics from the National Immunization Survey (NIS) show that this statement is incorrect. Offit cites an article by Saad B. Omer and colleagues published in the *Journal of the American Medical Association* in 2006 as evidence for this claim. However, that article investigates the effect of nonmedical exemptions from vaccination on the incidence of pertussis, and also the impact of lenient or more stringent mechanisms for obtaining exemptions on exemption rates by state. Thus, the figures used in the article by Omer and colleagues are not rates of vaccination, but rates of vaccination exemption, which are not the same. As a result, Offit cannot substantiate his claim that "the percentage of unvaccinated children has more than doubled" with evidence from the cited article. (Indeed, this article, along with evidence from the NIS, supports my earlier claim in chapter 1 that rates of exemption have increased the proportion of voluntarily unvaccinated children within the total group of unvaccinated children, which itself has diminished since the early 1990s.)[8]

Offit makes two more claims similar to this one. He argues that the Wakefield paper in *The Lancet* in 1998 led to a decrease in MMR vaccination in the United States: "Parents of a hundred thousand children chose not to vaccinate them."[9] While technically true according to the article that he cites, that article shows that while there was a slight uptick in "selective nonreceipt" of MMR between 1998 and 2000 (an increase of about 1.5 percent of US children), by 2004 selective nonreceipt of MMR had returned to 1995 levels.[10] In general, nonreceipt of MMR for any reason continued a downward trend, so that in 2004 it was at 8 percent of the population eligible to receive the vaccine. Because selective nonreceipt was generally steady throughout the study period, and overall nonreceipt declined, the proportion of children voluntarily not vaccinated is now higher within the total number of unvaccinated than previously. (This is more evidence supporting my argument in chapter 1.) Thus, Offit's statement, while technically true in the immediate aftermath of the Wakefield paper, implies that the paper had a more significant and long-lasting impact on MMR vaccination rates in the United States than is supported by the evidence. And later in the book he repeats his citation of the article on exemptions by Omer and colleagues, stating that "between 1991 and 2004, the number of unvaccinated children in states with philosophical exemptions more than doubled."[11] As already shown, this mistake equates exemption rates with rates of nonvaccination. Not only do nonmedical exemptions not match total rates of nonvaccination in any state, but many parents opt for personal belief or religious exemption (where available) in order to selectively vaccinate.[12]

These arguments inflame the discussion by subtly implying a problem more significant than, and slightly different from, the one that actually exists. Another argument that inflames the discussion occurs in his examination of Jenny McCarthy, J. B. Handley, and Generation Rescue, the organization that Handley founded and for which McCarthy serves as foundation board president. Offit spends pages attacking the vilifying language that Handley himself uses, after noting (and demonstrating) McCarthy's florid profanity. Then, he criticizes Handley's suggestion that the only way to determine if receiving multiple vaccines at one doctor's visit is not harmful to children would be to do a double-blind trial with unvaccinated controls:

> Handley was asking for a study of vaccinated and unvaccinated children. One result is certain: given recent outbreaks of Hib, measles, mumps, and pertussis, unvaccinated children would suffer and possibly die from preventable infections. No investigator could prospectively study children who are denied a potentially lifesaving medical product, and no university's or hospital's institutional review board worth its salt would ever approve such a study. Handley's proposal harkens back to a dark time in our history when—between 1932 and 1972—investigators prospectively studied four hundred African-American men from one of the poorest counties in Alabama to see what would happen if their syphilis went untreated. It was called the Tuskegee Study. Withholding antibiotics that could have cured them, it was probably the most unethical medical experiment ever performed in America. (162)

Offit is right that it would be unethical to create a completely randomized controlled trial of multiple vaccinations versus no vaccinations at all, given officially accepted safety profiles of vaccines. To deny vaccinations known to prevent disease, in the context of high overall vaccine receipt and acceptance, would be ethically suspicious. However, it would be possible to tweak Handley's suggestion and do a double-blind study of multiple vaccinations in one visit versus vaccines delivered singly, which would certainly be a more ethical study design than what Handley proposed.

What stands out as inflammatory in Offit's response, though, is his use of the Tuskegee example. The Tuskegee incident was egregiously racist and demonstrated that the study's designers and practitioners clearly valued the gathered evidence over the black men's lives. Offit chooses one of the worst ethical breaches in American medical science, the touchstone of current bioethics classes, to drive home his point. The entire purpose of this anecdote is to smear celebrity vaccine skeptics by connecting them to a prominent, and universally recognized, ethics breach based on racism.

To end the imaginary crisis—that is, a crisis in *belief* that is not based on evidence—Offit suggests we must reinvigorate trust in medical science as well as the individuals who conduct it and give their lives to vaccinate children around the world. He uses his last chapter, "Trust," to provide an overview of difficulties in changing religious and philosophical exemptions from vaccination, trends in medical practices and hospital systems requiring that both patients and personnel be vaccinated, and the challenge of reversing distrust in government. In the end, he suggests that "we have to set aside our cynicism about those who test, license, recommend, produce, and promote vaccines" (206), although how that will happen is unclear, given that it is difficult to know whom one can trust. By his own admission, well-meaning people can be wrong, and well-meaning people don't always make good scientists. At the end of the chapter, Offit tries to demonstrate that vaccine scientists and public health workers are fundamentally good people, people who can be trusted, by using the example of Patricia Heaton, a pediatrician who joined Merck "to lead its rotavirus program" (205). He provides examples of more good people arguing for vaccination in the epilogue, which ends with another plea to remember the "better angels of our nature" that were elicited after the September 11, 2001, terrorist attacks, when "we were united in our grief" (214). Thus, Paul Offit's solution to the problem of voluntary nonvaccination is to "recapture the feeling that we are all in this together, all part of a larger immunological cooperative" (214).

At least one question remains in my mind after reading *Deadly Choices*: Do we trust Paul Offit? His typically brash approach to the issues and his damning of everyone who does not agree with his version of the evidence are not calculated to bring skeptical readers to his side. I must admit to being biased against him before I read the book. In May 2010 I went, with a graduate student, to an "Immunize VA" conference in Richmond, Virginia. Paul Offit was a featured speaker. At one point during his talk, he suggested that vaccination refusal was caused by "mothers with PhDs who know too much for their own good." My female graduate student (a PhD candidate) and I (a mother with a PhD) looked at each other in horror as the audience tittered. At another point, he got a standing ovation when he mentioned that his hospital had passed a rule that personnel could be fired for not receiving a flu shot. My graduate student and I passed notes, somewhat dismayed that people should lose their jobs as a result of their beliefs. These feelings reemerged for me as I read *Deadly Choices*.

But I imagine that I am not alone in feeling a concern for the truth on reading Offit's book. It is not only that I found him playing fast and loose with a few statistics (I am sure I will be faulted for similar errors upon publication of this book), or that he used unnecessarily inflammatory language to set up his arguments or drive them home. It's that he told me, the reader, that I must trust again, but not how I am to establish or ascertain the conditions of others' trustworthiness. It is to his credit that Offit discusses a number of vaccination disasters, and that he does see a potentially beneficent role for vaccine safety advocates. But his central message to readers is that there are a whole host of folks that they cannot trust, including themselves when they seek information on the Internet or by watching investigative news programs. And he suggests that parental fears are imaginary, even though many parents who have these fears fervently believe that their children have been injured by vaccines or that they could be. So, if I were a vaccine-skeptical parent reading this book I might be offended by Offit's presumption that I need to trust only those experts that he dubs worthy, especially given that a former director of the NIH (Bernadine Healy) went on record in 2008 suggesting that current vaccines might have a role in causing autism in some children.

But if I were a vaccine-skeptical parent, I would probably see right off that Offit's book was not written for me, insofar as it tells me that I already believe in people who are not trustworthy, I don't know how to evaluate scientific evidence, and I am endangering everyone by even questioning the value of a vaccine for chicken pox.

The Panic Virus

Seth Mnookin, in *The Panic Virus*, provides a clearer argument and a more painstaking approach to telling the story of contemporary vaccination concern, although his overall message is quite close to Offit's. And his book, too, is not written for the vaccine-skeptical reader, although his mode of argumentation is less confrontational. Like Offit, Mnookin believes that the media are primarily to blame for rising concerns about vaccination, because, he argues, the scientific method is hard to convey in a typical sound bite or even in an investigative article. And he, like Offit, focuses squarely on the issues that are most visible to outsiders of anti-vax circles—the *DPT: Vaccine Roulette* documentary and resultant concerns about pertussis, MMR and autism, and thimerosal and autism. For Mnookin, celebrity antivaxxers, irresponsible news reporting, talk show hosts, and prominent leaders of autism organizations all peddle emotion over science, to the detriment of the rest of us.

The story Mnookin tells in *The Panic Virus* traces the development of two parallel tracks of public discourse about vaccines, from the 1980s onward. On one track there is a scientific and medical establishment increasingly sure that vaccines are safe, even after the tribulations of the thimerosal controversy and the June 2000 Simpsonwood conference. On the other track are vaccine skeptics, who increasingly press a link between vaccines and autism, either caused by the MMR vaccine or by thimerosal, or by some complex combination of both (complex because MMR never contained thimerosal, so one theory that combines these two causes involves the thimerosal preparing the child's body for an anomalous response to the MMR vaccine). The vaccine skeptics, Mnookin argues, are supported by the true culprits, the media, who keep the issues alive—in particular, journalists seeking a good story. Yet Mnookin argues that a "ratcheting up" of the rhetoric was undertaken in 2003 by leaders in the antivax movement, who felt increased persecution when government reports consistently refuted claims of vaccine-caused autism.[13] Thus while the media are the problem throughout *The Panic Virus*, vaccine skeptics are not blameless—especially those who are at the forefront of the so-called antivax crusade. According to Mnookin, they feed the flames of a dead controversy and convince hapless parents that the government, scientists, and even their own doctors are involved in a vast conspiracy to harm American children.

While Mnookin's targets occasionally shift, the same cast of characters that Offit brings forth is here: irresponsible reporters, distraught and gullible parents, and celebrity show-offs and other charlatans who dazzle while hijacking real people's emotions and concerns. This latter category includes Andrew Wakefield, Dr. Bob Sears, Robert F. Kennedy Jr., David Kirby (author of the 2005 book *Evidence of Harm*), and Congressman Dan Burton, who in congressional hearings in 2000 made a public connection between thimerosal and autism. These folks would have been unsuccessful, in Mnookin's view, if the media hadn't played along: "Wakefield might have provided the spark, and any number of other charlatans and hucksters might have fanned the flames, but it's the media that provided—and continues to provide—the fuel for this particular fire" (306). In particular, Mnookin blames lazy journalists: "The type of journalism that relies on the reporter's notion of what does or doesn't 'seem' correct or controversial is self-indulgent and irresponsible. It gives credence to the belief that we can intuit our way through all the various decisions we need to make in our lives, and it validates the notion that our feelings are a more reliable barometer of reality than the facts" (307). Mnookin follows this comment with one that links vaccine skepticism to denials of global warming. At an earlier point in the book, he suggests that bad journalistic coverage of scientific issues has many negative social consequences, including aiding and abetting "people's delusions and fantasies" (86). Mnookin follows this latter observation with a chapter about Morgellons disease, a highly contested condition in which individuals claim that fibers grow out of their skin, confirming his claim that federal money is spent on fictitious problems when the media fan the flames. This juxtaposition of issues suggests that vaccine skeptics are just like those who, from the perspective of the mainstream medical community, suffer from "delusional parasitosis" (95).

Early in the book Mnookin asks his central questions: "Why, despite all the evidence to the contrary, do so many people remain adamant in their belief that vaccines are responsible for harming hundreds of thousands of otherwise healthy children? Why is the media so inclined to air their views? Why are so many others so readily convinced? Why, in other words, are we willing to believe things that are, according to all available evidence, false?" (12). His answer is that vaccine skeptics are leery of modernity: they capitalize on anxieties about modern life and appeal to populist sentiment against elites (and thus against scientific expertise), as well as to subjective beliefs over objective science. He likens vaccine skepticism to the movement against the fluoridation of water in the 1950s. For Mnookin, these elements of vaccine skepticism are both the origin and result of a lack of trust in experts, and they convey "social anxieties about modernity and . . . faceless bureaucracies," just as the anthropologist Arnold Green argued about antifluoridation activism (33, 60).

In addition to these broad claims about why vaccine skepticism emerged in the late twentieth century with such apparent force, Mnookin provides a number of more specific explanations about why people believe things that are demonstrated by science to be false. He offers a series of psychological concepts meant to explain this phenomenon. He considers *cognitive bias*, "essentially a set of unconscious mechanisms that it is our feelings about a situation and not the facts that represent the truth," detailing later in the book a set of subtypes of cognitive bias, like *pattern recognition* and *clustering illusions*. He mentions *confirmation bias* as another way the unconscious mind works to move us away from facts toward feelings, as well as *cognitive dissonance, irrational escalation*, and the convergence of views in group situations called *availability cascades*, a term invented by Timur Kuran and Cass Sunstein to describe a "self-reinforcing process of collective belief formation by which an expressed perception triggers a chain reaction that gives the perception of increasing plausibility through its rising availability in public discourse." In addition, Mnookin argues that the Internet provides *information cocoons*, which allow people to seek out news they agree with rather than be subject to more common, and mainstream, information sources. Parents of autistic children, he suggests throughout the text, are particularly susceptible to this latter problem, as they stay up late at night to look for answers to their children's troublesome behavior (12–13, 15, 193, 194, 196, 198).

The Panic Virus also offers the reader science itself. Over and over Mnookin emphasizes how difficult the science of vaccines is, how hard it is to demonstrate the safety of vaccines, how hard it is to understand why doctors and scientists equivocate while still believing in the value of vaccination, and why parental concerns are misplaced. To be sure, he is critical of those scientists who do not seem concerned about real potential risks, writing that "regardless of the relative harmlessness of ethylmercury, there was a troubling self-assuredness that underlay health officials' blasé attitude toward thimerosal's potential risks, which echoed the complacency regarding the whole-cell pertussis vaccine in the 1970s" (122). Yet because of his sympathy for science and scientists, he is simultaneously critical of those scientists who should speak better and more clearly about vaccines *and* apologetic that much of the problem is inherent in the nature of science itself: "When officials at the CDC wrote that there was 'no data or evidence of any harm,' they meant to offer the strongest reassurance they could, given that they could never say definitively that thimerosal had *no* side effects—there was always the possibility that some piece of new evidence might emerge in the future. But to a public not well versed in the language of science the line read like an equivocation" (127; emphasis in original). Further on he presses a similar point about the difficulty of conveying the complexities of scientific insight and method: "The realities of the scientific method also present an uncomfortable challenge for anyone tasked with explaining to the public why this inherent open-endedness doesn't negate the high degree of certainty that accompanies widely accepted conclusions. The combination of ambiguity and authority implicit in science is hard enough to understand if you are sitting across a table from a scientist; it is an exponentially more challenging point to convey when filtered through media outlets that eschew nuance and depth in favor of attention-grabbing declarations" (159). Thus, part of the reason why people believe their feelings and manipulative celebrities rather than science is that the latter is just really, really hard to understand, and those responsible for conveying its universal truths to the general public are, to put it baldly, bad at it.

Like Offit, Mnookin provides some room for skepticism about his own analytic capacities, as he includes some serious errors in evidence meant to support his arguments. For example, he states that in 1954, during the Salk polio vaccine trial, "1.8 million children had been injected in 211 counties spread over forty-four states" (43), when in fact the figure of 1.8 million children was the total of all children in the study population. Only around 650,000 were injected with something—over 400,000 with the vaccine, and the remaining 200,000 or so with a placebo. The rest of the children involved in the trial were *observed controls* (that is, children injected with nothing whose health was tracked), who were part of the total number included in the counted incidence of disease. The importance of this error is that Mnookin uses it to suggest the substantial public confidence and trust in medicine at the time: "When . . . Jonas Salk announced that he'd developed a polio vaccine, millions of citizens had already been primed to do whatever they could to fight this national menace. Within days, parents were lining up to volunteer their children for what would be the largest medical field trial in history" (169). Inflating the number of children actually volunteered exaggerates this point.

No doubt there was tremendous support for the Salk trials, but in no area where the trials took place did the number of injected children (all volunteered by their parents) equal the total number of children available. Hundreds of thousands of parents across the country held their eligible children out. Thomas Francis, the study evaluator, was concerned that in the observation study too many of the volunteered children receiving vaccine would come from the middle classes, precisely the group of children more susceptible to polio than their poorer counterparts, thus distorting the study's findings.[14] Other errors by Mnookin include suggesting that vaccination rates are declining, especially for pertussis, and using statistics about exemption rates as proxies for rates of nonvaccination.[15]

I must admit that I found it odd that both Offit and Mnookin suggest that vaccination benefits women's liberation, as mothers, "no longer needing to spend weeks quarantined at home with sick children, have had a greater freedom to join the workforce."[16] One could also make the argument that because women's liberation in the United States has meant joining the work force rather than receiving maternity and family leave benefits, social and economic forces demand vaccines that will allow both parents to work without the need to attend to sick children. (And, as a result, it is the affluent who can forgo vaccination, as they are more likely to have a parent or caregiver available in the event that children become ill.) It is hard not to read these claims as paternalistic attempts to endear themselves to skeptical mothers, who, after all, might consider that if they weren't in the workplace, their children might just as well get sick and be cared for at home. The argument here is typical of Offit's and Mnookin's books overall—to make a point on the surface that doesn't really address the broader complications and meanings of illness, medical care, and public health prevention in people's intimate lives.

In the end, *The Panic Virus*, like Offit's *Deadly Choices*, can conceptualize vaccine skepticism only as the result of being taken in and manipulated against one's own best interests. Both texts focus primarily on showy organizations, glitzy and popular talk shows, and the issues focused on by the media; as a result, the Internet, the media, and celebrities and charlatans are the ones to blame. What these texts do not do well is explain why people, from their own accounts and experiences, come to believe in vaccine injury, the likelihood of vaccine risk, and officially debunked linkages between vaccines and conditions like autism. Mnookin's use of psychological categories to explain how people misunderstand the events around them is meant to suggest how *those other people are duped*, while we, the readers, are edified by the complexities of the scientific method and how easy it is to get things wrong. This is just a popular version of the "taxonomy of reasoning flaws" that are thought to beset antivaxxers as they troll the Internet for information.[17] Thus *The Panic Virus*, like *Deadly Choices*, is meant to explain vaccine skepticism to people who already think it is a problem needing to be solved by getting more people to vaccinate—both books show people who already agree with their premises that vaccine skeptics are gullible, emotional, antiscience, and fearful, easily swayed by irresponsible journalism and the lure of celebrity stories. They were published at a moment in which reporting on vaccination controversy was changing, and helped create the stupid, or deluded, antivaxxer as a staple of Facebook ridicule, news reporting, and television programs.

Both Seth Mnookin and Paul Offit blame the media for extending vaccination controversy beyond the point when the science was in question and for not reporting accurately on the evidence that existed at any given point. For these authors, the media perpetuate vaccination controversy when there is none—they see certain kinds of reporting as validating vaccine concerns, just as charlatans and poor medical researchers delude gullible parents. While they seem to understand the media's role in vaccination controversy differently than I presented it in chapter 2, they are really just demonstrating the same thing—they show, in other words, how the media, in focusing attention on just one aspect of vaccination concern, created a public perception of vaccine skepticism that was not only narrow, but actually skewed from the diverse contexts of its emergence and continued vitality.

Offit and Mnookin think of the media's role as negative, in that they think of it as *wrong reporting*, just as they think of vaccine skepticism as *wrong belief*. A different interpretation suggests that reporters created the stereotype of the vaccine-skeptical parent because of their commitment to science. Once the public health establishment repudiated links between thimerosal and autism and MMR vaccine and autism, journalists and other writers in the popular media represented frustrations similar to public health officials and clinicians concerning vaccine-hesitant parents and the threat of communicable disease. This understanding follows Elena Conis's claim that reporting on vaccination supported public health perspectives, as the media fell in line with public health goals and medicine's approach to the problem of parental belief.[18] In this view, the media's problem was not in being wrong about the science, as Mnookin and Offit claim, but in listening to scientists who were, and continue to be, tonedeaf about the sociocultural contexts of vaccination concern.

Mnookin and Offit have a point, that reporting has contributed to current vaccination controversy. But it isn't because "real science" is hard to report about, or even that journalists are overcommitted to a "both sides" strategy in reporting on public controversies. It's that the focus of reporting overall doesn't address, express, or represent the myriad concerns that people have about vaccines and the increasing medicalization of American culture. Since around 2005, news reporting on vaccination has followed the medicoscientific response to vaccine skepticism by insisting that vaccine refusers are wackos or selfish or just stupid. And this is why the issue of trust emerges as both important and nonsensical—important because clearly there is an issue of trust involved in understanding why some people do not agree with vaccine mandates or refuse to vaccinate themselves or their children, but nonsensical because the experts insisting that those same people need to trust science have just criticized them for being duped by the very people they *have* trusted. Offit and Mnookin take the scientific perspective in deeming vaccine skeptics wrong and wrongheaded. They insist that *their science* is dependable and trustworthy, without making an effort to understand vaccine hesitancy and refusal from the perspective of vaccine skeptics. As readers will see in future chapters, the issue of trust emerges in discussions of science denialism—and scientists again publish requests that ordinary individuals trust them, even in the context of books detailing how corrupt scientists have manipulated the facts.

Do we (sometimes or often) trust the wrong people, the wrong experts? Undoubtedly. How do we learn what is the truth? That is a key question at the heart of vaccine skepticism and public health in the era of alternative facts. In the next chapter, I look at two books written about vaccination controversy by parents to explore how they came to understand vaccination as a problem and what they think are the origins of vaccination concerns for modern families. Their explorations of vaccine skepticism in the context of their own parenting suggest that figuring out what is true *for them* influences their broader analysis. While I do not want to go so far as to say that facts are entirely subjective, as the arguments of this book proceed, I will be exploring how we can understand scientific facts to be influenced and how decisions about public health need to take this understanding into account. Without such an analysis, calls to trust science will not be heeded by a uniformly trusting populace.

4

Being a Responsible Parent

Accusations of bad, irresponsible, or simply inattentive parenting are rife in public debates about vaccination and vaccine refusal. A typical complaint about nonvaccinating parents is that they care only about their own, presumably privileged, children, and that they endanger the health of other children, either too young to be vaccinated, immunocompromised, or in some other way highly vulnerable to infectious disease and unable to be vaccinated. In the opposing view, nonvaccinating parents claim that others can be irresponsible, either sending sick children to school, ignoring the potential adverse outcomes of vaccination that put particular children at risk, or participating in a system that puts all children at risk of chronic, adverse conditions. Wherever you stand on vaccination, there's a way to blame a parent's behavior for bad outcomes.

In the media, the irresponsibility of nonvaccinating parents has become a commonplace, allowing, for example, Ginia Bellafante's article, excerpted at the start of chapter 2, to claim that antivaxxers refuse vaccines for their children just as they might not allow their children to eat

Oreos or watch the Disney channel.[1] Setting aside, for the point of this argument, that excluding Oreo cookies from a child's diet is no simple matter, this commonplace assertion grounds arguments for vaccination as the responsible choice for today's parents. By claiming that nonvaccinating parents treat vaccines (like Oreos) as trivial, news reporting and other public discourses frame a particular kind of responsible decision-making as the province of educated, thoughtful parents. Good parents, in other words, vaccinate, although now they do so not in blind obedience to medical authorities, but because they know it is the best choice for children.

This chapter discusses the issue of parental responsibility in the context of three recent books on vaccination controversy. The purpose here is to explore how expectations of parental responsibility animate vaccination concerns and practices. The three books are works of scholarship, although of differing kinds, and each explores parents' views of vaccination against the recent history of vaccination concerns. The books considered here all support vaccination, although differently from one another. Examined together, they demonstrate that embedded within vaccination controversy is another problem—knowledge-seeking parents and their sometimes unorthodox approach to mainstream medicine and public health. In juxtaposing these texts, I show that arguments about vaccinations and parents obscure other pressing questions about what we expect of parents in the information age. And I ask, pointedly, how provaccine authors struggle with the question of parental responsibility, and how the obligation to vaccinate aligns with contemporary expectations of knowledgeable use of medical treatment and informed medical decision-making.

I look at three texts: two scholarly studies and one extended nonfiction essay. Mark Largent's *Vaccine: The Debate in Modern America* and Eula Biss's *On Immunity: An Inoculation*, published in 2012 and 2014, respectively, are books that explicitly use the authors' ethos as parents to stage arguments about the meaning of vaccination controversy.[2] Although Largent is a historian and faculty member at Michigan State University, he introduces personal details of his experiences having his daughter vaccinated as an entry point for his research on vaccination. Published to artistic acclaim, Biss's *On Immunity* is written from a mother's perspective and offers a sympathetic approach to the concerns of new mothers about vaccination.[3] As a work of creative nonfiction, it takes as its starting point the experiences of mothers and the ways in which American motherhood prepares one to be fearful of a world that can be dangerous to infants.

Because these authors reference their ethos as parents, their conclusions, however close to Offit's and Mnookin's, seem more sympathetic to those parents who voice or act on their vaccination concerns. Yet this impression is somewhat deceiving. Both Mark Largent and Eula Biss reinforce the narrow focus on childhood vaccine risks that was established by the media after the turn of the twenty-first century. Both distinguish themselves from other unknowing or more easily manipulated parents who spurn vaccines altogether or peddle false claims. Indeed, their most significant arguments concern parents' obligation to *know*, to conduct research and deliberate about every health decision concerning their children. And threaded through their arguments is a moralism about parental knowledge and responsibility, one that reveals their positions to be deeply embedded in certain forms of privilege: being a university professor, being the daughter of a doctor, being white, being middle class, being able to choose one's doctor.

Those forms of privilege—identity markers and aspects of social status—are not in themselves a problem, but the way that they shape arguments about vaccination is. Interestingly, the sociologist Jennifer Reich's book *Calling the Shots: Why Parents Reject Vaccines* identifies the nonvaccinating parents (mostly mothers) that she interviews as part of this very same educated, affluent, and white middle class.[4] This is the third book that I discuss in this chapter. In Reich's argument, this privileged social position is something of a liability, as it shields these parents from understanding the implications of their decisions on poor and underprivileged children.

Taken together and analyzed against one another, these three books suggest that within vaccination controversy other concerns fester. How parents are to interact with state mandates and federal recommendations to vaccinate, how communities should uphold medical and social norms, and why vaccination is both a private and a public responsibility—these are the specific concerns within which parental approaches to vaccination are understood and evaluated. Parents understand and enact their responsibilities—to care for their children knowledgeably, to make good decisions about their health care, and to affirm medical norms and expectations independently, among other responsibilities—variously; not all parents come around to the same decisions with respect to vaccination.

Thus, parental responsibility itself becomes a problem in these texts, because it is both a mechanism for acceding to norms and a mode of resisting them. As a result, it represents an unresolved problem in vaccination controversy and a focus of attention on all sides.

Too Many Too Soon

Early in *Vaccine: The Debate in Modern America* Largent establishes his primary claim:

> It is not merely the nature of vaccines that disturbs parents; it is their sheer number. American children are now expected to get between twenty-six and thirty-five inoculations by the time they start kindergarten. To make matters worse, three-quarters of these vaccinations are administered in the first eighteen months of life, with as many as six at a single office visit. Every new vaccine added to the vaccine schedule adds yet another batch of potential side effects.[5]

This core problem—the expansion of the vaccine schedule for children following the passage of the Vaccines for Children program in 1993—is both the starting point and the recurrent justification for Largent's claims about the legitimacy of parental anxieties about vaccines. Indeed, he makes some broad claims to explain and support his argument—for example, "Most parents are much more willing to accept the consequences of a communicable disease than they are willing to accept the consequences of having made a child sick by giving them a vaccine" (27)—without presenting any evidence.

Throughout *Vaccine*, Largent focuses on the difficult position of reasonable parents who need to make decisions about their children's vaccinations, concluding that parents, given the context of a confusing public debate, must take it upon themselves to be educated about the risks and benefits of vaccines and to make each decision knowledgeably. Among the authors discussed in the previous chapter and this one, Largent is the most convincing in his criticism of public health approaches to vaccination. He argues that by not acknowledging parents' legitimate concerns about the expanded vaccine schedule for infants and children and insisting that all vaccines are equally necessary and equally safe, public health officials are needlessly encouraging the "vaccine-anxious parent" to traffic with more radical vaccine refusers. These anxious parents were initially set up for concern, he argues, by three main historical incidents (two of which were discussed in chapter 1): (1) the rise of alternative medicine, (2) reporting on Gulf War Syndrome, and (3) reporting on the Congolese origin of HIV/AIDS in the polio vaccine trials in the 1950s. Largent suggests that these early "sources of doubt" created a welcoming climate when the thimerosal and MMR controversies became public in the late 1990s, giving parents a specific focus for their personal concerns about the expanding vaccination schedule.

Arguing for the uniqueness of contemporary parental concerns about vaccines in comparison to historical antivaccination movements, Largent also distinguishes the "vaccine-anxious parent" from true antivaxxers. The latter are fringe believers in alternative medicine whose ideas became more palatable to the vaccine hesitant when the vaccine schedule expanded, stories about vaccine-caused Gulf War syndrome and HIV/AIDS circulated culturally, and thimerosal and MMR vaccine were identified as possible causes of autism. Largent provides detailed histories of both the thimerosal controversy in the United States and, in Britain, Andrew Wakefield's research on autism, vaccines, and gut disturbances, both of which came to public attention in the later 1990s. In both instances he targets the medical community as initially, and subsequently, "dismissive" of parental concerns, arguing that such dismissiveness forces concerned parents to pay attention to the more radical claims of true antivaxxers: "By virtue of their unwillingness to engage with parents' concerns and, for the moment, see past their rigid, normative notions of public health, physicians and public health officials have effectively handed the debate over to polemicists and thrown vaccine-anxious parents into the arms of anti-vaccinators" (83). Especially with regard to thimerosal, Largent explains why parental concerns still make sense, even in the context of a medical establishment that denies any danger—parents see mercury as mercury, he argues, and legitimately seek safer alternatives.

For Largent, the expansion of the vaccination schedule for infants and children provided two concrete kinds of problems for parents. First, children are subjected to multiple vaccines, as well as multiple shots, at well-child visits to their doctors, making it difficult to determine when side effects are associated with specific vaccines. Second, vaccines against serious diseases are undifferentiated from those that protect against more mild illnesses. Parents, he reiterates, will feel differently about the vaccines for measles and polio than they will about the vaccine for chicken pox, the latter of which, he implies, was approved largely because it saved families lost work time and kept children in school (21–22). In other words, he argues, the continued emphasis on the importance of all vaccines in the schedule distorts parents' reasoning about individual vaccines and does not acknowledge that specific concerns about particular vaccines may be valid. From the public health perspective, a concern about an individual vaccine might seem to indicate a concern about all of them, but Largent suggests that this view is an artifact of public health's defense of all vaccines as essential rather than understanding parents' more selective concerns. He writes, "There is a striking incongruence in the public debates about vaccines: critics attack *particular* vaccines—such as the vaccines against the chickenpox or HPV—and health officials respond with blanket arguments about the vital importance of vaccines *generally*. Such an approach allows authorities to respond to parents' concerns without addressing them" (166; emphasis in original).

Largent has a generous understanding of how easy it is to get a philosophical exemption from vaccination, implying throughout the text that parents have more choice in the matter than most parents might feel themselves to have. Indeed, he explains that he once got one when his daughter missed a vaccination because of illness and he couldn't get an appointment with her physician for a month. This explanation suggests that he lives in a state (Michigan) with an apparently easy mechanism for philosophical exemption, and underscores how important his own situation is to the broader claims that he makes in the book. Whether Michigan actually had an easy exemption mechanism at the time or it was simply easy for him, given his knowledge, status, and resources, is not clear from the text.[6]

In the end, he argues that parents must educate themselves with good information about the risks and benefits of vaccines, and then make their choices deliberately. Largent's portrayals of Jenny McCarthy and Dr. Bob Sears in the book are congruent with this perspective. Both McCarthy and Sears emerge as figures who have helped parents make sense of the confusing cultural and scientific situation with respect to vaccines, McCarthy because "she has an amazing ability to speak sensibly and compellingly about the issues of autism, vaccines, modern medicine, and the desperate state in which many mothers of autistic children find themselves" (147). In Largent's view, Bob Sears, author of *The Vaccine Book* and a physician in Orange County, California, provides a valuable alternative vaccination schedule for parents who want to vaccinate but who are put off by the ACIP-approved one. Both McCarthy and Sears are presented as resources for well-meaning and educated parents who are throughout the book represented as stymied by state mandates, health officials who are rigid to the point of seeming to be uncaring, and confusing scientific evidence.

The "us" created in the text is this group of affluent, educated, well-meaning, vaccine-anxious parents. Largent's primary arguments appear to be made possible by the privileges that his own position allows. He does argue explicitly that one of the things that makes vaccine concerns like his legitimate is that they are made by educated people, but he does not seem to acknowledge that taking personal responsibility for decisions about his child's vaccinations—so that they are a "conscious choice, rather than drifting into a decision that has been made by someone else" (175)—may be made possible by his class position, the state he lives in, the doctors he goes to, and even the schools his child attends. In effect, by arguing for parental choice in vaccinations, Largent is suggesting that vaccine mandates are not as constitutionally guaranteed as *Jacobson v. Massachusetts* has been interpreted to mean. In addition, he is suggesting that the refusal of parental choice by public health authorities exacerbates vaccination concerns rather than ameliorating them. In thinking that parental choice can be exercised easily by parents simply taking charge, he ignores those parents who might not have choices about their doctors, who might fear state involvement if they do not follow the law, or who may lack the literacy skills or resources to obtain a religious or philosophical exemption. In other words, he doesn't acknowledge the constraints that impede the decision-making power of others who do not share his demographic privilege.

What is most interesting about Largent's critique, however, is that he forcefully indicts medicine and public health as causing vaccination controversy by their callous responses to what he thinks of as parents' legitimate fears and concerns. At the end of the book, he suggests that vaccination controversy is an expression of a more general sense of "frustration with the condition of medical care in the United States today. Overburdened doctors and nurses, crowded waiting rooms, tremendously expensive insurance, massive profits made by pharmaceutical companies, and an elaborate maze of bureaucracy separating ill patients from the people who are expected to help them have all combined to alienate many parents from the medical establishment" (173). His basic position is that reasonable conversations about vaccination should treat parental concerns seriously, and public debate should acknowledge that politics and culture are party to the problem. Yet even though he puts the problem squarely in the public sphere, his solution is personalizing and moralizing—better parents, he implies, make active choices and don't "drift into a decision that has been made by someone else" (175). One could argue in response that doing things because other people with expertise have decided on them is a hallmark of modern societies. It is the very sign of trust that Paul Offit thinks we need to return to in order to end concerns about vaccines and what he thinks of as their imaginary threats to health.

Managing Maternal Anxiety

Eula Biss's *On Immunity: An Inoculation* makes an interesting intervention. The quote from the *Kirkus Review* on the inside front flap of the dust jacket states that *On Immunity* "giv[es] readers a sturdy platform from which to conduct their own research and take personal responsibility"—a somewhat odd recommendation for a book that ends with a call to communal responsibility. Indeed, *On Immunity* plays continuously on the individual's relation to the group, trying to ascertain how "people like me" (i.e., the author) can understand their responsibility to others. Biss treads this ground early on, in presenting a conversation with her son's pediatrician about his impending birth and whether he really needed the hepatitis B vaccine the day he was born. The doctor told her, to her ironic embarrassment, that the vaccine was really for "inner city" babies, "not something, he assured me, that people like me needed to worry about."[7] By the end of the chapter, she clarifies her perspective:

> When relatively wealthy white women vaccinate our children, we may also be participating in the protection of some poor black children whose single mothers have recently moved and have not, as a product of circumstance rather than choice, fully vaccinated them. This is a radical inversion of the historical application of vaccination, which was once just another form of

bodily servitude extracted from the poor for the benefit of the privileged. There is some truth now that public health is not strictly *for* people like me, but it is *through* people like us, literally through our bodies, that certain public health measures are enacted. (28; emphasis in original)

Throwing down the gauntlet early on, Biss insists that if "people like us" don't make their bodies available to public health through vaccination, they are endangering the lives of poor black children of single mothers without stable households. Of course, there is much to be said for a perspective on public health that understands one's own responsibility to others as a motivation for behavior. I don't mean to ridicule Biss's stance here. This is her way of suggesting how personal responsibility is also communal responsibility, a connection that she emphasizes later through a rather unusual statement about the inherent anticapitalism of vaccination: "But refusal of vaccination undermines a system that is actually not typical of capitalism. It is a system in which both the burdens and the benefits are shared across the entire population. Vaccination allows us to use the products of capitalism that are counter to the pressures of capital" (96).

However, I would like to suggest that the us/them dichotomy established in the longer quotation from Biss above is curious. Why are there "people like us"? Biss initially associates the phrase with the racist pediatrician, but then picks it up herself without irony to confirm a commitment to those black others who are at risk. "People like us," the rest of the book suggests, must find reasons to care about others who are otherwise outside of our field of vision. The friends with whom she considers the values of vaccination and the concerns of motherhood throughout the text are, we are led to believe, more "people like us." The life experiences of those others, *who also might have concerns about vaccination*, are absent from the text, which presumes that those very concerns are part of the neurotic experience of motherhood for "people like us." At no point in the text do those other mothers and their concerns make an entrance. Their purpose in the text is to represent those others whom the author imagines she is protecting by immunizing her son, but they do not represent anyone who might have something to say about the issues discussed in the book, or with whom she might even have a conversation about those concerns.

Instead, Biss talks to her friends and the mothers of children her son plays with, generating questions in part through these interactions, then seeks answers by interviewing scientific experts, reading books, consulting her family members (experts in medicine and philosophy in their own right), and attending conferences. Her voice is both naive and knowledgeable—she presents herself as curious but needing to learn about medicine, the body, and vaccination, with access to experts both in her own family and in the world at large, as someone who knows some stuff and who also knows how to find out about stuff that she doesn't already know. She's read Stoker's *Dracula* (*On Immunity* addresses, in large part, the novel *Dracula* and the ideas of blood, community, and infection that circulate within it), *Silent Spring* by Rachel Carson, Voltaire's *Candide*, Sontag's *Illness as Metaphor*, parts of Kierkegaard's *Works of Love*, books by the feminist science studies scholar Donna Haraway, vaccination and disease histories by Michael Willrich and Nadja Durbach, Marx's *Das Kapital*, and Lakoff and Johnson's *Metaphors We Live By*, among numerous other texts. Her thoughts about vaccination circulate through most of the issues and characters introduced by Offit and Mnookin—Wakefield, Robert F. Kennedy Jr., Dr. Bob Sears, the 2004 and 2011 IOM reports on vaccination and adverse events, Edward Jenner and the history of the smallpox vaccine, the swine flu debacle in 1976, concerns about environmental toxins, Barbara Loe Fisher, misinformation, the Internet, and Paul Offit himself—but she moves differently through these topics, as they generate questions for her as a mother and send her to libraries, experts, and her philosopher sister and physician father for answers. The personal— at times intensely personal—elements of the book's narrative bring the reader into an unusual affective space, where fears are understood to be generated by the vulnerability of children and the difficult decisions of the mothers who protect them.

Biss is not only the caring, observant maternal community member— she is capable of criticizing others. She cites mothers who think of their choice of nonvaccination as part of "a broader resistance to capitalism." Then she suggests that they are in fact demonstrating their "privileged 1 percent" status, "sheltered from risk while they draw resources from the other 99 percent" (107). She quotes Dr. Bob Sears as saying in *The Vaccine Book* that "tetanus is not a disease that affects infants, . . . Hib disease is rare, and measles is not that bad." Then she counters with evidence that "tetanus kills hundreds of thousands of babies in the developing world every year, . . . most children will encounter the bacteria that causes Hib disease within the first two years of their lives, and . . . measles has killed more children than any other disease in history" (107). These are just two examples of her explicit support for vaccination against the concerns of others who question it. The mothers who elicit more of Biss's sympathy tend to be mothers "not like us," whose experience makes their vaccine skepticism more compelling to her, such as the Vietnamese friend exposed to Agent Orange during the war: "After coming to this country, she did not vaccinate her children as infants, for a number of reasons, including her sense that it was not safe. . . . I could not ask her to risk her children for the benefit of the citizens of the country that had put her in danger. The best I could do, I determined, was hope that my own child's body might help shield them from disease" (88).

Biss argues that it was the experience of AIDS and its lasting impacts on health education that changed perceptions of immunity in relation to disease for her cohort of mothers:

> AIDS education taught us about the importance of protecting our bodies from contact with other bodies, and this seems to have bred another kind of insularity, a preoccupation with the integrity of the individual immune system. Building, boosting, and supplementing one's personal immune system is a kind of cultural obsession of the moment. I know mothers who believe this is a viable substitute for vaccination, and who understand themselves as raising children with superior immune systems. But children with superior immune systems can still pass disease. Pertussis, like polio and Hib disease and HIV, can be carried without symptoms. (137)

This is one moment where Biss almost approaches understanding her friends' perspectives from their point of view, but her moralizing finish to this passage, recounting one mother's surprise that healthy carriers can cause disease outbreaks, stops her from exploring this alternative account of the body's relation to others.

On Immunity appears to have two main purposes. One is to detail Biss's own struggles coming to terms with her decision to vaccinate her son, even though that decision seems to diverge from the practices of "people like us." The other is to show how much media reporting of science reinforces existing fears. In a passage that discusses how science has not, at least historically, been kind to women, she suggests, in keeping with long-standing feminist analysis, that the problem is about ideology triumphing over science—"it has been the refuse of science repurposed to support already existing ideologies." She continues: "In this tradition, Wakefield's study [the 1998 *Lancet* publication subsequently retracted] forwarded a hypothesis that was already in the air, a hypothesis that held particular appeal for women still haunted by the refrigerator mother theory [of autism]. Those who went on to use Wakefield's inconclusive work to support the notion that vaccines cause autism are not guilty of ignorance or science denial so much as they are guilty of using weak science as it has always been used—to lend false credibility to an idea that we want to believe for other reasons" (70). Later in the text she writes that "what gets reported back to us from the land of science is that which supports our existing fears" (140). Thus, for Eula Biss as for Paul Offit and Seth Mnookin, the media are primary culprits in distributing questionable scientific theories in sensationalistic and attention-grabbing reportage. Fear is at the basis of vaccine skepticism—and knowledge, like the knowledge-seeking practices she engages in and describes throughout the entire book, is what allays fears into manageable, daily practices of care and attention. When scientific studies—real or fabricated—contribute to and inflame existing concerns, we respond with questionable retreat into our own superior immunities, rather than, in the analogy from *Candide* that Biss uses to conclude her argument, tending our gardens together.

The Responsibilities of Privilege

Of the three books discussed in this chapter, only Jennifer Reich's *Calling the Shots: Why Parents Reject Vaccines* explicitly takes on the topic of parental responsibility from a critical perspective. In her concluding remarks, Reich specifically argues that a culture of mother blaming contributes to the "norms dictating that mothers should question more, ask more, and invest more," norms that accompany the intense responsibility of raising children in the information age.[8] In this way she shows how parental research concerning their children's health is constructed as a moral good in a particular context—one in which parents, even well-resourced parents, feel obligated to manage their children's lives and medical care in specific ways.

There is much to recommend in this detailed ethnographic study, which is one of only a few that succeeds in presenting the views of nonvaccinating families without caricaturing them as crackpots. For the study, Reich interviewed thirty-four parents with varying vaccination practices: full refusal, selective vaccination, and individualized vaccination schedules. She also interviewed health care providers and lawyers involved in vaccination injury compensation, analyzed online parenting and vaccination information websites, and observed the IOM members as they met to discuss vaccine safety. As a result, her book richly examines the salient cultural contexts in which parents make vaccination decisions. As she remarks in her introduction, most research on vaccine-refusing or vaccine-skeptical parents focuses on what they think. Her study, on the other hand, aims

> to put these views in a cultural, historical, and social context. I argue that these views represent broader cultural trends that support a view of medicine as personalized and individualized. These views are rooted in ideas about middle-class and affluent parenting that expect parents to heavily invest in their own children, even at a cost to others. This ideology of individualized parenting is tightly bound to economic and social trends that privatize individuals and their bodies into informed consumers. Parents tout their commitment to informed individual choice as a way of expressing their commitment to their children. (19)

I concur with the basic contours of this analysis, insofar as "personalized and individualized" medicine frames most representations of medical treatments (think drug advertisements) as well as people's own experience of medical care (being asked, for example, to work with physicians on treatment decisions).

Yet Reich's insistence that there is something specifically class-based about vaccine refusal and skepticism seems, to me, unsupported by evidence and the result of misunderstanding the role of social class and privilege in enabling parents to voluntarily opt out of vaccine mandates. Reich also consistently criticizes her nonvaccinating informants, belying an inability to understand their practices from their own point of view. She does two specific things that reveal her own normative bias: (1) she consistently refers to voluntary nonvaccinators as "free riders," suggesting that they are protected by the communities that they themselves endanger, and (2) she feels the persistent need to explain why her informants are wrong or misguided. As a result, while she depends upon these parents and their sincere efforts to explain their views and practices to her, she seems not to respect these views and practices, and does not understand the convictions that underlie them. Instead, she explicitly adopts the perspective of mainstream public health, and as a result she cannot see these parents as anything but *wrong believers* whose practices must be modified to ensure the health of society's most vulnerable, the sick and the poor.

At the crux of Reich's argument is the idea that public health through vaccination relies on herd immunity and, specifically, the cocooning of the immunocompromised and undervaccinated by those vaccinated and presumed immune. Nonvaccinators are a problem because they endanger these two vulnerable groups, and their ability to do so is related to their status. Reich argues that they can afford to go unvaccinated because others will bear the brunt of their health care decisions—with wealth and access to medicine, the voluntarily unvaccinated children can take risks that others cannot. Reich's response to this situation, like Biss's, is to emphasize the collective good and the communal responsibility of vaccination—to garner support for more public conscientiousness and less private investment of parental energy and thoughtfulness.

To get to this point, Reich reiterates throughout *Calling the Shots* that voluntary nonvaccinators are a largely affluent, white, and privileged group. There is an obvious advantage to this argument if you want to criticize vaccine resistance—it implies that wealthy white families freeload by exploiting their already unfair advantage over others, an element of their demographic privilege and lack of responsibility to others without those advantages who are more vulnerable (because of poverty or immune-system compromise) to vaccine-preventable diseases. Simply put, the argument criticizes nonvaccinating mothers for their lack of interest in the welfare of other people's children—the epitome of neoliberal carelessness and lack of concern for anyone except oneself and one's family.

That parents have created an individualistic and family-centered set of arguments justifying voluntary nonvaccination is not surprising—that is how rhetoric works. People ground their arguments in commonplaces that are generally accepted. Making arguments that go against community expectations of public responsibility demands that families utilize existing ideas that are generally accepted in other domains or that have been persuasive historically. Making an argument for voluntary nonvaccination on the basis of the unique somatic situation of one's children aligns vaccination practices with emerging discourses of precision medicine, as well as other trends emphasizing children's uniqueness (such as "different learning styles" in education circles). Indeed, the first time I heard someone talk about voluntary nonvaccination was at a dinner in which someone described not vaccinating her children as a "personal family decision." At the time, and knowing nothing about vaccination controversy, I took a completely mainstream view and thought to myself that vaccination was anything *but* a personal family decision. But in a society that increasingly sees government and community as secondary to individualistic pursuits, such a statement makes some sense.[9]

In research on H1N1 flu vaccination clinics, my research group identified parents who viewed vaccination decisions as personal. Indeed, we found "the use of a personalized rhetoric in vaccine refusal is a mechanism to assert the uniqueness of the self and family in the face of generalizing tendencies in public health practice."[10] The families we interviewed in this study were not wealthy, and none had exempted their children from routine vaccinations of childhood.[11] The Pew Research Center found in 2015 that parents with *less* education were actually more concerned about the safety of the MMR vaccine, while parents with more education felt more comfortable with its safety profile.[12] Thus it is not clear that Reich's repeated assertion that vaccine-refusing families are wealthier and more educated than vaccinating families is true. At the least, the accepted truism that affluent families are more likely to exempt their children from vaccination may not be a true gauge of the general population's actual concerns about vaccination. Exemption rates may track high socioeconomic status, but only because wealthier families may have the resources to successfully gain exemptions without losing necessary welfare benefits or incurring the attention of child protective services. In other words, constraints on poor parents may make acting on their vaccination concerns difficult.

Reich's effort to understand her informants and to explain their beliefs and practices is marred by her effort to demonstrate that they are wrong. As parents, she implies, their efforts are misplaced. She suggests that those who identify as researchers are hardly that, as they do not conduct the kind of systematic research characteristic of science and social science. In other words, she is extremely critical of the very "culture of individualistic parenting" that she seeks to understand.[13] Moreover, she sees the parents' efforts to manage their children's uniqueness and vulnerabilities through nonvaccination, select schools, and special diets as reinforcing the very privileges that separate them from the poor—a damning observation from a scholar with a clear social justice agenda. Indeed, she writes that "taking advantage of opportunities [to advocate for their children] involves obligations to invest in others' children too, obligations that are arguably higher for those who have the best access to high-quality food, healthcare, schools, housing, and resources" (239).

But from a different angle, these parents are just participating in normative experiences of parenting in the information age. Reich suggests as much in her use of the word "norm" to describe current social expectations of maternal information gathering quoted above. Indeed, current scholarship in a field called *biopolitics* suggests that such behaviors should be positively cast so as to recognize the individual subject as an "ethopolitical agent" who can enhance personal vitality and capacities through careful somatic management. As I will discuss later in the book, vaccine skeptics, seen this way, are ideal "biological citizens."[14] Yet for Reich, regardless of how they might be influenced by changes in medicine and parental norms, part of what is wrong with these voluntary nonvaccinators *is their social class*. What if we were to find that other parents, not so wealthy or so white, also harbored vaccination concerns? How would we understand their commitment to communities if many of them basically felt that their compliance with state mandates was not voluntary but the result of coercion? What if those same, less well-off families wanted *more social power to treat their children's individualized somatic identities*? What if they want some vaccination choices too?

Families that voluntarily forgo vaccination actively question public health truisms and resist what Reich terms a social contract: "Outside the vaccine context, there are few places where our social contract with each other is debated so regularly and openly" (238). For me, this is the stickiest point of her argument. While I understand that her purpose is to show how important this particular social contract is to maintaining the health of communities and their most vulnerable, I have a hard time understanding how, after interviewing families that do not accept the precepts of such an agreement and who do not see themselves as being obligated within such a contract, she could continue to uphold it as existing and foundational to people's compliance with vaccination mandates. Reich's interviewees refused to accept vaccination as part of a social contract that mandates that they be concerned about and obligated to others over and against their obligations to themselves and their own health. Making an argument that we need to find ways to bring voluntary nonvaccinators back into this particular view of a public health social contract seems to be ignoring how much they repudiate it. It is an interpretation that does not accept their understanding of themselves, their bodies, their health, and their social commitment as valid. And it is an interpretation grounded in the perception that parents who hold to such views and engage in practices that ensue from such views are irresponsible.

All three of the authors discussed in this chapter make their arguments on the basis of parental responsibility. This coherence of argument suggests that parental responsibility, not only vaccination concern, lies at the center of vaccine debates today. Yet the authors are not fully aligned with one another. Mark Largent ardently defends parental anxieties about vaccines and his critique of health officials who "respond to parents' concerns without addressing them."[15] He and Eula Biss agree that parents must take responsibility for their vaccine decisions regarding their children, Largent explicitly through argument and Biss implicitly through the trajectory of her essay, in which she worries through decision-making and knowledge-gathering, presenting herself as someone who learns to trust the experts and be a responsible community member through her research and her experiences. Unlike Largent, Biss does not criticize scientists or doctors—she is much more like Offit and Mnookin in this regard.

Jennifer Reich criticizes parental responsibility when it does not cohere with public health management of herd immunity through vaccination. In the case of her interviewees, parental research that leads to voluntary nonvaccination for themselves and their children is dangerous and worrisome, threatening the health of the less fortunate and demonstrating a stratified society in which the wealthy don't care much about the health of others. Such research, she implies, isn't really research but the ferreting out of information that conforms to already held beliefs or that supports the individualistic and individualizing practices of a privileged class.

Responsibility is necessary and good, therefore, unless the enactment of it leads to behaviors that contravene socially normative expectations. Parental responsibility for making medical decisions for their children thus seems somewhat precarious, never fully assured to cohere with legal mandates or public health expectations. Parents have access to more health information now than ever before, thanks to the Internet and an increasingly collaborative medical culture in which shared decision-making is a norm and patients are often asked what their preferred treatment will be. But parental use of that information, heralded on one side as a way of exerting their responsibility and reviled on the other as a fake kind of research that puts other children at risk, is not wholeheartedly accepted. It's only good if it leads to results that are already accepted as appropriate by public health and medicine.

Trusting others with the health of one's children creates uncertainties that are exacerbated in the information age. To deal with these uncertainties and the difficulties of trust they engender, parents turn to a variety of sources, including Internet sites, social networks, celebrities interviewed on television talk shows, popular books, and their doctors. They do research and contribute to a context that the anthropologists Melissa Leach and James Fairhead describe as divided by two different kinds of science: "clinical/personal versus epidemiological/population." In their words, "These are grounded in the different conceptual and political worlds: the world of parents, intimately concerned with their own children, their personalized immunity, and their sense of personal responsibility and need to choose for their children's health, versus the world of public health policy makers, emphasizing the societal good and political importance of mass vaccination."[16] To suggest that parental research is only good or worthwhile when it ends up aligning with the epidemiological or population health type of science does a disservice to those parents who are engaged in expected norms of biopolitical citizenship of the twenty-first century but come up with different answers to their questions. Vaccination controversy shows us that disagreement about health outcomes and the advisability of bodily interventions can produce discordant approaches *within science*. How, as a society, we deal with these circumstances of fundamental disagreement reflects how well our social contract is working. But the question is not how to make vaccine skeptics agree to a public health social contract that they repudiate. The question is how to approach vaccination in such a way that the epidemiological or population view is understood not to be a self-evident truth, but one way among many of understanding evidence and establishing policies.

Of course parents use tools at their disposal to advocate for their own children. Mark Largent argued as much when he described getting a personal belief exemption from vaccination in order to manage his daughter's school attendance in the context of a fully booked pediatrician's schedule. *Of course* middle-class parents have more tools at their disposal than poorer parents, and many white parents have resources that are less available to parents of color. These are self-evident facts in a society stratified by class and race. All three of these texts raise these issues in various ways. The concerns raised in this chapter about socioeconomic status and the responsibilities of parents to protect not only their own children but other children cut to the heart of public health policies and laws concerning vaccination.

But instead of showing us how terrible nonvaccinating parents are because they don't care about other people's kids, I want to suggest that the emphasis on privilege masks the more fundamental problem of parental decision-making and responsibility. Reich gets at this when she suggests mother blaming has to stop as one part of changing the current climate within which vaccination decisions are made. But her numerous suggestions for change focus on bringing parents around to the epidemiological or population perspective, in the context of a limited acknowledgment of vaccine-skeptical sentiments. I think that we need more attention to the problem of parental responsibility altogether.

How is it, I want to ask, that parents taking on this responsibility in a fully socially normative manner can be excoriated for believing the wrong things? Is the expectation of parental responsibility—especially the responsibility to do research and to understand medical procedures and published results of experiments—just a way of managing parents into socially acceptable roles and practices? Are parents who do not comply with the expectation that they will engage actively and knowledgeably in the medical care of their children lazy or indifferent—unless that medical care is vaccination, in which passive compliance is expected and valued? How informed of vaccination practice are parents supposed to be, given that there is no real informed consent to the procedures, simply a CDC-approved information sheet given out to parents as a routine element of the interaction?

Vaccination is the perfect phenomenon in which to situate the study of these broad questions about responsibility in the information age, because it is a mandatory public health practice largely disseminated through private doctors' offices and individualized to specific children through a complex schedule and varying state laws. It represents the fragmented nature of our health care system in the United States, and it raises questions about how much knowledge is necessary or good to be a responsible parent, especially when such knowledge turns some away from socially normative practices of well-child care.

Put another way, a broader social anxiety expressed through vaccination controversy and the discourses that constitute it may concern the relation of parents to the bureaucratic authority of the state. This problem is not new. The question of parental authority over family health was also central to resistance to smallpox vaccination in the Victorian and Progressive eras.[17] Trust emerges in this context as something created by knowledge—one trusts the bureaucrats or medical authorities when one's own research confirms their mandates. Yet for those parents whose research suggests otherwise, the state and medical authorities roll out corrective and persuasive measures—more scientific defenses of vaccination, a signed "vaccination refusal form" forcing parents to acknowledge the dangers of nonvaccination, punitive actions linking welfare entitlements to children's vaccination status, among other measures. Trust, of course, is not likely to be created through these kinds of mechanisms.

The rest of this book explores the questions raised in this chapter, through discussions of denialism, scientific facts, medicalization, and the viral imagination in fiction and film, before turning, in the last chapter, to the novel findings of my research group's interview studies. The discussion will demonstrate, I hope, the difficulties of using references to *science* as a monolithic source of truth to dispel controversies that are inherently social, value-laden, and rooted in people's worldviews. Indeed, the notion that science itself produces truths that are indisputable is a theme that I explore. Doing so in the era of "alternative facts" has been an interesting exercise. In my view, "alternative facts" have always existed, and current political contexts have brought to the fore the shifting grounds of agreed-upon reality. Rather than using science as a club to bludgeon socially salient versions of reality, we might, alternatively, explore the implications of disagreement in a democratic society, in which citizens must decide on mechanisms to manage different points of view.

5

IS VACCINE REFUSAL A FORM OF SCIENCE DENIAL?

Science denial seems to be all around us. There are AIDS denialists, climate change denialists, and vaccination denialists, among others. All of these folks apparently don't believe in facts that everyone else accepts as true: HIV causes AIDS, global warming is caused by human activity, vaccinations are the single most important preventative health strategy ever invented and save millions of lives every year. That is, pundits claim, there exists a widespread group of science haters or scientific illiterates out there, people who either refuse to believe or don't know how to believe in science itself.

What does it mean to make these claims about science denial as a phenomenon and to identify vaccine skeptics as science deniers? Recent rhetorical studies look at how denialists make their claims. Emma Bloomfield finds three basic patterns characteristic of denialist discourse: targeting the other as a villain; discounting evidence; and shifting the responsibility of proof to the other.[1] I found when working on AIDS denialist discourses that some typical rhetorical patterns prevail—"the scattershot presentation of evidence and argument, the attack on all truth claims associated with mainstream positions, and the suggestion of a concerted and organized conspiracy."[2] Yet these approaches, while identifying specific argument strategies, don't address what the charge of denialism does in public debate itself. Bloomfield may be right that deniers themselves try to "shut down productive discussion," but the countercharge of denialism tries to do the same.[3]

In this chapter and the next, I focus on denialist labeling and the implications of arguing that others are denialists. I am not interested in ensuring agreement that so-called deniers are wrong or establishing how to change their views, in part because this strategy appears to be ineffective but also, more importantly, because it is fraught with epistemological problems.

The term *epistemology* refers to theories of knowledge. In philosophy, epistemology is distinguished from *ontology*, which refers to the nature of being or reality. Basically, epistemology refers to how we know things, as well as how we know that we know things: how, in an argument or justification, knowledge is used or presumed, or what knowledge is thought to be. An *epistemological problem* is one that gets the knowledge part of an argument or claim wrong—it misconstrues who knows what, how knowledge is created or sustained in a particular circumstance, or why people agree with some knowledge claims yet dispute others that are seemingly credible.

Every time we insist that a denier is wrong, we are making a knowledge claim. What I explore here is how often those claims rely on incorrect assumptions about how we know things and why we believe in certain forms of evidence. We can avoid this problem by paying attention to what the accusation of denialism *does to the conversation*—how it construes the facts of the case and what solutions to the disagreement are implied by its articulation. In this chapter and the next, then, I address the epistemology of making denialist claims—asking, for example, what forms of knowledge are understood to be valid when claiming that someone else believes the wrong thing—and I suggest why a different approach to the so-called truth about vaccines might be profitable in the context of the particular controversy in which we find ourselves.

By taking this position, I am not claiming that science has no validity, or that assaults on science are inconsequential. What I am trying to do is to shift the ground of the debate from one in which scientific truths are known and valued ahead of time and all questions about them are a priori assaults on those evident truths. Considering what arguments about denialism *do* is a strategy to reorient a controversy in which current antagonists speak past one another. It is a rhetorical approach that values context and situation over absolutist claims about truth.

Charges of denialism often imply a cultural situation in which wrong beliefs proliferate—I want to explore what that implied situation is, and how it may, or may not, really be causing vaccination skepticism. In addition, labeling someone a science denier suggests that person shouldn't be trusted in general because they harbor wrong beliefs. Those wrong beliefs are part of a larger pattern, a denial of scientific facts, which, the argument goes, everyone should be able to recognize as true and valuable. As a result, exploring charges of denialism involves considering how we understand right and wrong beliefs about science in a democracy, that is, in a society defined by civil engagements over diverse beliefs and political positions.

I start with the term *denialism* and explore its history. *Denialism* was first used to describe those who refute the Holocaust, a historical event. Denialism's origins in academic and public fights over the reality of the Holocaust are meaningful in relation to claims of science denial: they provide a context for understanding what history is, how historical evidence is understood to support shared notions of reality, and why some people believe in unorthodox and seemingly damaging ideas about the past. Then I consider what science denial is—that is, how it is portrayed and argued for in public debate, setting up an explicit contrast with historical denialism. I show that popular discussions of science denial utilize psychological rationales for explaining its durability and cultural force. We saw some of these psychological rationales in the discussion of *The Panic Virus* in chapter 3. This reliance on psychological theories is almost always inadequate for understanding why specific forms of resistance to scientific evidence emerge culturally and stick with us.

The discussion in this chapter leads directly to the next, which explores the history and epistemology of scientific facts and considers how public controversies over science denial may affect how people understand and come to trust certain forms of scientific evidence. Drawing on the idea of cultural construction and a historical approach to facts allows us to see how the problem of *interest* or *bias* is an ever-present threat to public acceptance of science. Situating vaccine skepticism in the context of ongoing public debates about the reliability of government-sponsored scientific inquiry allows us to see how trust in science has been compromised. The call, then, to *trust science* (as we saw at the end of Offit's *Deadly Choices*) is difficult to accommodate to a situation in which manipulation, corruption, and interest have made it unclear who can be trusted. And the way instances of historical and scientific denialism generate responses about the importance of *facts*, *truth*, and *trust in the scientific method* suggest that the most salient element of the critique of denialism—that denialism is *politically motivated*—is routinely ignored in the public discussion about how to counteract its most deleterious effects on the common good. Considering the political, or ideological, basis of denialism forces debates about climate change, vaccines, and HIV/AIDS into the realm of *values*, which, in my view, is where they should be.

Holocaust Denial, Poststructuralism, and the Question of Truth

Holocaust deniers do not believe that the genocidal killing of European Jews by the Nazis occurred during World War II. The historian Deborah Lipstadt shows that Holocaust denial emerged in Europe directly after the war ended and "found a receptive welcome in the United States during the 1950s and 1960s—particularly among individuals known to have strong connections with antisemitic publications and extremist groups."[4] Whereas "until the beginning of the 1970s, Holocaust denial in the United States was primarily the province of these fringe, extremist, and racist groups," she writes, denialist ideas took hold because from the 1960s on poststructuralist ideas began to erode traditional conceptions of historical truth (65, 81). Thus, while Lipstadt and other historians identify anti-Semitism as the primary motivation for Holocaust denial, they argue that it is made possible by "relativistic approach[es] to the truth [that] permeated the arena of popular culture, where there is an increasing fascination with, and acceptance of, the irrational."[5]

Poststructuralism is a term that refers to a variety of critical methods, typically found in philosophy, linguistics, and literary analysis. What Lipstadt and others are referring to is a particular form of poststructuralist analysis, called *deconstruction*, that emphasizes the undecidability of textual interpretation. Undecidability refers to the difficulty of settling on one singular meaning for any given linguistic expression. For deconstructionists, language is fundamentally ambiguous, and writing always presents internal contradictions of meaning. Deconstructive interpretation often shows how various meanings compete with one another throughout a text, emphasizing the arbitrary nature of our interpretive choices.

Poststructuralism is often confused with *postmodernism*, a trend in architecture and the arts that emphasizes the local contexts of meaning in a broader, and chaotic, world. Postmodernism heralded the end of "grand narratives" and emphasized the fragmentary and contingent nature of artistic expression and interpretation. One can understand poststructuralism, and deconstruction more specifically, as philosophical trends within postmodern sensibilities. Poststructuralist approaches to historical analysis do challenge traditional approaches to the truth, insofar as deconstruction puts unitary truth in question by emphasizing incommensurable conflicts of meaning within texts. Yet by putting truth "under erasure," deconstruction doesn't do away with the idea of truth—it is not a form of nihilism, although some critics do make this claim. Deconstruction suggests that truth is not self-evident and that multiple truths compete for legitimacy in any given discourse.

It is striking that two prominent books on Holocaust denial, Lipstadt's *Denying the Holocaust: The Growing Assault on Truth and Memory* and Michael Shermer and Alex Grobman's *Denying History: Who Says the Holocaust Never Happened and Why Do They Say It?*, suggest that a relatively abstruse philosophical trend laid the groundwork for the acceptance of Holocaust denial across a broad swath of the US population. To my mind, Lipstadt provides a better discussion of poststructuralist ideas than Shermer and Grobman, beginning with the notion that "various scholars began to argue that texts had no fixed meaning."[6] Lipstadt connects this philosophy of the radical ambiguity of textual meaning to other trends that seemed to lead to an obsession with irrationality (she refers to recurring conspiracy theories about John F. Kennedy's death) and to the debasing of history when "history is rewritten for political ends and scientific historiography is replaced . . . with 'ideological conformity'" (19). For Lipstadt (as well as Shermer and Grobman), poststructuralist approaches to facts and meaning make it difficult to establish shared notions of history: "These attacks on history and knowledge have the potential to alter dramatically the way established truth is transmitted from generation to generation. . . . No fact, no event, and no aspect of history has any fixed meaning or content. Any truth can be retold. Any fact can be recast. There is no ultimate historical reality" (19).

Lipstadt, Shermer, and Grobman see both poststructuralism and Holocaust denial as assaults on the practice of history. For them, a particular form of heinous belief and its spread throughout certain populations show that traditional notions of history are crumbling, to our peril. Shermer and Grobman in particular discuss the practice of history at length—what constitutes good history and how to differentiate "legitimate revision" from "denial."[7] There is a significant focus in their book, *Denying History*, on boundaries and rules, that is, what allows one to distinguish good history from bad. (This response is remarkably like mainstream responses to vaccine skepticism and refusal—that vaccine skeptics are scientifically illiterate and, therefore, can't distinguish reputable science from pseudoscience.) Lipstadt herself won't appear with Holocaust deniers publicly because such appearances confer legitimacy to their claims. To appear on television or in other public contexts discussing the Holocaust with deniers would suggest that there are facts on the "other side," and propose that the other side is simply interpreting the facts differently. For Lipstadt, that portrayal of the situation is unacceptable. Like scientists in vaccination controversy, the historians discussed here do not accede that there is a public debate about the Holocaust. Instead, there is the truth and there are deniers.

In this argument, reliable and objective practices produce or reveal historical truths. Yet these historians must deal with the fact that the practice of history is a subjective endeavor: "The obstacle confronts all scientists, but in most fields the built-in self-correcting mechanisms of science help separate fact from fiction. Not so for most historians, whose subject of study is in the past, making the testing of hypotheses difficult."[8] The problem of interpretation haunts these texts, whose authors want a surefire way to show that Holocaust deniers are wrong, but over and over again run into the problem of subjectivity in understanding the past.

It is important to note that neither Lipstadt nor Shermer and Grobman are arguing that poststructuralism *caused* Holocaust denial. Rather, they argue that poststructuralist ideas undermine shared notions of what counts as the truth, thereby creating a context in which radical challenges to the evidentiary record of the Holocaust can be accepted. In other words, they are saying that poststructuralist ideas make ordinary people vulnerable to the manipulations of fringe extremists. Similar ideas have been put forward about the role of the Internet in spreading antivaccination ideas. Anna Kata argues, in "A Postmodern Pandora's Box: Anti-vaccination Misinformation on the Internet," that postmodernism, with its critique of authority and expertise, lays the groundwork for the spread of antivaccination ideas on the Internet.[9] In particular, she writes, "postmodernism does not accept one source of 'truth'—a philosophy adopted by the antivaccination movement. . . . The Internet acts as a postmodern Pandora's box, releasing arguments that are not easily dismissible" (1715). These interpretations agree about the erosion of shared understanding of the truth across several cultural domains. For many historians and scientists, this phenomenon is dangerous, because traditional notions of how to tell that something is true disappear, as a function either of a philosophical trend (poststructuralism or postmodernism) or of a medium (the Internet).[10]

These authors are right to suggest that poststructuralism presents a challenge to traditional history. However, their response—to demonstrate that the Holocaust did happen and, in the case of Shermer and Grobman, to argue for a kind of scientific historical method that depends on a "convergence of evidence" to establish historical facts—means that they have conceded, in a sense, to the deniers' challenge to remain "in the realm of proof, or *forensic* rhetoric."[11] For these authors, the historical problem of questioning the Holocaust (or any fixed truth) demands the response that history is the practice of discovering the reality of the past (Lipstadt's version) or that history is a scientific discipline based on a reliable and systematic method of gathering and interpreting evidence (Shermer and Grobman's version). To my mind, another response, albeit more in keeping with poststructuralist philosophy, would be that the ambiguity of textual meaning and, therefore, the relative ambiguity of documentary evidence suggest that we establish the truth on other grounds. Some evidence is better than other evidence, but the way we decide which evidence is convincing is variable, ambivalent, and constructed—not guaranteed by method or specific forms of evidence.

That is, poststructuralist approaches, and deconstruction in particular, can *help* us to understand the contingencies that influence how we understand and evaluate evidence. Poststructuralism suggests that our decisions about textual and other forms of evidence, in the face of their inherent ambiguity, are choices contingent on a variety of circumstances, including trust, disposition, prejudice, knowledge, and language. The evidence does not "speak for itself," because speech (as well as writing) is inherently ambiguous. We stabilize inherently unstable meanings by recourse to contextual factors that are external to documentary and textual evidence.

In my estimation, stronger arguments against Holocaust denial are available when one *accepts* the subjectivity of historical understanding—and the related contingencies of deciding what is true. Interpretation and the implications of particular interpretations are precisely what is at issue. Accepting historical subjectivity allows us to pinpoint what is objectionable in Holocaust denial: the ideological nature of resistance to the Holocaust, that is, anti-Semitism. Starting with the corrosive effect of anti-Semitism—its pervasive influence on the way history is understood, evidence is arrayed, and human experience is represented—provides a way to see denial as a politically motivated vehicle for prejudice against Jews. But starting with anti-Semitism is starting with an interpretive position rather than with the evidence; by accepting the existence of anti-Semitism, I am already understanding Holocaust denial through its lens.

Seeing Holocaust denial as a specific result of anti-Semitism allows us to understand its particular moral implications, indeed, the way that denialism in this instance deflects moral accountability. Some deniers argue that all suffering in wartime is horrific—suggesting, in other words, that the Final Solution was just part of the regular business of war. Holocaust deniers argue that the death of millions of Jews and others in Nazi concentration camps is either (1) a fiction perpetrated by a conspiracy or (2) what is to be expected of the circumstance. That is, Holocaust deniers appear either to repudiate the existence of evidence persuasive to the majority or to argue that such evidence is immaterial because it points only to the ordinary violence typical of war. Either way, Holocaust deniers refuse to accept a *moral* understanding of Nazi concentration camps and the Final Solution—they evade that moral understanding through denial.

Denialism's diminishment of documentary evidence and its downplaying of the horrors in survivor narratives contribute to this moral problem, but, in my view, establishing proper historical method will never fully refute historical denial that is a cover for moral bankruptcy. If Holocaust denial is caused by anti-Semitism, then improved method won't effectively counter it because poor method isn't the problem. Ideology is.

Science Denial and the Question of Belief

For the law professor and psychologist Dan Kahan, *denialism* is not only not a helpful or accurate descriptor for vaccine skeptics; it is a form of labeling that contributes to, rather than explicates, voluntary nonvaccination.[12] He argues that putting vaccine skeptics in the same category as those who don't believe in evolution or climate change is a very questionable communication practice, because it lumps together different groups of people: "Critics of mandatory vaccination are small in number and their hostility to vaccines is generally unshared by the majority of the population. Positions on evolution and climate change, by contrast, are highly charged symbols for cultural groups" (54). Creating a broad category of *science denial*, in his view, can actually strengthen the phenomenon you are trying to counteract. Kahan promotes science communication practices that are based on understanding how the cultural context influences decision-making in the context of risks. Analyzing controversies over the rollout and implementation of Gardasil, the Merck vaccine for HPV, Kahan demonstrates how poor communication practices actually created resistance to vaccination by polarizing the population, which led to increased "pressure to conform their perceptions of risk to those that distinguish their group from competing ones" (54). Portraying vaccine skeptics as denialists "needlessly risks provoking the same cultural cognition dynamics that impeded reasoned public engagement with the HPV vaccine" (54). He notes earlier that "misleadingly implying that increasing numbers of parents are fearfully refusing vaccination could create exactly such fear and resistance" (54). In this way Kahan shows how denialist labeling, as an argument strategy, can backfire against those trying to increase trust in vaccination.

Yet discussions of science denial inevitably gather together climate change deniers, AIDS denialists, and creationists (among others), as if the same issues are at stake in each controversy, as well as the same mechanisms of denialist expression. Focusing on those mechanisms of expression, or rhetorics, Mark Hoofnagle of the *Denialism Blog* states outright that "denialism is the employment of rhetorical tactics to give the appearance of argument or legitimate debate, when in actuality there is none."[13] In my discussion of denialism in my 2011 book, *Viral Mothers*, I explored specific rhetorical tactics that made AIDS denialism an available oppositional discourse for global breastfeeding advocates, and my analysis supported the idea that denialism functions as a rhetorical resource for people wanting to produce a "cultural challenge to authority and what is perceived to be hegemonic belief."[14] Yet in arguing that denialist arguments can be shown to share common rhetorical characteristics, I was not then and am not now trying to suggest that they are based on a similar resistance to science in general, as the term *science denial* implies. Denialist claims are more profitably examined in the specific contexts in which they are expressed. Resistance to the scientific consensus on each of these issues—evolution, HIV/AIDS, climate change, and so on—expresses a distinct set of cultural concerns. The rhetorical similarity of method should not be confused with the actual things that worry people.

The lumping together of various resisters leads to predictable ways to counteract so-called science denial. *I Fucking Love Science*, a popular science blog, does this in introducing the idea of inoculation theory, which guides the teaching of science by refuting common misconceptions.[15] Michael Specter's 2009 book, *Denialism: How Irrational Thinking Hinders Scientific Progress, Harms the Planet, and Threatens Our Lives*, argues that people act out of irrational fears against valuable medications, genetically modified foods, vaccinations, race-based approaches to medical treatments, all the while using supplements for which there is no scientific support.[16] Sara Gorman and Jack Gorman, coauthors of *Denying to the Grave: Why We Ignore the Facts That Will Save Us*, look specifically at what they call *health science denial*, using a similar approach identifying psychological impediments to reason.[17] Andrew Shtulman, in *scienceblind: Why Our Intuitive Theories about the World Are So Often Wrong*, uses the notion of *intuitive theories* to explain why so many of us don't rely on actual scientific concepts to explain the natural world—and so often get causality wrong.[18] By characterizing skepticism about these modern developments as science denial, critics see a kind of cultural blindness to the value of science that is rooted in psychological mechanisms that, while normal, impede rational thinking that appropriately utilizes scientific evidence.

In putting the origin of science denial inside of individuals' heads, instead of the cultural context in which they live, denialism's critics suggest strategies to overcome it that are essentially psychological—appealing to people's emotions, developing science's own charismatic leaders, and counteracting poor decision-making patterns. By putting science deniers together, critics suggest that what joins them is denial itself, not the specific arguments that they muster, the concerns they express, or the charges that they make against mainstream scientific positions and the evidence that is supposed to persuade them. Specter suggests that the "march of technology" is culturally necessary and those who are opposed to it base their decisions on fear: "Denialism is often a natural response to this loss of control, an attempt to scale the world to dimensions we can comprehend."[19] Gorman and Gorman refer to evolutionary psychology:

> Many of the thought processes that allow us to be human, to have empathy, to function in society, and to survive as a species from an evolutionary standpoint can lead us astray when applied to what scientists refer to as *scientific reasoning*. . . . In this book, we explore the psychology and neurobiology of poor health decisions and irrational health beliefs, arguing that in many cases the psychological impulses are *adaptive* . . . but are often applied in a *maladaptive* way.[20]

Shtulman's reliance on intuitive theories allows him to show how they are "coherent," "widespread," and "robust"—and therefore more difficult to dislodge than simple "factual errors" about scientific processes.[21] These psychological approaches suggest that deniers just need to change their minds, because the problem is the way that they think. "Inoculate" them against denialist beliefs, debunk their misconceptions, demonstrate their irrationalities, or simply teach them better from an early age: these strategies aim to fix the thought processes of deniers, who are imagined, fundamentally, to misunderstand both how science works and why scientific facts should be trusted.

The creation of the broad category *science denial* and the use of psychological theories to address its adherents' wrong thinking are linked strategies: these writers and researchers are able to identify universal psychological problems as the cause of science denial by labeling it as such. The psychological approach aims to identify and repair the general psychological processes that lead people to think incorrectly and therefore to resist the reasonable scientific information presented to them. But you can only take this approach—that there are general psychological processes that support people's wrong thinking—if there is a general problem to be solved, a problem that is not defined or circumscribed by specific criticisms or concerns. These strategies allow those who are trying to argue for science to do exactly what Dan Kahan has argued against—putting strange bedfellows together so that they appear to be the same. Of course, Kahan himself has a psychological rationale for this behavior (his concept of *cultural cognition*), but the point still stands. *Science denial* as a concept justifies the psychological approach that emphasizes wrong thinking and an inability to be rational, just as the psychological approach is strengthened if the problem is generalizable rather than specific.

Yet science is not a monolith. That, of course, is its strength—the fact that scientific ideas are debated, experiments are conducted to test hypotheses, and results are interpreted variously and sometimes overturned. Discussion, dissension, and disagreement within scientific circles are strengths of modern scientific endeavor, as they are meant to lead to better science through the normative model of experimental refutation. It is normal for scientists to try to refute each other's claims—to disagree with one another just enough to devise experiments meant to test prior results—as a way of confirming important findings and moving science toward consensus. When ordinary individuals—nonscientists—participate in this endeavor, they are sometimes called *citizen scientists*. Often, however, their credibility is undermined by claims that they are not scientists and therefore not qualified to evaluate scientific findings.[22] Who, then, is qualified to make claims against scientific orthodoxy? And how are beliefs attached to our own understanding of scientific credibility and what makes an argument about scientific findings persuasive?

Many AIDS denialists are scientists, and some are doctors. Many climate change deniers are also scientists, although the blogs are quick to point out that they aren't climate scientists, just as they are quick to point out that few (if any) AIDS denialists are retrovirologists. This problem of the high educational level of many supposed science deniers bedevils critics' arguments. If one has to be some kind of superexpert to understand the particular science involved—a particular kind of scientist, rather than just a scientist—then ordinary citizens' belief in climate change, or the fact that HIV causes AIDS, or that the earth has been around for more than a few thousand years is based on *trust* rather than actual scientific reasoning. Indeed, the idea that we must trust climate scientists, 97 percent of whom believe in global warming, against our individual experiences of cold winters (for example), demonstrates the significance of trust in experts as a crucial element of the public discussion. I'm not arguing that we shouldn't trust climate scientists in this regard; indeed, I do. What I'm suggesting is that my trust in their statistics and interpretations of those statistics is not necessarily rational. It is based on my sense that they are likely to be telling the truth, because the science of climate change is not something I understand deeply.

To be honest, for me a singularly persuasive element about climate change arguments is the effort that we must make to rectify global warming—that is, the narrated warnings about dire futures. The effort is so enormous—including drastically reducing automobile travel, air conditioning, and air travel (as brief examples)—no one in their right mind would contemplate it if not absolutely necessary. I once attended a conference session at which the physician giving a presentation on health and environmental issues said that the real figure for energy use decrease in the United States to counteract global warming is somewhere around 75 percent. That shocked me. I can imagine a 25 percent reduction, perhaps even a 50 percent reduction, but 75 percent? How would I wash my clothes, my dishes, myself in that scenario? Thus, I am persuaded by the general, television-worthy evidence of warming, for sure, but in the context of my sense that only committed and truth-telling people would tell stories that include dire predictions about human survival. I don't have a way of understanding the data that would allow me to say that I know by actual study of the evidence that climate scientists are correct. I am persuaded, then, because I think that climate scientists would tell such stories only if they were truly afraid of the consequences of not doing anything to reduce global warming. I believe in *them*.

My reasoning is open to criticism—I can imagine someone suggesting to me that only doomsday aficionados would create such a dire scenario and narrate it publicly, probably to elevate their own stature and enhance funding streams to their labs. I myself tend toward doomsday scenarios and depressive fiction—my husband and I loaded up on canned beans and other nonperishables in the weeks ahead of Y2K, sure that the grid would go down, and we would have to fend for ourselves and our two children with our camp stove. I thought that Ebola was likely to spread like wildfire across the United States in fall 2014, because I misunderstood how difficult it is to actually infect someone with Ebola. I like sad novels and movies, and I read stories about disasters like the Shackleton shipwreck and climbing deaths on Mount Everest. Does that mean I am predisposed to accept dire global warming scenarios? It's entirely possible, although I'm not aware of any studies that try to link attitudes toward climate change with reading habits or depressive outlooks. While writing this book I lived in a state where a former attorney general tried for years to gain access to email messages from a climate scientist who used to work at a state university. The attorney general was trying to prove that state funding was used fraudulently. It was an entirely political gesture, especially because the scientist didn't even work in the state anymore, and it helped to convince me that the effort to repudiate climate science was not on the up-and-up.

My point here is that belief in evidence is culturally situated; it is not just an effect of cognitive processes. It is both inside and outside of us as individuals, and is affected by politics, culture, social networks, temperament, and the way we understand scientific evidence to be related to personal experience. Psychological approaches that identify wrong beliefs and the supposedly improper processes that lead to them ignore what really bothers people in the specific instances of their resistance to mainstream scientific evidence and arguments. Thus, while there may be people whose worldview is completely opposed to the practices and philosophy of modern science, in general science denial appears to be a poor way to address the specific beliefs of vaccine skeptics.

Vaccine Skepticism as Science Denial, Wrong Thinking, and Culture

Michael Specter titles his chapter in *Denialism* on vaccine resistance "Vaccines and the Great Denial."[23] Like other authors on vaccine skepticism, Specter runs through the usual suspects in his chapter—the 1998 Wakefield article in *The Lancet*, the IOM report on immunization safety in 2004 that exonerated both thimerosal and the MMR vaccine of causing autism, Jenny McCarthy and Generation Rescue, Barbara Loe Fisher and the National Vaccine Information Center, RFK Jr. and "Deadly Immunity," representative Dan Burton, the differences between ethylmercury and methylmercury, among other individuals and topics. Yet because Specter's general topic is denialism, his interpretation of vaccine skepticism is somewhat different from what we have seen already in books by Paul Offit, Seth Mnookin, Mark Largent, Eula Biss, and Jennifer Reich. Making his arguments within a larger set of claims about science denial has some interesting consequences.

For one thing, suspicion of science becomes the origin, not the effect, of vaccine resistance. For example, in discussing how AIDS activism changed expectations about medical treatment and shared decision-making, Specter writes, "The rise of such skepticism toward the scientific establishment (as well as the growing sense of anxiety about environmental threats to our physical health) has led millions to question the authority they once granted, by default, not only to their doctors, but also to organizations like the National Academy of Sciences" (65). He explicitly brings up the issue of trust, but then derisively suggests that "because this is the age of denialism, evidence that *any* pharmaceutical company has engaged in venal behavior means they *all* have" (65; emphasis in original). Indeed, he writes later in the chapter, "Instincts evolve. We have become inherently suspicious of science, so when a drug company or researcher does something wrong, fails to show data that could be harmful, for example, or when there's an issue having to do with the safety of a particular product, it feeds into the underlying suspicion and permits people to say, 'Ah! All of science is bad'" (87).

For Specter, irrational fears of progress fuel suspicion of science and denial of its contributions to modern life. In general, he defends the mainstream position that fear of disease has diminished as a result of successful vaccination programs, and only the return of disease will cause parents to trust vaccines again. At the end of "Vaccines and the Great Denial," he asks, rhetorically, "How many American children will have to die in order to make the point that vaccinations are vital?" (101). Interestingly, he himself acknowledges that a similar argument is made by Jenny McCarthy, a figure he criticizes for her outsized influence on vaccine skepticism. He quotes McCarthy as saying, "I do believe sadly that it's going to take some diseases coming back to realize that we need to change and develop vaccines that are safe. . . . If you give us a safe vaccine, we'll use it" (94). That he agrees with Jenny McCarthy on this point is not made clear at all in his text, because Specter's purpose is to demonstrate that her views and those of other vaccine skeptics are based on the irrational fears of science denial.

Thus, as I argued more generally in the previous section, creating a category of disbelief that causes various forms of resistance to science's evident progress and success allows Specter to avoid understanding how specific circumstances motivate parents and others to question vaccines. His characterization of science denial also suggests the kind of solution that many science denial critics propose to counteract the problem—correct misconceptions with facts, although gently, because denialists don't give up their views easily.

Gorman and Gorman make similar arguments throughout *Denying to the Grave*, although they make their case through evolutionary arguments about the adaptive functions of particular forms of decision-making that interfere with optimal scientific reasoning. Shtulman is similar in arguing that "there is a fundamental disconnect between the cognitive abilities of individual humans and the cognitive demands of modern society."[24] The Gormans' conclusions set out somewhat contradictory methods for counteracting the poor, emotion-laden decision-making processes that ordinary people use—they recommend better education in statistics and scientific method for children, at the same time acknowledging that people respond to emotions and narratives more positively than to statistics and reason. The problem for the Gormans is that they believe reason and the scientific method should trump personal experience, emotion, and individuality absolutely. They suggest that those very things that make us human—our tendencies toward empathy, emotional connection, and a reliance on experience rather than abstraction in making decisions about self and family—are the things we must guard against.

Shtulman likewise argues that scientific reasoning is as important for the social good as moral reasoning in terms of how we interact with our fellow human beings.[25] Indeed, he argues that we must "think like scientists" in order to "reap the benefits of science" in the modern world (253). All of these authors understand science to stand against personal experience and the anecdotal and narrative forms of human connection that make life meaningful. In a sense, these authors ultimately argue that we need to learn to be less like we are naturally, to fight against what are portrayed as natural modes of thinking and doing, in order to follow scientifically determined steps toward better health and well-being.

Yet in a philosophical system that separates emotion from reason and depends on reason to establish what counts as a fact and the way we create facts, emotion will always come in second as a factor in decision-making. Gorman and Gorman write repeatedly about locations in the brain that regulate emotion and get fired up when faced with a charismatic leader. But identifying brain structures and neural mechanisms is a sideshow. Enlightenment philosophies influence our values, the theoretical and experimental practice we call *science*, and what counts as a fact. That is, Enlightenment philosophies are the basis for the split between reason and emotion that makes arguments like the Gormans' possible. But they constitute only one way to slice the cake of human nature.

That what makes us human is also what makes us fallible and poor estimators of risk is an old story. Beware the poets and Sophists—they will manipulate you. Use reason and careful, deductive thinking to determine truths that are universal. Such thinking goes against our nature but can be learned and practiced. We must guard against our natural tendencies and teach our children to discipline their own minds for better outcomes. Yet again and again we go against our best intentions—we buy the lottery ticket (because it is fun to have a little hope), we neglect sunscreen (because we like a tan), we drive rather than fly (since in a car we are behind the wheel and feel in control, even if it is actually more dangerous).

I do agree with Specter and the Gormans that wrong thinking contributes to misperceptions of risk. When my daughter was about to go to France for eight months, directly after a terrorist incident at the Rouen cathedral (about an hour from where she would be living), my elderly mother expressed her concerns. "Mom," I replied, "every time she drives on Interstate 81 to visit her boyfriend in Charlottesville she puts herself at greater risk than living in France right now." That is just one example—an easy cherry pick to demonstrate how much terrorism occupies our imaginations while routine dangers go unnoticed. But I would argue, with Mary Douglas and Aaron Wildavsky, that a more profitable approach looks at how risk perceptions are keyed to protecting core cultural institutions (such as automobile infrastructures).[26] We don't see those risks because they are masked by our reliance on the things that are actually dangerous to us. One doesn't need a psychological theory to demonstrate why we are blind to them—a cultural explanation is available.

Why is culture a better explanatory framework than the mind? For one thing, cultures differ, and thus the explanations that are based on understanding them as the contexts for belief are grounded in people's lived experiences, not generalized theories about reasoning or neurological mechanisms. And we have extensive ethnographic data about how people's lived experiences shape their realities. As Melissa Leach and James Fairhead have shown in their 2007 book, *Vaccine Anxieties: Global Science, Child Health, and Society*, understanding of vaccination risks and benefits differs in different cultural contexts.[27] When you use cultural-ist frameworks to explore people's beliefs and practices (in other words, when you indulge in anthropological thinking), you have to address the specificity of what people believe and why it arises in a particular time and place. In other words, you have to pay attention to what is actually in front of you, rather than using it, through inductive reasoning, as an instance of a larger pattern (such as science denial) that transcends the particular circumstance.

Such an approach is evident in Nicoli Nattrass's book, *The AIDS Conspiracy: Science Fights Back*. Nattrass is specifically interested in under-standing AIDS denialism in South Africa, which leads her to pay close attention to the situation there in the 1990s and early 2000s. The ap-proach she uses understands both global and local contexts as influenc-ing: "The idea that AIDS conspiracy theories travel easily while adapting to local conditions is consistent with what scholars of urban legends call 'ecotypification.' In this approach, contemporary legends have two 'an-chors,' a 'legend kernel that remains constant across social situations' and the 'details of ecotypification rooted in local settings.'"[28] She also acknowledges that there are divergent reasons for why people subscribe to conspiracy beliefs or denialist positions, and that these encompass both culture and psychology: "History and social context matter—but this is far from the only thing that determines whether particular individuals choose to endorse AIDS conspiracy beliefs or not. Individual psychologies, experiences, and social circumstances act to shape why some individuals in the same broad sociohistorical context find AIDS conspiracy beliefs compelling, while others do not" (42). Nattrass argues that symbolic fig-ures like the "hero scientist," "living icon," "cultropreneur," and "praise singer" play key roles in persuading people to adopt denialist positions, as does a "cultic milieu," which is a "fluid countercultural space in which alternative therapies and conspiracy theories flourish" (3–5).[29]

In the end, Nattrass draws an analogy between AIDS dissident scientists and the "hero scientist" of vaccine skepticism—namely, Andrew Wakefield. While I don't agree fully with her analysis, or the terms she relies on, she provides a compelling interpretation of how conspiracy theories, denialist assertions, and what she calls "the AIDS conspiratorial move" operate in the cultural sphere and especially in South Africa. Her questions attend to the specific circumstances of AIDS denialism and conspiratorial accusations, trying to address the problem of why people believe in things that kill them (or why they refuse to believe in things that will help them to live).

Without an understanding of the cultural forces she identifies, as well as the contexts in which they play a role, interpretations of denialism seem unanchored to specific circumstances. For example, in addressing South African AIDS denialism, Nattrass writes:

> The post-apartheid context was also one in which the power of science was being felt in more intimate ways, not only with regard to the HIV epidemic, with its complicated testing and treatment regimens, but also in the genetic engineering of food. This may also have generated new insecurities, perhaps with ramifications for how people think about the origin of HIV. For example, in a focus group discussion among AIDS conspiracy believers in Cape Town, . . . comments suggest a distinct ambiguity toward science in that it is both distrusted (for meddling with nature) and recognized to be powerful, perhaps even to the point of developing a cure for HIV. But even so, the process of scientific experimentation is clearly perceived as fraught with danger. (20–21)

Here the relation between a concern about GMOs and concerns about HIV as the cause of AIDS is not one of similarity but of articulation— the one establishes a disposition that affects how people think about the other. They are related, but not the same. The complexity of concerns, then, is acknowledged, and the ambivalence evident in some people's approach to science is recognized in their statements, rather than dismissed as simply not acknowledging the positive power that science plays in everyone's lives. Thinking through the cultural context—thinking through a culturalist approach that takes people's beliefs seriously—provides a richer understanding of the situations that result when some people refuse to believe things that the majority know to be true. It does so by paying closer attention to what bothers people, as well as what they believe, and it situates those concerns and beliefs with respect to both broader trends and the particular locations in which they are expressed.

Are Michael Specter, Andrew Shtulman, and Sara and Jack Gorman wrong that psychological mechanisms play a role in various forms of resistance to scientific information and argument? I don't know. In the context of a psychological framework, their arguments make sense, and the Gormans especially offer important, though qualified, suggestions about how to change people's minds when they are engaged in practices that are bad for their health. They also demonstrate, somewhat convincingly, that education in science should engage children in actual scientific thinking rather than less meaningful, rote activities. But the main problem with the psychological approach that dominates these three books is that it identifies the wrong problem at stake in vaccine skepticism. Making the specific resistance to vaccination just another instance of something called science denial repudiates the actual concerns of many people, not just those who forgo vaccinations. And it separates scientific endeavor from the realm of belief and emotion, when, in fact, beliefs and emotions are crucial to the way people engage in and support (or repudiate) science.

One of the Gormans' key examples about poor science education in elementary schools—an exercise in leaf collecting that Sara's older sister had to engage in as a child—is laden with negative emotion: the memory of the assignment is "pain and agony," and there was no knowledge gained from it. Sara Gorman reports that she "never forgets this because the project tortured Rachel."[30] Yet this report is entirely anecdotal—the authors do not indicate that they interviewed Rachel's classmates to see if their reported experience was similar, even though it is plausible that other children loved the assignment, and perhaps one or two actually became plant biologists as a result. The point here, just as in my previous discussion of my personal belief in climate change, is that *beliefs* cannot ever be fully subject to reason; they are always at least partially, if not fully, based on experience and influenced by emotions or other affective responses. I don't know if leaf collecting has a valid backing in biological education; I am not a science educator. I remember having to do a similarly torturous insect collection for a ninth-grade biology class. I am sympathetic to the experience recounted by the Gormans, but that is largely an effect of my own *experience*, and not my understanding of the role of collecting in the biological sciences or how biological facts are created and sustained.

For Michael Specter, Sara and Jack Gorman, and Andrew Shtulman, science denialists engage in *wrong thinking*; they believe in facts that are not true, that is, in things that are not properly facts. It is easy to see why these writers focus on the purported psychological mechanisms that encourage people to believe in things that are simply wrong. If the problem is wrong thinking, then people can be educated to *think better*—and better thinking will be scientifically based, mindful of ordinary psychological pitfalls. Such thinking will lead to decisions that cohere with the scientific and medical mainstream; in that sense, such decisions will be correct. In this way, making vaccine skepticism a form of science denial and defining *science denial* as the result of identifiable cognitive errors allow these authors to suggest how to correct denialism without calling anyone stupid. And people's cultural affiliations—the contexts that sustain such wrong thinking—are not maligned. The Gormans are especially attuned to this potential problem, emphasizing that we all engage in behaviors that result from common psychological misperceptions. What this explanation does not account for, however, is profound disagreement with regard to the facts of the matter. What if people's beliefs are simply, and basically, different?

Vaccine skeptics don't believe in the same facts that vaccine proponents do. Earlier in this chapter I showed how some historians were committed to demonstrating that good, systematic, and scientifically accurate history produces convincing evidence of the factual nature of the Holocaust. These historians believe that their methods offer evidence of a shared past that everyone can believe in. Yet Holocaust deniers clearly discount such evidence, suggesting that the production of that evidence is tainted by improper influence. That most of us understand the deniers' concern to be evidence of anti-Semitism doesn't change the fact that the deniers simply don't agree. They do not share the mainstream consensus about the facts of the Holocaust.

I am not suggesting that the facts of the Holocaust should be in question because deniers claim that they are. What I do want to suggest is that the question of denialism—historical and scientific—appears to hinge on what constitutes a fact and how people are brought to believe in certain facts as true. In the next chapter, I will explore this problem by looking at the history of "the modern fact," as Mary Poovey puts it, as well as how doubt can be manipulated so that trust in the scientific enterprise is diminished.[31] Here I want to conclude by returning to the question of denialist labeling that I began with. I have tried to show that people believe different things; that belief in scientific evidence is not given in the scientific method but a product of context and, importantly, the influence of affective factors; and that culture is a more fruitful explanatory framing for health beliefs and practices than psychology because attention to culture forces us to identify the specific concerns that people have and understand how those concerns are related to their lived experiences. If we accept my arguments as plausible accounts of people's engagements with science, how do we understand vaccination resistance in relation to what many people think of as science denial?

Holocaust denial teaches us that motivations and bias matter. It also shows that purified method does not guarantee agreement. Indeed, one might go so far as to say that Holocaust denial demonstrates the contingency of the truth—how much historical truths rely on people agreeing to them through belief in the process and quality of historical explanations. That kind of belief is forcefully emotional and binds its adherents to specific narratives. It is, in many ways, the way all of us believe in things.

If science is unnatural, as the Gormans and Shtulman suggest that it is, in that it depends upon nonintuitive modes of thinking and very specific forms of structured inquiry, then to be a science denialist one must merely be an ordinary person. What goes by the name of science denial in most public discussion is really a demonstrated *lack of trust in orthodox science and scientists.* That is a very different thing. Denialism, as I have argued elsewhere, is a critique from the margins toward the center.[32] It is in this sense that vaccine skepticism can be understood as a form of science denial: it is generally a counterhegemonic position, taken up by those who knowingly resist the mainstream view of infectious disease and its deleterious effects on health. Yet *denialism* as a term is most often used to deflect attention *from* the actual beliefs of people who resist mainstream or orthodox views *toward* their supposed modes of wrong thinking.

If scientific thinking is unnatural, if it goes against adaptive human behaviors, if it is difficult and must be trained into people, then it is a mode of wrong thinking that nevertheless produces certain results that are valuable to us. Gorman and Gorman write that "our brains are not designed for linear risk perception even though that is how the world really is" (241). Indeed, they write that people "favor stories over statistics" (228). If the latter claim is true, and the first part of the former claim is true, then the latter part of the former claim is false. The world is *not* really linear—but linear thinking is helpful in framing certain modes of understanding the world. Stories and statistics define different ways of framing and presenting evidence. They have different uses, and our preferences for one over the other are based on temperament, education, practice, and experience, as well as our goals for using evidence in any one specific instance. *Science denial*, as a concept and a label, is used by those who disdain the messy interrelations of emotions and reason, of subjectivity and science, in human experience and decision-making—by those who think, like Plato, that the poets can be banished from the state without loss. How science became associated with facts stripped of interest, how it manages the ongoing problem of interpretation, and how its findings might be understood as cultural constructions are the subject of the next chapter.

6

WHAT ARE FACTS, AND
HOW DO WE TRUST THEM?

I had already finished the first draft of this book when the White House adviser Kellyanne Conway used the infamous phrase "alternative facts" to refer to (then) White House press secretary Sean Spicer's seemingly dubious claim about the size of Donald Trump's presidential inauguration crowd. Conway made the comment on NBC's *Meet the Press* on Sunday, January 22, 2017, and it immediately went viral. CNN reports the exchange between Conway and the host of *Meet the Press*, Chuck Todd, as follows:

> "You're saying it's a falsehood. And they're giving—Sean Spicer, our press secretary—gave alternative facts," she said.
> Todd responded: "Alternative facts aren't facts, they are falsehoods."[1]

The opposition between facts and falsehoods in this exchange seems clear, especially when one looks at photographs of the crowds at Obama's first inauguration and those taken of Trump's. If photographs are documentary evidence of crowd size, Spicer's claim that Trump's crowd "was the largest audience to ever witness an inauguration, period" is patently wrong. Conway's spin was not successful in altering media reporting on the question of inaugural crowd size, and her euphemism for "lies" continues as an Internet meme to this day.

Indeed, the psychologist Andrew Shtulman, author of *scienceblind: Why Our Intuitive Theories About the World Are So Often Wrong*, uses Conway's *Meet the Press* interview as the opening gambit in a short piece for NPR's *Cosmos & Culture* blog, claiming that "alternative facts" about science are treated with cultural complacency, since they cohere neatly with people's "intuitive theories" about how the world works. Listing vaccine skepticism as one of the outcomes of the primacy of alternative facts in people's misunderstanding of science, Shtulman states that intuitive theories operate to "prevent us from learning more accurate theories of the world, blinding us to counter-evidence and counter-instruction" that come from the world of science.[2] As we saw previously, the argument here is that misconceptions about reality (i.e., real facts) are the result of normal psychological processes that nevertheless cause people to believe in erroneous things (i.e., alternative facts).[3]

As unappealing as it is to even appear to come to the defense of Kellyanne Conway, I feel it necessary to state that there have always been alternative facts. Perhaps politicos have been less blatant in their use of them, and presidential advisers have, historically, tried harder to hew to documentary evidence, but people have always subscribed to differing accounts of reality. Even historians, it must be said, disagree about the meaning of evidence, the actual causes of past events, and even the events themselves. Philosophers, literary critics, and science studies scholars have been the primary academic investigators of the theoretical implications of radical contingency, and the influence of their findings was most forcefully felt in US scholarship in the last quarter of the twentieth century. That influence goes by the label *poststructuralism*, which I discussed in the previous chapter. A poststructuralist (and specifically deconstructionist) approach would immediately question the apparent dichotomy between real and alternative facts and suggest that the opposition is necessarily unstable. Real facts, any deconstructionist would tell you, rely on the notion of alternative facts in order to be accepted as true, and, as a result, alternative facts reside *within* the concept of real ones. Truth is always haunted by its necessary, repudiated, other.

I am not going to spend a chapter discussing alternative facts, nor will I argue that people's actual alternative facts—those that go against the consensus—are true. The point here is to indicate that facts themselves are not given in reality. They are, instead, the result of shared understanding, a consensus that accepts them to describe the world. That we moderns depend upon the nonintuitive nature of scientific experimentation and reasoning to create facts that we then accept as descriptive of reality suggests how far we have come to distrust our own experiences in favor of abstractions presented to us by experts. This phenomenon itself is a feature of modern social formations.[4]

Alternative facts as a phrase may gauge a current threshold to countenance differences of view. It is easy to jump from Conway's cynical use of the phrase as a defense of an unpopular president to questions of so-called science denial. But understanding why people believe different things matters in studying a cultural controversy seemingly grounded in scientific evidence. I start with the assumption that the dichotomy "facts versus falsehoods" is not a productive way to understand why people do not believe in things that scientists and the scientific establishment take to be true.

To move from this assumption to a more productive understanding of vaccination resistance in relation to scientific evidence, in this chapter I focus on the idea of the fact itself as a cultural construction, and how the fact, when viewed as an epistemological category, can shed light on why *real facts* are not always trusted. Looking at facts as culturally contingent units of knowledge allows us to understand better how they can be put into question in certain ways, why others can be influenced by this questioning, and how differing views that depend on variable acceptance of facts might be addressed more successfully. At the least, such an exploration may suggest why correcting wrong views with right ones is a largely unsuccessful exercise in addressing the problem called denialism, and why trust is a consistent feature in calls to believe in the facts that scientists present to the rest of us.

Facts as Cultural Constructions

In the previous chapter, I showed that some historians are concerned that a poststructuralist approach to knowledge undermines collective confidence that certain things actually occur and can be accounted for with reliable evidence. My response was that poststructuralist arguments can cement, rather than break, consensus about historical events by demonstrating that it is not the facts themselves, outside of cultural context, that determine what we believe. Paula Treichler helpfully parses this issue in the chapter "AIDS, HIV, and the Cultural Construction of Reality," in her magisterial book, *How to Have Theory in an Epidemic: Cultural Chronicles of AIDS.*[5] Her discussion explores how to think about facts as materially real and as cultural constructions.

Treichler's discussion of cultural construction is one way of translating the idea of linguistic indeterminacy that is characteristic of poststructuralism to the realm of science and the notion of scientific facts. Treichler writes:

> The concept of cultural construction can be understood as follows. It is a way of talking about how knowledge is produced and sustained within specific contexts, discourses, and cultural communities; it takes for granted metaphor and other forms of linguistic representation; it presupposes that ideas are produced out of concrete contexts and have concrete effects; it takes for granted hermeneutical activity; it is a complex of ideas and operations sustained over time within a given community; hence, it is institutionalized. . . . Although meaning is indeed arbitrary and fluid, this does not mean that it is arbitrary and fluid within a given signifying system. The predictability and stability provided by a given history, society, culture, and set of disciplinary conventions are anything but arbitrary. (173)

In this passage, we see how the indeterminacy of meaning does not mean that anything goes. Instead, meanings are stabilized by contexts (history, society, culture, and disciplinary conventions). What is important here is the idea of *facts as objects of knowledge*, which within the framework of cultural construction means *facts that are produced through specific practices*. It does not mean that facts don't exist, or that they are fictional in the sense of not being real. Rather, it means that facts exist *for us* in relation to the practices by which we come to know them as such.

In the context of a scientific concept, *cultural construction* refers to the practices (like experimentation) and the discourses (like journal articles) that establish that concept as something real. Treichler spends some time discussing scientific naming practices. HIV, for example, is an acronym that stands for the name of a virus: the human immunodeficiency virus. HIV became an established fact when particular experimental practices made it possible to isolate it as a virus, name it as a particular kind of virus, and establish how it acts on the human immune system to cause illness. Its naming was controversial given that Robert Gallo and Luc Montagnier disagreed about the kind of virus that it was and therefore initially gave it two different names. What it really *was*—that is, what kind of virus—was made true, in part, through the naming.[6] Furthermore, Steve Epstein, in *Impure Science: AIDS, Activism, and the Politics of Knowledge*, demonstrates that only when highly active antiretroviral treatments (HAART) were successful in 1996 did HIV really become the focal point of AIDS treatment—immunotherapies fell away as virology took precedence over all other practices to address HIV disease, in part because research in virology had developed the only successful therapy to date.[7]

HIV as a *thing in the world* can thus be shown to be reliant on the discourses and practices that describe and define it. This does not mean that HIV *as a thing* does not exist or does not cause AIDS. Rather, it suggests that there are a number of conventions and activities that are formally needed to recognize an entity not yet named or understood as something that exists. Before HIV became the recognized cause of AIDS in the medical community, there were many other potential causes. Research, and research practices, as well as successful pharmaceutical therapies, made HIV into the recognized thing that causes AIDS. Its existence as that thing before it was recognized as such does not detract from the understanding that its status as a *fact*, something that we understand to be true, depends on these knowledge practices and naming conventions. Calls to deny the existence of HIV or to question its causal relationship to AIDS often rely on a return to the beliefs and frameworks that preceded the establishment of HIV as the virus that causes AIDS in the scientific community—theories about recreational drug use among gay men in the United States, for example.

Treichler argues that acknowledging how facts are created in specific cultural contexts does not make them fictional or unreal. The concept of cultural construction does not do away with notions of truth or the responsibility to act in the world. Instead, she writes, "a serious commitment to a constructionist model undermines rather than reinforces relativism or pluralism. . . . The use of the concept *cultural construction* intensifies the responsibility to make choices."[8] She also writes, "Cultural constructions are not lies. . . . To be sustained, a lie requires the invention of an alternative universe" (174). Acknowledging the cultural construction of facts—in science and in history—makes us more aware of the grounds on which we agree what the facts are and what they mean to us. It makes us more conscious of our decision-making, the cultural contexts in which those decisions take place, and the evidence that is used to make them. To refer again to the historical reality of the Holocaust, and to use Treichler's terms, the Holocaust is a historical phenomenon that is "a reality that is too costly to give up" (173). Believing in the historical reality of the Holocaust, we can *at the same time* acknowledge it as a construction *and* argue that deniers are lying, because their stories must create an alternative universe to explain away the facts that most people accept as true.

Facts create cultural questions not only because they are things that we must agree to, things that are made up in the process of experimenting, naming, and contextualizing, but also because facts are very particular kinds of things. Facts as concepts have a history. While facts in the classical period might have been abstractions that everyone took to be true, facts from the scientific revolution onward have been epistemologically linked to the experimental methods of natural science. To understand why people adhere to and defend different facts about what seem to be the same phenomena, we can consider the history of what we call a fact and the problems that can be identified in the concept itself that are a result of this particular history. Understanding the history of the fact as an idea seems an appropriate way to address, or begin to address, why people believe in different things. At the least, this seems like a good thing to do in the era of alternative facts.

What Is a Fact?

Mary Poovey, in a detail-filled book titled *A History of the Modern Fact*, suggests that facts as we know them are troublesome "epistemological units."[9] Indeed, in her view, facts are not the end of an argument about what is real and what is false, but the beginning of one: "Disputes over the relation between facts and values, arguments over how data are gathered and packaged, and quarrels about the very possibility of objectivity can all be seen to derive, at least in part, from the peculiarity written into the epistemological unit of the modern fact."[10] Beginning her analysis with the late sixteenth century, Poovey shows how numbers came to represent both accuracy and virtue—to be accurate in one's accounts was to demonstrate civic virtue, first for merchants and then for everyone. Numerically rendered facts eventually became the basis for the administrative state in the nineteenth century—the bureaucratic reliance on statistics and statistical norms to govern. Poovey's two most important assertions, at least for my purposes in this chapter, are (1) that numerically rendered facts are seen to be disinterested (unbiased), but may not be so, and (2) that the relation of facts to generalizations is troubled by what philosophers call the problem of induction.

I'll take the second point first. For those readers who, like me, have to look up *induction* and *deduction* in order to remind ourselves of their meanings, induction is the invention of general rules and theories from observation and empirical methods (the rule from the instance). In induction, theories are developed from facts, usually a large number of facts that are collected over time. Deduction, on the other hand, is the use of general rules and theories to explain the meaning of what is observed. In deduction, facts are distilled from theories (the instance from the rule).

The *modern fact*, as Poovey renders it, is an epistemological unit that inaugurates and extends the problem of induction. What is the problem of induction? Modern facts are representations linked to material circumstances, what Poovey calls "observed particulars." From the scientific revolution onward, "observed particulars" are aggregated through experimentation to point toward larger generalizations. The relation of facts to generalizations is at the core of the problem of induction, which concerns how we know that an individual instance, an observation, will be repeated so as to demonstrate a rule. In other words, when does an observation become a fact, and when do those facts aggregate to become something larger than their discrete occurrences over time? In Poovey's words, the problem of induction is "the peculiarity of seeming both true to nature (in some sense) and amenable to generalization"—it is the problem of drawing a general conclusion from a number of individual cases (10).

The theory of evolution is a paradigmatic example of induction at work. Charles Darwin collected observations over the course of five years (1826–1831) on his round-the-world trip on the HMS *Beagle*. The theory of evolution by natural selection was the result of trying to understand, in general, how the variation in species that he observed could be explained. Further refinement of the theory has been developed through molecular biology and genetics, which explain the precise mechanisms through which natural selection occurs to favor particular genetic variations over others.

If induction is the way that theories are developed through observation and the collection of facts, deduction describes how theories are tested by experimentation. Sara and Jack Gorman show that theories allow scientists to postulate null hypotheses that can be refuted. The null hypothesis is a claim that can be falsified; usually it is rendered in the negative (there is no difference between x and y) or carefully calibrated to be demonstrably wrong. Deduction through experimentation produces facts through that process, showing either that the null hypothesis is true (there is no difference between x and y) or that it is false (there is a difference between x and y). In induction, the facts are puzzles that scientists have to account for through existing theories or by inventing new theories, while in deduction, facts are experimentally produced to refute or uphold the theories that exist.

To get at the first assertion listed above, that facts seem to be disinterested but might not be, we can turn to Poovey's account of how the scientific revolution and changes in mercantilist accounting procedures altered traditional notions of what a fact was. She shows that from the late 1500s through the early nineteenth century, facts came to be partly wrested from their original meaning of *things known to be true* to the outcome of "systematic knowledge" that we now call *science*. As the scientific revolution developed, facts outside of systemic theories of natural philosophy could not be corroborated. Thus, "ancient facts, which referred to metaphysical essences," no longer counted as facts, while "modern facts [were] assumed to reflect things that actually exist, and they are recorded in a language that seems transparent. Since the early nineteenth century, this transparent language has been epitomized as numerical representation" (29). Furthermore, "the enhanced prestige of numbers, to which double-entry bookkeeping had already contributed, played a complex role in th[e] transvaluation of values: to the extent that numbers were considered disinterested because transparent to their object, so too were those [people] who produced numerical knowledge" (71).

Thus, numbers robbed observed particulars of their embeddedness in particular sociocultural situations—the statistical representation of facts strips them of any interest (or cultural value) that might inhere otherwise. Yet while Poovey writes of "the success of the long campaign to sever the connection between description and interpretation," and observes, "that numbers seem to guarantee value-free descriptions speaks to the triumph of some of the accounts of numerical representation I chronicle," she also says that "many of us believe description, whether numerical or not, never was—and never can be—freed from the theoretical assumptions that seem implicit in all systematic knowledge projects" (xxv).

This last idea is particularly important in understanding accusations of denialism. The problem of *interest* in the modern fact—in other words, the question of whether it is possible to render facts purely descriptively or if there is always a cultural influence inherent in them—haunts denialist controversies. Arguments for and against Holocaust denial forward the notion that bias influences the other side's claims. For mainstream historians, the evidentiary record is full of facts that speak to the true existence of gas chambers, murder, and intent that characterize the accepted historical account of the Holocaust. But deniers argue that such an account is *interested*, framed by a systematic attempt to promote Jews and their interests. The same problem occurs over and over in various forms of so-called science denial—that there is an "orthodox" AIDS science that denies the possibility of alternative explanations, that climate change is a hoax meant to take down the United States, that evolutionary theory is an assault on Christian values and belief, that medicine is so committed to vaccination as both a disease-preventing strategy and a pharmaceutical moneymaker that it is unwilling to acknowledge its true risks. Poovey suggests that it is the "peculiar nature" of the modern fact to both initiate and sustain these kinds of arguments, because the modern fact encloses but does not solve this problem of interest: "This debate [over the question of whether numerical representation removes interpretation from description] simply voices the peculiarity written into the epistemological unit that has dominated modernity" (xxv).

As a result, all parties to denialist arguments accuse the other side of undue interest, and on all sides facts are put forward to bolster these claims. Mary Poovey's discussion offers an important insight into why these kinds of controversies are not amenable to claims made on the basis of facts. Her work suggests that in modern contexts we believe that facts solve problems by indexing reality, but those very facts carry with them the problem of unacknowledged interest (that is, bias) as an essential aspect of their existence.

In the nineteenth century, Poovey shows, one answer to this problem from within science was to accommodate uncertainty within scientific method. A British scientist, John Herschel, insisted that the answer to the problem of induction was to refine scientific method to include an understanding of its limits. In this way, scientific experimentation was assured authoritative status by "factoring the limits of epistemological certainty into the method of science itself" (320). What Poovey means is that the problem of induction, or the relation of the particular to the general, was addressed within scientific practice by a refinement of methods, an acknowledgment of the possibility of human error, the development of methods to address that error, and continued attention to "the limitations of the knowledge that [empirical] laws generated" (321). This view—that attention to the limitations of knowledge production within science serves as a hedge against bias—is evident in Nicoli Nattrass's final statement about how the "pro-science advocacy movement" can succeed against emerging and sustained forms of denialism: "Keep an active and credible presence on the Internet, both with regard to exposing cultropreneurs and promoting evidence-based medicine. In so doing, they [science advocates] need to educate people while also acknowledging that scientific practice is contested, socially structured, and can be biased and shoddy. . . . Recognizing and exposing the limitations not only builds credibility by acknowledging reasonable concerns, but assists in the broader project of promoting good science."[11] Whether this is true—that is, whether acknowledging limitations creates and sustains trust in scientific knowledge—is taken up in the next section of this chapter. In Nattrass's statement, however, we can see that scientists rely on the acknowledgment of limitations as a guarantee of their disinterestedness and as support for the strength of their claims.

Poovey shows us, then, that the modern fact, the backbone of the contemporary scientific enterprise, still involves significant tension between what is observed and the conclusions that can be drawn from observation in relation to generalizable laws. The particular and the general do not always sit well together. For example, the observed particulars of the clinical context sometimes go against the general rules that are established by the gold standard of medical research, the randomized double-blind trial. Evidence-based medicine (EBM) relies on the latter to demonstrate the benefit of medications and treatments, but such evidence sometimes conflicts with what is learned through years of clinical experience. Public health and medicine rely on generalizable findings for population-based recommendations—for evidence of treatment value, as well as treatment harm—but it is well known that individually people respond differently to treatments, with significantly different clinical outcomes. Every person has an individual experience that does not necessarily coincide with the norms established through randomized experimentation. The ordinary facts of people's lives, in other words, are not always confirmed by scientific method, and people do not routinely apply deductive thinking to decision-making.

With respect to vaccination controversy, the observed particulars of some parents' experience conflict with the results of population-based analyses that are trumpeted by medical and public health inquiry into vaccine injury. A typical self-report of vaccine skepticism starts with a story that "something changed" after a child was vaccinated, even if the statistical analysis of evidence of adverse events demonstrates that across the population, vaccination cannot be identified as the cause of that observed problem.[12] Parents may understand their family's health and well-being through a personalized lens.[13] I will discuss this point later in the book when I address the interview data that my research team has collected. The point here is that what counts as a fact leading parents and individuals toward particular health care decisions is not always, or not even primarily, a *scientific* fact. And if it is one, it may be a scientific fact calibrated for the circumstances of an individual's, or a family's, experience. Facts in these cases are decidedly, and acknowledged to be, interested, pertaining to the family and its influence on the individual. When one begins with facts understood in this way, it is then easy to think that perhaps all facts retain a kind of interest specific to their origins and their purpose.

Do modern facts still exert such pressure in the postmodern era? At the very end of *A History of the Modern Fact*, Mary Poovey states that "postmodernism and the postmodern fact simply set aside the problem of induction," although the modern fact is not wholly displaced by this new view (327–28). Certainly, in science and biomedical research, the modern fact would seem to continue its triumphant reign. Postmodern convictions of the cultural contexts of human knowledge production and their suspicion of the paradigm of discovery that dominates the sciences have not necessarily transformed basic scientific practice. Poovey does suggest early on in the text that mathematical modeling is a postmodern tool, stressing as it does systematic and generalizable knowledge at the expense of observational evidence and the observed particular. Modeling, of course, extends the abstraction of numbers to another level, as it removes prediction and the idea of a norm from reality altogether, suggesting that algorithms and formulas can tell us more about what is to come than an observation of the world around us. Global warming is an example of a modern fact that is the result of observation—the measurement of rising atmospheric temperatures—as well as a contentious controversy that results from (postmodern) modeling of the effects of climate change.

To my mind, Poovey reveals a problem inherent in the way that we understand evidence and its role in establishing our view of reality. She shows why many of us are ambivalent about evidence-based medicine and its seeming disregard for the things that we observe in our own lives or those patterns that our doctors see in their clinical practices that do not translate into results in randomized controlled trials. In this sense, we have not fully moved to a postmodern context in which we are willing to jettison the factual basis of our own experience and those around us whom we trust. Even modern facts are problems for many of us when the broad systematic scope of statistical generalization does not cohere with what we have experienced as reality. Statistics about the unlikelihood of vaccine injury are not necessarily helpful when parents think *their* child has been injured by a vaccine. While some parents will take that information as evidence that something else has occurred to change the child's health, others will disregard that information or advocate against it. Understanding why will take more than telling them that they have the facts wrong.

Variant approaches to facts do not mean that facts don't matter to those who dispute them, that people are stupid, or that manipulation is at stake, although any one of those things might be true in a particular instance. Both Mary Poovey and Paula Treichler suggest that variant approaches to facts can be understood as the result of different ways of assessing the interest inherent in particular arguments that make use of those facts. In acknowledging the problem of induction, or the responsibilities of cultural construction, these authors suggest that unacknowledged interest is a shadow within what we think of as value-free units of information. One could argue that denialists pick up on those shadows and exploit them in predictable ways, to suggest that those facts are not facts because they are made in the interest of particular narratives or orthodox positions. To respond to these claims, one can simply double down and insist that facts are facts, but I would suggest that we see now in public controversies over vaccination that such a response is unproductive, enhancing stalemated positions rather than ameliorating differences of opinion or contributing to improved understanding.

If we acknowledge, instead, that interest inheres in facts, that descriptions are tinged with interpretation, that numbers are not value-free representations of observed particulars, that the relation between evidence and the systematic ways we interpret evidence is complicated by our methods in ways that we can't fully bracket from our results—if we acknowledge, in other words, that facts are both humanly produced *and* represent our best efforts to produce truthful accounts of the world—then we might begin to have conversations in which the accusation of denialism is an invitation to discuss the problem of values and belief that underlies current debates about evidence. This kind of acknowledgment is not the same as the acknowledgment of limitations that is thought to correct the problem of induction with regard to scientific experimentation. Instead of acknowledging, and then bracketing, the social contexts of scientific evidence and the potential for bias, this approach relies on fully situating our use of that evidence in the context of our lives, our values, and our experiences.

To understand what this approach might look like, we need to consider the question of trust. Poovey implies that scientists believe that attention to methodological limitations in science creates conditions of trust for scientific facts, and Nattrass explicitly states that acknowledging these limitations "promot[es] good science" with the public.[14] In the discussion that follows, I interrogate this idea. Trust is indeed precisely what is at stake in vaccination skepticism, and we have already seen in the work of Paul Offit and Seth Mnookin that calls to trust science and scientists are a staple of vaccine promotion in the face of such skepticism. What I hope to show is that there already exist plausible arguments about why many of us don't trust either scientists or science about these questions. In part, it is this lack of trust that makes alternative facts attractive.

Doubting Science and Creating Trust

To explore the question of trust as integral to a discussion of denialism and the idea of scientific facts, I turn to Naomi Oreskes and Erik Conway's book *Merchants of Doubt: How a Handful of Scientists Obscured the Truth on Issues from Tobacco Smoke to Global Warming.*[15] They make a unique argument about science denial in this book, suggesting that denialism is an effect of a calculated attempt by a small group of prominent scientists to forward a political agenda. They look at cigarettes, acid rain, the strategic defense initiative, the ozone hole, global warming, and what they call "the revisionist attack on Rachel Carson." In making their argument, they are more like critics of Holocaust denial than critics of science denial, as they show a particular political agenda to be motivating a purposeful effort to repudiate widely accepted facts. They thus imply that members of the public who agree with these politically motivated scientists are manipulated by them and, therefore, not really fundamentally antiscience in their basic beliefs. In this way, their argument about science denial is more like the argument put forward by Offit and Mnookin that people don't trust the real experts because they are manipulated by the media to believe the wrong people.

Journalists do not come off well in *Merchants of Doubt*; they are repeatedly represented as conforming to the journalistic rule of balanced reporting, which Oreskes and Conway argue is not appropriate to the coverage of scientific discovery or consensus:

> While the idea of equal time for opposing opinions makes sense in a two-party political system, it does not work for science, because science is not about opinion. It is about evidence. It is about claims that can be, and have been, tested through scientific research—experiments, experience, and observation—research that is then subject to *critical review by a jury of scientific peers.* Claims that have not gone through that process—or have gone through it and failed—are not scientific, and do not deserve equal time in a scientific debate. (32; emphasis in original)

They also reiterate, like Mnookin, that "science is hard . . . and nothing is ever *entirely* clear," using this refrain to suggest that ambiguity of results and uncertainty over causes makes scientific consensus difficult to credit with authority and trust (71; emphasis in original).

Oreskes and Conway have a complex story to tell about the efforts of a small group of scientists to question the scientific consensus about cigarettes, cancer, and developing environmental concerns, but their overall arguments are relatively simple. They argue that these scientists used a constitutive element of scientific inquiry—doubt—and exploited it to suggest repeatedly that there was no scientific consensus concerning these issues, and, therefore, no regulatory action on the part of government was necessary. In the authors' view, exploiting doubt was a particularly astute strategy, because

> doubt is crucial to science—in the version we call curiosity or healthy skepticism, it drives science forward—but it also makes science vulnerable to misrepresentation, because it is easy to take uncertainties out of context and create the impression that *everything* is unresolved. This was the tobacco industry's key insight: that you could use *normal* scientific uncertainty to undermine the status of actual scientific knowledge. (34; emphasis in original)

The "merchants of doubt" were right-wing anticommunists, and their motivation was a commitment to a self-correcting free market system. Oreskes and Conway identify specific ways in which the same scientists—many of them well connected and prestigious in their own fields—manipulated established scientific consensus and misrepresented risks to the public, often through governmental reports or statements from appointed commissions. In the end they argue that "the network of right-wing foundations, the corporations that fund them, and the journalists who echo their claims have created a tremendous problem for American science. . . . Scientists have faced an ongoing misrepresentation of scientific evidence and historical facts that brands them as public enemies—even mass murderers—on the basis of phony facts" (236).

This last claim about mass murder is a reference to an attempt in the early 2000s to smear Rachel Carson's claims that DDT causes cancer, and thus to argue that the decision to ban DDT caused unnecessary deaths in Africa and elsewhere from malaria.[16] Oreskes and Conway suggest that the attack on Carson was a crucial element of the overall strategy: "The construction of a revisionist history of DDT gives the game away, because it came so long after the science was settled, far too long to argue that scientists had not come to agreement, that there was still a real scientific debate. The game here, as before, was to defend an extreme free market ideology. But in this case they didn't just deny the facts of science. They denied the facts of history" (229–30). Here we can see explicitly how Oreskes and Conway's arguments dovetail with those of critics of Holocaust denial.

Merchants of Doubt is a plea to trust real scientific experts instead of politically motivated ones. The version of science articulated here is reminiscent of Paula Treichler's comments about the responsibility to act in the context of cultural construction: "Sensible decision making involves acting on the information we have, even while accepting that it may well be imperfect and our decisions need to be revisited and revised in light of new information. For even if science does not give us certainty, it does have a robust track record."[17] Yet reading this passage and others in *Merchants of Doubt* that argue for trusting scientific experts and their expertise, I am struck by the inherent contradiction in the argument that Oreskes and Conway are making. For example, they write, "But without some degree of trust in our designated experts—the men and women who have dedicated their lives to sorting out tough questions about the natural world we live in—we are paralyzed, in effect not knowing whether to make ready for the morning commute or not" (273–74). We must trust others, I agree, but after reading their book, how do I know whom to trust? Trust experts, but the experts that the government has relied on lied to you; trust science, but science can be manipulated for political gain; trust the scientific method, but the scientific method is inherently uncertain and open to doubt; trust scientific consensus, but that too can be manipulated and made to appear less authoritative than it really is. Don't trust journalists, even though they might be the way you get most of your scientific information.

Distrust appears to be created by the system, and by that I mean the relation of scientific endeavor to the government (through funding and through appointments), the purposes of science communication to the public, and the status of science as an elite activity that is "hard" and thus not immediately accessible to ordinary citizens. Manipulation is also endemic to the system, or at least I can't be sure when I am being manipulated—especially because to create the story that Oreskes and Conway tell, they had to do a tremendous amount of research, something only academics or independent scholars have the time and inclination to do. The rest of us mostly rely on news reporting, but according to them even the *New York Times* and the *Wall Street Journal* have peddled the lies put forward by the denialists they investigate. Thus, while Oreskes and Conway end where Offit does, with a plea to trust experts and their expertise, they also undermine that final argument with the force of all their previous discussion about greed, exploitation, corruption, and the cynical manipulation of the facts. They offer no concrete advice about how to determine whom we should trust, as degrees, professional position, and past accomplishments appear to have no bearing on when scientists will turn away from their disinterested commitment to the truth and allow politics to infect their judgment and public statements. The one thing I think I can do after reading *Merchants of Doubt* is to avoid the scientific opinions of right-wing think tanks, but I was predisposed to that view before I read the book.

If people are being manipulated to distrust science in general or certain kinds of scientific positions or discoveries, we still need to understand why they agree with information that others believe is false. The answer in *Merchants of Doubt*, as in *Deadly Choices* and *The Panic Virus*, is that these folks just don't understand science. Yet after reading *Merchants of Doubt*, I think a better answer to this question is that it is difficult in these circumstances to know whom to trust. If Oreskes and Conway are correct—and I am persuaded by their evidence and analysis that they are—then, from the 1950s through to the present day, American citizens and others have been subjected to what amounts to a disinformation campaign about scientific evidence for environmental threats to our health and well-being. In the context of such a campaign, distrust seems a reasonable response.

The bioethicist and author Carl Elliott might agree. In a terrifying article called "Pharmaceutical Propaganda," he details ways in which pharmaceutical companies create demand for their products by funding patient awareness and support groups, publishing bogus research, and manipulating regulatory agencies.[18] Particularly chilling are his comments about how bioethicists themselves are caught up in these activities and relationships. The ordinary criticism of such behavior is to identify conflicts of interest that individualize the problem, but he offers "corruption" as a more accurate term. In all of the instances of corruption that he identifies, *undermining* is the primary effect—undermining of real news, undermining of peer review and scholarship, undermining of "the notion that academics are free of vested interests in the topics that they teach" (102–3). In the end, all of this undermining is really "undermining of social institutions that depend on trust. Institutions are difficult to build, but they can be surprisingly easy to destroy" (103).

In the particular case of vaccination skepticism, such distrust would also seem logical. After all, as with the tobacco industry, we have an entire industry that provides its own studies of safety and efficacy, funds its own researchers, is selective about what research is disseminated to the public and to regulatory agencies, and guards its proprietary evidence closely. I'm speaking of the pharmaceutical industry and the specific companies that make vaccines. We also have government agencies—the FDA and the CDC—that authorize committees to evaluate evidence, allow vaccines to be produced and used, recommend that vaccines be put into the formal schedule, and advocate vaccine use widely. There are people on those committees and in those agencies who have developed vaccines and whose research concerns vaccines. While one could argue that they have the expertise to make decisions about vaccine safety, efficacy, dissemination, and use, one could also argue that they are invested in continued funding for scientific research in vaccines and vaccine acceptance overall. In other words, they are *interested*, and insofar as they are interested rather than disinterested, they may be unable to make the dispassionate judgments necessary to convincingly demonstrate that objective expertise prevails in decision-making in these contexts.

I am *not* making those arguments. *Merchants of Doubt* suggests to me that these are plausible positions for ordinary citizens to take. I agree with Oreskes and Conway that the events that they investigate in the book constitute an assault on good science and on the reputation of scientists in general. The problem is that anyone who has grown up during the period that they examine might be persuaded by these events that confidence in science in the abstract is quite difficult. It makes a certain kind of sense that vaccines would be the target of suspicions—as a specific instance of a more generalized distrust.

But I am also not arguing that certain individuals are susceptible to these suspicions and that their concerns are therefore not really valid but only the effect of this unfortunate historical circumstance. I am not arguing that vaccine skeptics are somehow trapped by their history and manipulated by the historical situation that makes trust in science difficult. Both of these kinds of arguments are ways of explaining away vaccine skepticism as a form of science denial.

What I am arguing instead is that vaccine skepticism is linked to these broader historical trends; concerns about vaccines gain traction when they are articulated in the context of these trends, just as belief in AIDS conspiracy theories in South Africa might have been related culturally to concerns about genetically modified foods. In my view, distrust of science does not cause vaccine skepticism (or, at least, it does not cause all vaccine skepticism). Instead, the distrust of government-sponsored science that was inculcated by the controversies that Oreskes and Conway treat or the situations that Carl Elliott describes creates a cultural situation in which concerns about vaccines are articulated as concerns about the reliability of the scientific data that support vaccine use. Vaccination concerns emerge and are persuasive, one might say, because there is a cultural context that facilitates certain ways of expressing them.

Readers might note here a similarity to the idea that poststructuralism can lead to problems of denialism by undermining the standards of truth, or the argument that postmodernism facilitates vaccination resistance for similar reasons. But I am making a different argument. Both of those arguments use a general or universal statement to explain specific concerns—in this sense, they are deductive. I am arguing that a specific concern gains cultural legibility when the context offers a way to express it, and especially when there are opportunities to articulate it in relation to other concerns. This argument does not fall on one side or the other concerning the efficacy or risks of vaccines. Instead, it links certain kinds of decisions about vaccine reception to a troubled sociocultural context, a context in which distrust of government and of science is, if not rampant, a consistent cultural theme. In this way, my approach is fundamentally inductive—I am trying to develop a theory to fit the observations I have made. My argument also suggests that calling on folks to trust science and scientists, without a reasonable discussion of how that trust might be developed, is an empty gesture.

Some research shows, indeed, that trust in medical science itself is perceived as a risk—at least to vaccine skeptics. Pru Hobson-West, a British sociologist, has studied what she calls "vaccine critical groups," and has found that trust in expert authorities is often explicitly targeted as a risk with respect to vaccination. Trusting in experts is dangerous: "Trusting blindly can be the biggest risk of all."[19] Instead, these groups emphasize the need for individuals to educate themselves in order to trust their own decision-making: "Rather than trust in experts, the alternative scenario is of a parent who becomes the expert themselves, through a difficult process of personal education and empowerment" (212; see also 208). Hobson-West argues that her findings demonstrate methodological limitations of existing approaches:

> Trust in self is not assumed to be automatic or pre-existing [by these groups]. If future research found that this kind of discourse was widely articulated then reference to a crisis of trust in authority is perhaps more accurately described as a crisis of faith or a crisis of deference. This suggestion has important methodological implications: quantitative attempts . . . to rank who the public trust assume that trust is like a commodity or finite resource, that it is switched back and forth between competing sources of authority. Such research is extremely limited in its ability to capture discourse of deference, personal responsibility and expertise, or indeed, unknowns. One contribution of this paper is therefore to show a range of discourses which might be missed through an overly prescriptive approach to risk or trust. (212)

Hobson-West's conclusion here suggests that these attempts to shore up mainstream science and the medical practices that depend on it are hindered by a misunderstanding of both what actually bothers people and who can really be trusted with their best interests.

To put it starkly, it is as if there are two different realities. In one reality, the manipulators are successful yet easy to recognize, and reliable science is both obvious and straightforward (although hard to do and communicate). In this scenario, experts can be trusted when they are properly identified and their work appropriately vetted. Science, methodologically secured by recognized limitations, bracketing, and experimentation regulated by null hypotheses, can be relied upon. The other reality is darker—the manipulators have infiltrated our most trusted institutions, and the truth is partly an outcome of their efforts. Nothing—not even scientific research—is quite what it seems. When the system is this corrupt, you can trust only yourself. So you do your own research, and what you come to trust is based on what you can discover. That's the way to be a responsible person, and parent, in a world of alternative facts.

The next two chapters explore some of the scholarly and popular criticisms that emerge from this darker view, which, I might add, is aligned with the standard critical stance of academics (which may be why it is something that I notice and seem to understand). I focus on the antimedicine movement, which parallels, in terms of chronology, the events discussed in *Merchants of Doubt*. Antimedicine proponents make powerful statements about how allopathic medicine and its alliance with pharmaceutical companies do more harm than good. Antimedicine provides a counterpoint to science denial arguments, in that it presents a considered challenge to the biotechnical orientation of medicine, argues that medicine as a profession has moved away from the core aspects of traditional doctoring, and provides evidence that medicine has now become dangerous to people's health. In this way, antimedicine suggests that certain forms of so-called science denial are principled and reasoned arguments against the development and practice of medicine as a science.

7

Medicalization and Biomedicalization

Momentous changes in medicine over the second half of the twentieth century caused deep concern among scholars about the widening social and cultural reach of medicine. This chapter introduces the sociological discussion of *medicalization*, which is a term referring to medicine's infiltration into arenas of ordinary life that were previously not the concern of doctors or other health professionals. The medicalization thesis emerged forcefully in the last quarter of the twentieth century, in the middle of a period of tremendous changes in the practice of medicine. From the perspective of 2018, it is sometimes hard to identify with these concerns, because we have become used to the very scenarios that are anticipated in these critiques. Indeed, we are so much more medicalized now than critics originally thought possible that their warnings seem, from the vantage point of the present, rather simplistic attempts to stave off the inevitable.

The medicalization thesis focuses on the social impacts of this expansion and normalization of medicine's purview and social authority, including problems associated with the use of drugs to treat behaviors or forms of embodiment that did not use to be considered illnesses. The sociologist Adele Clarke and colleagues extend this analysis to the current period, identifying the present scenario as *biomedicalization*, what she understands to be a technoscientific intensification of medicalization.[1] Although most approaches to medicalization are negative—criticizing, in other words, the expanding purview of medicine in the ordinary lives of modern people—there are some more positive approaches that emphasize the opportunities that current medical technologies offer us to improve our bodies and lives.

The arc of this chapter begins in the 1960s with the elaboration of the medicalization thesis and the critique of medicine that it offers, following it through to its expression as biomedicalization and, as the sociologist Nikolas Rose has elaborated, *biological citizenship* and *somatic individualism*.[2] These latter modes represent more positive approaches to medicalization, but they are not simple accommodations to enlarging norms of medical treatment. Rather, they express an optimism about forms of identity, embodiment, and life that are made possible by widespread internalization of some medicalized norms. In chapter 8, I introduce the ideas of a group of critics who extended the medicalization thesis in two ways: (1) an antimedicine position, directly questioning the value of medicine's role in overseeing patients' health; and (2) medical exposés that have proliferated since the early 2000s, considering critiques of medicine's evidentiary basis and the role of pharmaceutical companies in promoting questionable therapies. Through this chapter and the next, we see that scholars and physicians alike have considered whether and how medical treatments developed in the second half of the twentieth century are good for people (or not).

Taken together, then, these two chapters trace a robust theme in American culture: distrust of medicine articulated through critiques of medicine's (1) ever-expanding social authority, (2) increasing capacity to define proper ways to be healthy, and (3) risky practices that rely on corrupt relationships and shoddy regulatory mechanisms. By the end of chapter 8, we will see that medicine's critics are asking questions like the following: Are serious side effects worth minimal extensions of life expectancy? Is widespread screening and preventative use of medication appropriate if a majority of people never would have become ill at all? Are economic benefits of illness prevention appropriate as reasons to vaccinate or recommend other preventative measures? What is an acceptable lower threshold of risk for a preventative practice? These chapters raise these and other critical questions about medicalization, demonstrating an existing cultural uncertainty about the increasing capacity of medicine to save lives in the context of its expanding social authority and the potential and actual negative effects of its therapeutics.

I start, however, by showing how changes in medicine are exemplified by my father's and his father's experiences as physicians in the twentieth century.

A Personal Perspective on the History of Twentieth-Century Medicine

The elaboration of the medicalization thesis began in the 1960s, paralleling the major growth of medicine after World War II as a profession based increasingly on scientific laboratory evidence. In this period, both private and public investment in medicine grew rapidly, expanding clinical practice, laboratory research, and pharmaceutical invention. As a result, the medicine of the second half of the twentieth century was significantly different from that practiced in the first half. For example, in the second half of the century doctors used antibiotics to fight bacterial outbreaks and infections, vaccines became routine elements of well-child care, and an enlarging pharmacopoeia was applied to previously untreatable diseases. Few of us can deny how important medicine became to most people's lives during this period in the United States. Now, from our earliest hours as babies to the final days of our lives, medicine dominates our embodied experience, and influences (indeed shapes) how we understand the good life. Old age is now saturated with medical attention—indeed, aging itself is understood by many to be a disease process necessitating medication, treatment, and changed behaviors to forestall its bodily effects.

These enormous changes affected the experience of being a doctor as well as the experience of being a patient. My father, now retired, was a pathologist, attending medical school during World War II and beginning his practice in the mid-1950s.[3] He participated in the rapid expansion of scientifically based medicine during this period. His father, my grandfather, was an immigrant who came to this country as a teenager and was educated here. He practiced as a community doctor from 1921 to 1967, the year that he died. My father remarked to me that my grandfather offered services that are rarely available today, such as evening office hours and house calls. His office was in his home. He worked as a school physician part-time, until the 1940s, to supplement his income as a family doctor. His fees were minimal. New medications like antibiotics and drugs for high blood pressure improved his patient care. Yet even though he worked into the 1960s, his role as a physician in working-class neighborhoods in Philadelphia did not change much.

My father's practice of medicine illustrates some of the important postwar changes to medicine as a profession. My father trained in hospital pathology, at the time called "laboratory medicine," and worked in this field for forty years, 1949–1989. He noted to me that the biggest change in his field during this period was the automation of clinical lab procedures, which resulted in faster and more accurate test results. As lab tests increased in number and complexity over this period, so did the income of the hospital pathologists, who were now paid for work performed rather than a set sum. More pay was welcome to him, as I have three siblings, and my mother did not work outside the home, but this change demonstrates how medicine became more of a business. Other changes to pathology practice also reveal medicine's emerging business orientation.

For example, the number of autopsies performed decreased over this period, partly, my father told me, because doctors felt they knew what caused death as a result of better diagnostic testing, partly because of fear of malpractice (since autopsies often reveal missed diagnoses, even with good testing), and partly because they aren't paid for, and unpaid services diminish when medicine becomes more business-like. In a 1973 article on the history of autopsy, the authors identify diagnostic testing as the cause of the decrease in autopsies, but for another reason: the increased number of tests that pathologists oversaw and the significance of those tests to the financial health of hospitals meant that the pathologists simply had less time to perform autopsies. Another factor was the rise of experimental research in medicine, which became the primary method of acquiring medical knowledge.[4] Interestingly, because his lab had a relationship with the

University of Pennsylvania medical school, my father also saw diminished interest in pathology among students over the course of his career—while pathology was seen in the 1940s and 1950s as the center of the new scientific medicine, it became less important over time, and was no longer "the main basis of medicine."[5]

My father's perspective on wholesale changes to medicine from the 1940s through the 1980s is clearly framed by his specialization in hospital pathology, yet his anecdotal account points to how traditional patient-centered medical practice was transformed in this period. Dissection, for example, was an iconic medical practice framing the modern understanding of the body and disease since the late Middle Ages. The history of dissection is related to the history of autopsy, with both reappearing in the thirteenth and fourteenth centuries in Europe after a period of disuse.[6] The fact that autopsies are no longer performed very often because no one pays for them, because they might expose physicians to charges of malpractice, and because the scientific practices of medicine have moved from investigating the embodied signs of illness and decay to experimental methods and extensive diagnostic testing says a lot about the values and systems that manage medicine today.

One of the primary reasons my father went into medicine was because it offered, in the 1940s, an independent professional opportunity, important for Jews, who experienced significant anti-Semitism in education and employment.[7] Yet the development of medicine institutionally and bureaucratically has meant the loss of such independence, just as the reliance on evidence from large randomized trials has diminished the value of clinical expertise. The growth of insurance, medical costs, and, as a consequence, managed care has transformed the role of the individual doctor from discerning and autonomous professional to a health care team member who answers to other authorities. Yet this loss of individual autonomy has occurred in tandem with the increasing cultural influence of medicine and ideas about health more generally. We can see this anecdotally in widespread health information and reporting in newspapers, on the Internet, and in the encouragement of healthy behaviors by employers, government agencies, and community groups. We feel it as we are barraged with information about how to live healthy lives, how to eat and sleep and exercise, on a constant basis. Indeed, it often feels as if health is the purpose of life, and not the other way around. This effect is just one element of the transformation of medicine and society that my father and grandfather participated in as physicians in the twentieth century.

The Medicalization Thesis

Criticism of the social status of medicine and its enlarging cultural purview occurred initially in what is called the *antipsychiatry* movement. The basic premise of antipsychiatry arguments was that because mental illness is always diagnosed as behavioral deviance from social norms, it is necessarily cultural and political. In the introduction to *The Cultural Crisis of Modern Medicine*, John Ehrenreich writes that in the 1960s, psychiatrists began "diagnosing a wide range of behavior—from antiwar behavior to black 'rioting' to being a 'hippy'—as psychotic. The very medical notion of psychosis became suspect, tinged with political and social judgments. Psychiatry stood exposed, not as a science and not as unequivocally benign, but simply as a mode of social control operating to preserve the social status quo."[8]

Antipsychiatry involved prominent psychiatrists like R. D. Laing, who argued that mental illness was a "sane" response to a "sick society," and Thomas Szasz, who claimed that mental illness was a "myth."[9] Novels like *One Flew Over the Cuckoo's Nest* by Ken Kesey, later made into a film with Jack Nicholson, contributed to public awareness of these concerns.[10] The antipsychiatry genre came to include memoirs like Susanna Kaysen's arresting *Girl, Interrupted* (later a movie with Winona Ryder and Angelina Jolie), which castigated organized psychiatry for institutionalizing her in the late 1960s for being a normal, albeit confused and depressed, teenager.[11]

In the 1970s, the critique of psychiatry was picked up by sociologists, who began describing medicine's social control more broadly. Irving Zola described *medicalization* in 1972 as a situation in which medicine

> is becoming the new repository of truth, the place where absolute and often final judgments are made by supposedly morally neutral and objective experts. And these judgments are made, not in the name of virtue or legitimacy, but in the name of health. Moreover, this is not occurring through the political power physicians hold or can influence, but is largely an insidious

and often undramatic phenomenon accomplished by "medicalizing" much of daily living, by making medicine and the labels "healthy" and "ill" *relevant* to an ever-increasing part of human existence.[12]

This sociological critique focuses on how medicalization narrows socially acceptable normal behaviors and bodies, as well as how it "focuses the source of the problem in the individual rather than in the social environment; it calls for individual medical interventions rather than more collective or social solutions."[13] Thus, the medicalization thesis raised flags about medicine's enlarging role in the social life of modern citizens, suggesting that while advancing medical knowledge contributed to rising levels of health within the population it also changed the nature of ordinary life. This change occurred through a process that altered what counted as normal living as well as the social experience of illness.

Zola identified four social processes that contributed to medicalization:

1. The "expansion" of medicine's authority into various practices like eating, sleeping, and sex
2. Medicine's guild-like "control" over certain techniques and practices, like surgery and drug prescribing
3. Medicine's increasing supervision of "taboo" subjects like personal problems, pregnancy, and alcoholism, among others
4. The use of arguments referring to health to define social goods[14]

The first social process, the expansion of medicine's authority into areas not previously considered medical, is the most common understanding of medicalization today, but it is instructive to consider how the other three enable the first to be established. For example, John Ehrenreich distinguishes two types of critique that influenced the medicalization thesis at the time—one that focused largely on disparities between well-off and poor citizens, and one that focused on the cultural mechanisms of normalization and control.[15] While the former critique assumes that the problem with medicine is lack of access to medical care for many individuals, the second suggests that the problem is medicine's enlarging social footprint and capacity to set norms and expectations for social behavior. This second critique, which Ehrenreich calls the *cultural critique*, is clearly in line with commonly accepted definitions of medicalization, such as Zola's first social process pointing to medicine's expansion. Interestingly, Ehrenreich's cultural critique suggests that lack of access to medical care keeps some people outside of medicalizing norms.

Foucault and the Medicalization Thesis

Michel Foucault, the famous French thinker whose work is required reading for anyone wanting to understand the formation of modern knowledge, institutions, and bodies, is often referred to in discussions of medicalization. Foucault participated in the scholarly discussions around medicalization in the 1970s, although he differs in his understanding of its origins. He did not locate our current forms of medicalization in the post–World War II period. Instead, he went back to the end of the eighteenth century to identify a shift in medicine's relation to the body, disease, and society. Yet despite this historical distinction, Foucault's writing in the 1950s, 1960s, and 1970s about madness, sexuality, and medicine all contributed to the critique of medicine that the sociology of medicalization was engaged in. Here I briefly present some of the most iconic ideas in his work on the topic. In the next chapter, I discuss his relationship to Ivan Illich and contributions to antimedicine themes.

For Foucault, the eighteenth century marks a shift in what he calls *biopower*, social power that takes the body and its capacities as its focus. The emergence of modern biopower is linked to changes in governance structures—when the body of the king no longer serves as the basis for government, and the king's power shifts from the right to kill to the promotion of the life of the populace, a characteristically modern form of biopower develops. Modern biopower, Foucault argues, comes in two forms—*discipline*, in which the individual body is subjected to specific practices to encourage its adherence to norms, and *biopolitics*, which refers to management at the level of the population. In his early work, Foucault investigated instances of biopower in the formation of soldiers' and schoolboys' bodies, the incarceration of criminals and the insane, the development of clinical medicine, and the history of sexuality, identifying the eighteenth century as a pivotal moment in which there is a transformation to modern forms (although in the history of sexuality the

decisive shift occurs in the nineteenth century). His views on medicalization fit this pattern, suggesting that what sociologists have argued began
in the 1940s in tandem with the tremendous growth of medicine was
really an effect of much earlier changes.

Foucault's most identifiable statement about medicalization appears in
his essay "The Politics of Health in the Eighteenth Century," which was
published in two slightly different versions.[16] He begins both versions
by questioning whether one can argue that medicine is split between its
private and collective attributes, the doctor-patient relationship and public health (to pin down this distinction somewhat reductively). Without
coming to a conclusion on this question—indeed, by discarding the question posed in this way and reorienting it—Foucault spends the rest of the
essay defining the "politics of health" that support changes in medical
practice in the eighteenth century. In the 1979 version of the essay, he
writes:

> In this history [of the medical profession], the eighteenth century marks an
> important moment. Quantitatively, it saw the multiplication of doctors, the
> foundation of new hospitals, the opening of free health clinics, and, in a gen-
> eral fashion, an increased consumption of treatment in every class of society.
> Qualitatively, the education of doctors was more standardized; the relation-
> ship between doctors' practices and the development of medical knowledge
> was a bit better defined; a little bit greater confidence was accorded to doc-
> tors' knowledge and effectiveness; thus there was also a diminution in the
> value that one attributes to traditional "cures." The doctor separated him-
> self a little more clearly from other caregivers, and he began to occupy a
> more extensive and more valorized place within the social body.[17]

In other words, medicine as a profession began to modernize. These professional and institutional changes were related to two important broad
societal changes—social welfare that targeted the ill, not just the poor,
and the development of surveillance techniques to measure rates of illness,
health, and death in national populations. Because modern states expect
children to become adults as part of the healthy population, the family
became the locus of practices to promote health. As a result, the family's
structure as a kinship system took a back seat to its role in assuring "the
best possible conditions [for] a human being that will gain maturity."[18]
The dual result of these two movements was that the family became

a primary mechanism of medicalization in modern societies and health became a moral imperative of families.

In many ways, the overt discussion of medicalization in "The Politics of Health in the Eighteenth Century" is uncommon in Foucault's work. Foucault's typical approach to medicalization is not to name it as such but to show what its effects are. In Foucault's famous book *The History of Sexuality, Volume 1: An Introduction*, he does not explicitly discuss medicalization. Nevertheless, the book's argument about the "deployment of sexuality" involves an implicit critique of the medicalization of sex. Understanding this critique is crucial to understanding medicalization itself, as Foucault's approach involves the reader in recognizing his or her own investments in a medicalized perspective and experience.[19]

Foucault made his general argument in *The History of Sexuality* in a double movement. First, he said, since the Victorian period we have believed that sexuality is repressed and that liberation is to be had if we allow ourselves a freer expression of it. However, he argued in a second move, the reality of the situation is that, in the Victorian period and after, we have been obsessively talking about sex and thus participating in a "discursive explosion" that creates, rather than subjugates, sex. Our focus on sex has not been because it is buried and needs to be unearthed, but rather because a distinctly modern mechanism of biopower operates in relation to it. Rather than by forbidding its expression, sexuality is managed by regulating the discourses through which it is talked about. That is, *producing* discourses about sex, not *denying* them, is the primary mechanism through which sexuality is simultaneously created and socially regulated.

One effect of the movement to codify, investigate, and regulate sexual behaviors was the medicalization of sex, starting with those versions of perverse sex thought to endanger others (and later, the self). Early in *The History of Sexuality, Volume 1*, Foucault tells the story of a "farm hand from the village of Lapcourt," who, in 1867, was caught having sex ("obtained a few caresses") with a little girl. In telling the story, he compares it with a previous time, in which these "bucolic pleasures" were tolerated, even sought out, by "alert children." In the mid-nineteenth century, however, the man is "turned over first to a doctor, then to two other experts who not only wrote their report but also had it published." Identifying the investigation as "a judicial action, a medical intervention, a careful clinical examination, and an entire theoretical elaboration," Foucault suggests that what happens to this farm hand is an instance of medicalization: "Acquitting him of any crime, *they decided finally to make him into a pure object of medicine and knowledge*—an object to be shut away till the end of his life in the hospital . . . but also one to be made known to the world of learning through detailed analysis" (31–32; emphasis added).

The subject of sex makes it difficult to see this initially as an example of medicalization, but it is one, and a caustically criticized example at that. How do we know? This is the only time in the text that Foucault provides a full story to illustrate a point. To defend his other arguments, he refers to historical developments or specific texts for evidence. And in relating this narrative he changes his tone, and that tonal shift reveals his rhetorical strategy. He begins with a typical opening phrase for a story—"One day in 1867"—and continues with sympathetic language describing the "simple-minded" "farm hand" and his game of "curdled milk" with the little girl. Foucault overemphasizes the innocence of the encounter, using phrases like "everyday occurrences," "inconsequential bucolic pleasures," "timeless gestures," and "barely furtive pleasures" to press the point that these were either not noted in the past or were considered to be perfectly fine ways to spend an afternoon. But his presentation is ironic—in this day and age who really believes that sex with little girls is a good, or even neutral, activity? The distance between his rhetoric (positive and lush) and his topic (despicable and distasteful) forces the contemporary reader into an untenable position, either condoning the molestation of little girls or calling a cognitively disabled man perverse.

Medicalization is key in seeing this sexual activity as a violation of the little girl. And in showing the reader how his or her understanding of the scene is already inflected by the medicalization of sex, Foucault demonstrates that we are *already* within the framework that he is trying to explicate.[20] It works like this. Foucault's presentation of the scene demands that we ask ourselves how we know that it is a violation, a bad kind of sex that is dangerous. We know because of the study of men like this, the knowledge produced out of his case and those of others like him—a farm hand who, at the wrong place and time, got a hand job from a little girl. The circularity of the epistemology is the entire point. This is one of the most difficult aspects of the medicalization thesis—the recognition that we are already normalized to experiences and perspectives made possible by the very process we are criticizing.

Biomedicalization, Biological Citizenship, and the Moral Regulation of Health

Adele Clarke and colleagues suggest that medicalization spread from 1945 to 1985, but then a new formation, which they call *biomedicalization*, emerged.[21] Biomedicalization is a radicalization of medicalization, an outgrowth of technoscientific applications to medical practices that have transformed health care and the experience of illness in the late twentieth and early twenty-first centuries. In a 2010 book, Clarke and colleagues distinguish these two movements this way—*medicalization* describes "extensions of the jurisdiction of medicine" and *biomedicalization* describes "extension of biomedicine through technoscience"—keeping to the description of medicalization that characterized its initial discussion in the sociological literature in the 1960s and 1970s.[22] In developing the concept *biomedicalization*, they try to capture a set of changes to the practice of medicine as well as to the experience of illness and the self that characterize the period we live in today.

Clarke and colleagues follow the tradition of science and technology studies in using the term *technoscience* to describe the intertwined social impacts of science and technology development in the second half of the twentieth century. The efflorescence of technoscience in the 1960s, in part through Cold War competition with the Soviets, led to the emergence of biomedicalization in the 1980s. While *medicalization* emphasized control over bodily processes within the domain of medical intervention, *biomedicalization* focuses on prevention through the evaluation of risk and technical manipulation of bodies and practices—it describes not just normalization, but the forward-thinking optimization of bodies through material transformation.[23]

Clarke and colleagues identify five processes that characterize biomedicalization and differentiate it from the basic expansion of medicine socially:

1. A new political economy of medicine and health, through which knowledge, technology, services, and capital are created and circulate

2. An "intensifying" focus on health, optimization, and enhancement, in part accomplished by new surveillance mechanisms
3. The increasingly "technoscientific nature" of medicine (one example is a shift from "case-based" and "locally controlled" patient care to "outcomes-based care" that is managed centrally)
4. A transformation of the production and management of medical knowledge, information, and consumption
5. The transformation of bodies in the service of producing new identities, both individual and collective[24]

Biomedicalization can be traced by looking at economic, governmental, cultural, medical, and knowledge sectors, and also at all the things that people do or think about doing to their bodies as a way of producing and managing identities.

A few examples might be helpful in explaining the difference between medicalization and biomedicalization. Carl Elliott, in *Better than Well*, writes extensively about the social anxiety drug Paxil, which many people claim has made shyness into a psychological disorder.[25] That claim is, in part, a claim about medicalization, a claim about how a personality distinction that was once perfectly ordinary became a disorder in the expansion of psychiatry. Perhaps an even better example is psychoanalysis itself, which transformed psychiatry from the late nineteenth century through the 1960s, changing it from its original focus on psychotic behavior to neurosis, which brought many more people into doctors' offices for what was originally called "the talking cure." That shift is pure medicalization, bringing people who previously might have been unhappy but considered normal to seek the supervision of doctors.

The development of new antidepressant drugs in the 1980s changed this situation, biomedicalizing it. Now millions of people not only identify as depressed or socially anxious (a change attributable to medicalization), but millions also take these medications (such as Prozac, the most famous, as well as Paxil) in order to *be more like themselves*: "Enhancement technologies put me in touch with my true self."[26] Biomedicalization defines this latter shift, in which a technoscientific development (new medications), in conjunction with new diagnostic criteria and mechanisms (a change in the definition of "major depressive disorder" in the *Diagnostic and Statistical Manual of Mental Disorders* in 1980 and the shift in prescribing to general practitioners), leads to a transformation in the way that people think about their selves. People have always taken drugs to manage the stresses of ordinary life (think cigarettes, alcohol, opium, morphine, cocaine, Valium, Miltown), but the development of new medications in conjunction with changing diagnostic criteria enables people to enhance, optimize, or simply regulate their personalities and psychic experience.[27]

In another example, through the 1960s, vaccine development was relatively simple: whole bacteria or viruses were inactivated or attenuated, and the resultant material was injected into the body or given by mouth (in the case of the oral polio vaccine) to induce immunity. As Elena Conis has shown, the development of vaccines for the so-called mild diseases of childhood—rubella, measles, and mumps—caused the medical community to change its perspective on these illnesses in the 1960s. Once they became *vaccine-preventable diseases* (or VPDs), their complications were investigated more fully, and researchers and public health professionals presented them as more threatening to individual and public health than they had previously.[28] In this sense, these diseases themselves became medicalized in new ways as a result of the development of relatively straightforward vaccines—while they were not new diseases, their significance and relation to medicine changed as the result of vaccine development. Furthermore, childhood visits to the doctor also changed, as these became instances to give vaccinations. The well-child visit to the pediatrician emerged in the twentieth century as an example of the medicalization of child-rearing (amply documented by Rima Apple in *Perfect Motherhood: Science and Childrearing in America*), and the vaccination schedule that was established in the 1960s, 1970s, and 1980s cemented this trend.[29]

Biomedicalization affected vaccine development in the 1980s and 1990s as a slew of new vaccines (among them, hepatitis B, varicella, pneumococcal disease, rotavirus, and acellular pertussis) were created and licensed. More rolled out in the early 2000s, including vaccines for the four strains of the human papilloma virus, or HPV, that cause most cases of cervical cancer. Many of these vaccines do not include the entire bacterium or virus. Rather, they depend on complex production techniques (for example, recombinant methods) to identify and exploit key proteins on the bacterium or virus to spur an immune response but not bombard the immune system with antigens. As a result, vaccine proponents frequently point out, while children today receive more vaccines than they did 50 or 100 years ago they are injected with fewer antigens overall.[30] This argument is meant to suggest that the vaccines are more refined, safer, and less likely to cause bad reactions.

These technoscientific advances in vaccinology have led to an explosion in vaccine development, as well as the inclusion into the recommended schedule of vaccines to prevent diseases that are not thought to be as serious as even the previously considered "mild diseases" of childhood. Chicken pox is a good example.[31] Prior to the introduction of the varicella vaccine in the United States in the mid-1990s, chicken pox was thought to cause slightly over 100 deaths annually in the United States, and most of those deaths were in individuals with compromised immune systems.[32] The recommendation for universal childhood varicella vaccination was based on a variety of factors; prominent among those were economic considerations that highlighted indirect costs, such as parental lost wages. Lawrence Altman, medical reporter for the *New York Times*, summarized a CDC study referred to by federal officials in the announcement: "By the study's calculations, if all indirect costs of preventing chicken pox were included, such as a parents' lost wages, there would be a return of $5.40 in benefits for every $1 spent on the vaccine. But if only direct costs were considered, like hospitalization, the total benefits would only be 94 cents for every dollar spent on a chicken pox vaccine."[33] The study itself emphasizes the role of indirect factors in assessing the vaccine's overall impact on American society:

> The main goal of a routine varicella vaccination program is to prevent suffering from chickenpox or from major complications rather than to save lives. Since varicella causes very few deaths despite many chickenpox cases, a mortality-based outcome measure may underrepresent the program's cost-effectiveness. We have not attempted to place a value on the intangible costs of pain and suffering from varicella or to convert costs of morbidity from chickenpox and nonfatal complications into quality-adjusted life-years. Instead, the results allow the reader to explicitly evaluate these goals of a varicella vaccination program.
>
> We conclude that, at a cost of $35 for each vaccine dose, a routine varicella vaccination program for preschool-age children will not save money from the health care payer's perspective, but would still be desirable and would save money from the societal perspective. It has an acceptable cost per life-year saved compared with other established health interventions.[34]

Federal vaccine recommendations are complex processes utilizing scientific data from human subject trials as well as the results of mathematical modeling and policy considerations that take into account social as well as personal costs of illness. Over the decade after the initial recommendation in 1995, varicella vaccine was mandated for school entry in almost all states.[35] This linkage between vaccine development and the political economy of vaccine delivery, in connection with the legal establishment of the school-entry mandate, is an example of biomedicalization at work across several of the domains indicated by Clarke and colleagues. We have a biotechnical replacement for a previous embodied ritual of childhood, one that entails the control of infectious disease, the optimization of family sick leave, the minimization of expense to society (if not to the individual), and the necessity to record another milestone of child development in an electronic medical record and a school immunization file.

Clarke and colleagues' focus on the late twentieth century as a particularly important, and radicalizing, moment in medicine is shared by other sociologists. Nikolas Rose focuses on the impact of genomics on personal and collective practices to optimize embodiment. Using the term *biological citizenship* to refer to care of life (*bios*) through the body as an implicit social demand, Rose highlights the practices that individuals engage in to regulate themselves and produce new "vital" futures from bodily self-management:

> The maintenance and promotion of personal, childhood, and familial health—regimen, personal hygiene, healthy child-rearing, the identification and treatment of illness—became central to forms of self-management that authorities sought to inculcate into citizens and hence to their own hopes, fears, and anxieties. . . .
>
> By the second half of the twentieth century, health had become one of the key ethical values in such societies. . . . Encouraged by health educators to take an active interest in their own health, and "activated" by the new cultures of active citizenship, many [actual or potential patients and their families and advocates] refused to remain "patients," merely passive recipients of medical expertise. They became consumers actively choosing and using medicine, biosciences, pharmaceuticals, and "alternative medicine" in order to maximize and enhance their own vitality. . . . Health, understood as an imperative, for the self and for others, to maximize the vital forces and potentialities of the living body, has become a key element in contemporary ethical regimes.[36]

From this general understanding of biological citizenship, Rose identifies an emerging paradigm he calls *somatic individualism*, which he describes this way:

> We are increasingly coming to relate to ourselves . . . as beings whose individuality is, in part at least, grounded within our fleshly, corporeal existence, and who experience, articulate, judge, and act upon ourselves in part in the language of biomedicine. . . . We see an increasing stress on personal reconstruction through acting on the body in the name of a fitness that is simultaneously corporeal and psychological. Exercise, diet, vitamins, tattoos, body piercing, drugs, cosmetic surgery, gender reassignment, organ transplantation: corporeal existence and vitality of the self has become the privileged site of experiments with the self. (25–26)

I'm sure that many of us can see at least some of our own practices defined under this banner. *Somatic individualism* resonates with *personalized medicine*, which is a consistent and implicit promise of medicine in the twenty-first century, although it has yet to be realized in a significant way. It enables a particular ethical ideal—to be a good citizen one works on the self, improves the self, regulates the self, and manages illness and health through specific individualized practices that enhance vitality and fitness. *Somatic individualism* is a positive configuration of desire, opportunity, and self-making.

The process of biomedicalization that seems most directly related to emergent forms of biological citizenship is the last one indicated by Clarke and colleagues—work on our bodies that is connected to the management and production of identity. Rose offers a positive interpretation of biomedicalization and the practices it enables. He believes that new genetic medicine offers opportunities for individuals and groups to forge innovative vitalities and, as a result, new futures. He refuses, in other words, to cast the current situation as one in which the individual is regulated solely by others, through medicalization. It is not that all is rosy or good—there are worrisome implications in terms of the regulation of the self and others that should give us pause. For example, Rose writes, "Our somatic, corporeal, neurochemical individuality now becomes a field of choice, prudence, and responsibility"—not necessarily a happy picture, as we are all *obligated*, to a certain extent, to use biomedical information *for health* (40).

For Rose, the biological sciences create a context in which uncertainty must be managed in the pursuit of health. Those individuals who do so are the subject of demands from the cultural system (to be healthy, to use medical information and practices to better the self), as well as active participants in creating new models of embodiment, identity, and citizenship. His thinking relies implicitly on technoscientific transformations that Clarke and colleagues investigate—genetic medicine is nothing if not the application of extremely advanced scientific information and technical procedures to the lived experience and self-understanding of ordinary people who, if the advertisements I see on TV nightly are any indication, avidly conduct in-home genetic tests to determine not only their possible disease states but also their ancestry. Thus, the *somatic individual* is someone who carefully manages the self as a (medical) body, someone who relies on the networks, political economy, knowledge practices, and embodied opportunities that biomedicalization offers in the late twentieth and early twenty-first centuries.

Biological citizenship and its attendant form, *somatic individualism*, are incredibly valuable concepts in the context of critiques of medicalization and biomedicalization because they offer terminology that helpfully explains how individuals and groups respond to cultural changes in the realm of medicine, therapeutics, and biotechnology. Whereas Clarke and colleagues tend to present a relatively traditional sociological critique of biomedicalization, Rose embraces people's engagement with the rhetoric and pragmatic opportunities of medicine in the current moment. Both of these arguments rely on normative ways of viewing what people *do* in the context of a bio/medicalizing society. And, it turns out, what we do with this knowledge is the key element in how we think about these emerging norms.

The medicalization thesis identifies a problem (increased social authority of medicine) and its consequences (less personal freedom, more social surveillance, increased medication usage, linkages between moral meanings and disease incidence, and profound changes in the way we experience our bodies and their idiosyncrasies, to name a few). But critiques often don't offer much in the way of solutions. The recent edited volume *Against Health: How Health Became the New Morality* is a case in point.[37] The book attempts a jeremiad against health as the "new morality," but is stymied, in the end, by the question of what it all means.

After identifying how the current moment is a crucial point in the history of health's hold on the individual and collective imagination, the coeditor Anna Kirkland writes, in the book's conclusion, "If we take seriously the concerns assembled here, it is clear that both what we do and the ways we think must change," adding that the "most important way that this volume proposes to change our way of thinking about health is its insistence that we become more self-aware about our moral impulses even if we doubt that it is possible (and maybe not even desirable) to distinguish them from more objective conclusions."[38]

Thus, the solution to the problem of medicalization, the problem of health "as a new morality," is *awareness*. This conclusion is scarily close to Carl Elliott's discussion of the PR focus on awareness of illnesses as a way to sell pharmaceuticals (in his caustic contribution to *Against Health*).[39] The problem is real though—the medicalization thesis suggests that the expansion of medicine is bad for us, but offers only awareness as a possible solution, because although we might realize the extent to which we are medicalized, it is difficult to turn down a treatment protocol that might be beneficial personally.

A few years ago, I had a conversation with my brothers about statins, the cholesterol-lowering medications that my ninety-three-year-old father swears have helped him make it into his tenth decade. I told my brothers, both of whom were on statins at the time, that I distrusted guidelines that significantly expanded the number of people who should go on statins to reduce the risk of a heart attack or stroke.[40] My argument was that this was a ploy to put everyone in the world, or close to it, on cholesterol-lowering drugs—in other words, that it was an instance of medicalization.

My older brother looked at me incredulously and said that it seemed as if I was using a broad social critique to repudiate a treatment that might, in the individual case, be beneficial. His position is that we are intelligent medical consumers and that the information at hand (drug efficacy and an accurate cholesterol test) is valuable and can be intelligently discussed with a doctor to come to a personalized treatment decision. My position is that if you start down that rabbit hole, medicalization wins. To my older brother, my position is stupidly against health. (My younger brother, also on a low-dose statin at the time, largely stayed out of the conversation.

We did, after all, have this conversation while on a boat on Long Island Sound, so there were more pleasant things to pay attention to.)

While my older brother would probably think the entire book *Against Health* is a little much, he might agree with Anna Kirkland's statement toward the end of the conclusion that "challenging health—being against health in certain ways—will actually promote better conversations in pivotal moments like those that occur in the doctor's office."[41] That, at least, is what he was trying to persuade me of when we had our disagreement about statins—don't use a social critique to dissuade you of the benefits of medicine; just use it to your advantage in your personal relation with your doctor as you make important health decisions. He was really arguing for a mode of somatic individualism—use the information available as a mechanism toward optimization. Don't repudiate the means available to assure yourself a healthy future. Don't think of the tests as limitations but as opportunities.

But is this really possible? Can we just use knowledge to better our own awareness and personal interactions with our doctors, as a way of smart bodily management? Does medicalization really let us off the hook in this way, to use an understanding of its negative cultural effects to our own personal advantage? In other words, does the medicalization thesis just let us be better medical consumers? More active rather than passive? In other words, what is the point of understanding medicalizing and biomedicalizing processes and outcomes?

The sociologists Simon Williams and Michael Calnan provide a complex answer to these questions in their 1996 article, "The 'Limits' of Medicalization? Modern Medicine and the Lay Populace in 'Late' Modernity."[42] The simple way of rendering their discussion is to say no—the medicalization thesis is not, primarily, a mechanism to realize how to be better health care consumers. Instead, it sheds light on reconfigurations of medical practitioners, patients, knowledge, and policy. Williams and Calnan suggest that while early theorists portrayed medicalization as a "dependence on modern medicine, or the 'fabrication' of 'docile bodies,'" such characterizations produced a "largely 'over-drawn' view of medical power, dominance and control in the late modern era." In their view, recent sociological explorations of the risk society and modern social formations demonstrate a "critical and dynamic relationship between modern medicine and the lay populace," one in which a "'critical distance' is beginning to open up." As a result, they anticipated an emergent set of problems concerning doctors' roles in society, their social power, their responses to questions about their expertise and the limitations of their knowledge, and the issue of trust in experts in the context of "a society in which all knowledge is seen as provisional [and] doubt becomes a defining feature of modern critical reasoning": "Will medicine increasingly come to acknowledge its limitations and the contingent nature of its knowledge base, or will it instead simply shift towards more 'defensive' forms of medicine and 'damage limitation' as rear-guard action to growing public criticism and demystification of science and technology?" (1617–18).

I raise this discussion of Williams and Calnan's 1996 article at the end of this chapter because it suggests an alternative to what seems to be a rather disappointing conclusion to the value of understanding medicalization. I do not think that medicalization teaches us to be better health care consumers. The medicalization thesis illuminates a pervasive and ongoing theme of modern discontent—concerns about specialized expertise, loss of individuality and control, and increased surveillance and managerial regulation that characterize medicine in late modernity. Williams and Calnan state that "a critical re-configuration of professional power and dominance [with respect to medicine] is beginning to take place. At present [in 1996], however, the precise nature and extent of these changes remains largely open to question" (1618). If we are to try to find an example of a social phenomenon that represents this reconfiguration, or that speaks to it, vaccination controversy is a pretty good one. As Williams and Calnan point out, "Medicine's close association with the body may mean that it has become a focal point around which many of these broader social concerns and anxieties have condensed" (1618). The timing of their argument is prescient, especially when considering their anticipatory conclusions about forms of "critical reconfigurations" in relation to the growing influence of vaccine skepticism in the late 1990s and early 2000s.

Williams and Calnan write that "the increasing lay emphasis upon the 'un-natural' aspects of modern medical technology may represent a symbolic struggle over the human body" (1618). In the next chapter, I consider this symbolic struggle as it is addressed in the work of anti-medicine social theorist Ivan Illich and the iconoclastic physician Robert Mendelsohn. They extended the arguments of the medicalization thesis to concerns about medicine's actual dangers, focusing on its expansive social presence and transformation of ordinary life but also bringing attention to its disease-creating potential or, in Illich's terms, its *iatrogenic* capacities. Like Williams and Calnan, these critics anticipated the "critical reconfigurations" of society that medicine provoked, seeing in medicine's rise a troublesome loss of authenticity or a challenge to the limits of expertise. Antimedicine offers an opportunity to situate vaccine skepticism in the currents of a critical, and dark, twentieth-century perspective on medicine and its supposed triumphs, leading into a discussion of medical exposés that constitutes the second half of the next chapter.

8

Antimedicine in
Theory and Practice

While I was working on the first draft of this chapter, my husband and I went on a road trip to visit family. At some point we all got talking about medications—what we're on, why we're on them, and what they do. As a group, we were a pretty typical bunch of middle-class, middle-aged-to-elderly white Americans. We had a lot of medications in the house, both self- and doctor-prescribed, as well as theories and practices about taking them. The older members of the group tended to take more medicines. At least one of us is alive because of medical treatments all but unknown fifty years ago. All of us could be described as good biological citizens managing our health and optimizing our potential. We monitor our symptoms, hoping that the side effects of drugs and supplements won't be worse than the conditions we are trying to prevent or treat, and we accept or resist medications based on personal experience, somatic responsiveness, and perceptions of the reliability of the advice.

Within our family group, our relationship to these forms of medicalization differ—my husband and I are more skeptical of widely advertised prescription medications (like statins and antidepressants), more reluctant to take drugs regularly, warier of testing too much in the effort to find something wrong. Nevertheless, it struck me that all of us were taking our medications on trust—trusting the physicians who prescribe them, the companies that make them, the news articles about them, the informational websites that we consult, the scientific studies that we read, and the books that we buy to improve our knowledge about ourselves.

Antimedicine critics tell us why we should trust less and resist more. *Antimedicine* is related to the medicalization thesis but is not precisely the same. As I showed in the previous chapter, the sociology of medicalization focuses on aspects of ordinary life that are brought under medical authority, either socially or professionally. Antimedicine is similarly concerned with the expanding purview of medicine, but targets the more specific effects of medications and treatments. Like sociologists of medicalization, antimedicine critics will criticize the social effects of medicalization—loss of personal freedom and autonomy, for example, in a society that increasingly narrows its normative expectations for healthy behavior—but they also identify specific dangers of medical practices and procedures. In other words, antimedicine critics argue that medical treatment itself can be dangerous and that medicine must be limited in order to protect people's true health.

There are three basic kinds of antimedicine arguments. One, exemplified by the intellectual iconoclast Ivan Illich, is an extension of the medicalization thesis, criticizing the social authority of medicine but zeroing in on its iatrogenic capacities. (*Iatrogenic* is a word of Greek derivation meaning "doctor-caused" or "caused by medicine or treatment.") This critique is broad, sociological, and theoretically informed. Another is a more consumer-oriented antimedicine, arguing that much of contemporary medicine is costly and often unnecessary, sometimes damagingly so. This is a position that is likely to be put forward by physician authors. Finally, there is the antipharmaceutical crowd. They argue that current medical practice is overly influenced by the existence of drug treatments and the marketing efforts of drug companies. Some of the critics in this group go so far as to accuse the pharmaceutical industry of corruption and fabrication of research results in an effort to increase profits. This last group of antimedicine critics is made up of physicians, academics, and medical journal editors. The second and third groups often publish their ideas in the form of exposés of mainstream medicine and pharmacology.

The doubts about medicine that are promulgated by all of these critics are reminiscent of the problems of trust that I have pointed to throughout this book. The arguments that antimedicine critics make are meant to persuade us that there are ways to be healthy other than following the advice of physicians or the enticing advertisements of drug companies. In other words, they try to instill doubt in the practice of medicine as we encounter it now—in terms of both our own doctors and our expectations of life and what we do to be healthy. And while none of these critics says exactly the same thing, each does argue that medicine's development leads to various forms of ill health. The message that all of them put forward is that a healthy skepticism of contemporary medical practice, and, especially, of contemporary medicines themselves, is in order. Taken together, antimedicine critics are concerned not only that medicalization has transformed our relation to health, but that medicines taken as prescribed might very well kill us. Of interest, then, are their recommendations for how to avoid this fate.

Ivan Illich and the Limits of Medicine

Ivan Illich's iconic book, *Medical Nemesis: The Expropriation of Health*, was initially published in 1975, with the American edition coming out in 1976.[1] As an antimedicine text, *Medical Nemesis* is a cultural reference point for this unorthodox, yet influential, position. Illich himself is something of a cultural reference point, as he had an unusual career as a public intellectual. Trained in the Catholic priesthood, he served only briefly as a parish priest.[2] He was appointed to a number of visiting professorships in the United States and Europe, notably at Pennsylvania State University and the University of Bremen. At the latter location he was part of a group including the historian Barbara Duden, who with Illich initiated a unique approach emphasizing the radical dissimilarity of bodies in history. Illich's most famous works are *Deschooling Society* and *Medical Nemesis*, although *Tools for Conviviality*, according to Carl Mitcham, is his most general theoretical statement.[3] Although Illich's writing touched on many issues, for our purposes here it is enough to say that he offered wide-ranging criticism of modern developments that end up damaging, rather than improving, human relationships and human experience. In particular, he criticized institutions that promote a philosophy of the managed life.

For Ivan Illich, medicine's transformations in the twentieth century led to dangerous clinical, social, and cultural circumstances, which he identifies as various forms of "dis-ease." Early in *Medical Nemesis* he defines different forms of *iatrogenesis*, or illness caused by medicine. For Illich, *clinical iatrogenesis* is medicine's intrinsic dangerousness, the known and unknown "side effects" of treatment that sicken people. *Social iatrogenesis* is the way in which "medical practice sponsors sickness by reinforcing a morbid society" in which individuals seek treatments as consumers rather than actively working for social and political transformation.[4] It is at this level that health is "expropriated" through "overmedicalization." *Cultural iatrogenesis* is for Illich the deepest level of medicine-caused illness, in which people's innate capacities to confront and experience suffering, illness, disappointment, pain, vulnerability, and death are displaced by medicine's "pernicious techniques" (33).

Culturally and structurally, for Illich, medicine serves as a "radical monopoly," which means an institution that "disable[s] people from doing or making things on their own" (42). Radical monopolies are things, practices, or institutions that become important in themselves, rather than for the services they render. As a result, social forces then consolidate to sustain their existence, further disabling and alienating people from their own capacities. A classic example of a nonmedical radical monopoly is the automobile, which comes to actively displace other forms of transportation, whereupon local and national infrastructures are created to serve it. As a result, people come to depend on automobiles and no longer on themselves (their bodies and strength) for transportation, and the built environment does not allow people to walk to stores or easily transport purchased goods home on foot.

As a radical monopoly, medicine also becomes an end in and of itself, rather than serving primarily as a tool for healing. In the context of this critique, doctors are no longer healers with both practical and ritualistic roles to play, but technicians who work for impersonal institutions. Personal relationships, the most meaningful and trust-laden interactions that form the basis of successful treatment, deteriorate in the context of medicalization. Medicine, which used to promote natural healing by working with the body, is now a practice located in a faceless bureaucracy without commitment to individuals or their personhood.

Illich's own discussion is of course far richer than this brief summary can portray. He expresses nostalgia for previous historical periods during which, he claimed, healthier relations with doctors obtained. Much of his argument is targeted against technology, which makes doctors into technicians and patients into its servants. Medicine reduces autonomy all around—doctors lose their historical stature and authority, and patients no longer control their bodies, their environments, or their will. Cultural, social, and personal human experiences are turned into technical matters that are managed bureaucratically. In Illich's view, this change weakens people's individual and collective responses to life and illness. As an example, what he would consider the normal expression of pain in culture is tolerable *because it has cultural meaning*. Cultural iatrogenesis, however, robs pain of its intrinsic cultural meaning so that the patient can only request that it be stopped: "There is no historical precedent for the contemporary situation in which the experience of personal bodily pain is shaped by the therapeutic program designed to destroy it" (139).

Lest it seem that Illich is throwing the baby out with the bathwater, he is not against all medical discovery and advancement. I include here a long quotation from *Medical Nemesis* in which he sets out his argument that medical progress is a problem when it goes beyond "a certain level," although he doesn't fully specify how we are to determine that point:

> The destructive power of medical overexpansion does not, of course, mean that sanitation, inoculation, and vector control, well-distributed health education, healthy architecture, and safe machinery, general competence in first aid, equally distributed access to dental and primary medical care, as well as judiciously selected complex services, could not all fit into a truly modern culture that fostered self-care and autonomy. As long as engineered intervention in the relationship between individuals and environment remains *below a certain intensity*, relative to the range of the individual's freedom of action, such intervention could enhance the organism's competence in coping and creating its own future. *But beyond a certain level*, the heteronomous [subject to the authority of others] management of life will inevitably first restrict, then cripple, and finally paralyze the organism's nontrivial responses,

and what was meant to constitute health care will turn into a specific form of health denial. (220; emphasis added)

This lengthy excerpt shows that in Illich's view the problem is how medicine's expansion enlarges the authority of bureaucratic managers by limiting the freedom of individuals and their capacity for autonomous action, including bodily healing. Paradoxically, he notes, the extension of health care to all, instead of lessening illness, expanded the numbers of those who needed treatment, in part through a redefinition of health, which "broaden[ed] the scope of medical care" (222).[5] (In the United States, the shift to managed care in the 1980s and 1990s was supposed to control costs, but it had the opposite effect, perhaps for a similar reason.)

In the preface to the 1995 edition of *Medical Nemesis*, retitled *Limits to Medicine*, Illich reflects on some of his own limits when writing the original text:

I unwittingly prepared the ground for a worldview in which the suffering person would get even further out of touch with the flesh. I neglected the transformation of the experience of the body and soul when well-being comes to be expressed by a term that implies functions, feedbacks, and their regulation. . . . You can obliterate the experienced sensual body of the past by conceiving of yourself as a self-regulatory, self-constructing system in need of responsible management. . . . I did not sufficiently stress [the health care system's] subtle structures which pattern our response, turning us into subsystems.[6]

This comment echoes the *biomedicalization critique*, discussed in the previous chapter. It is not only the expansion of medical care that is the problem, but the redefinition of humans and their needs. Once "systems thinking" takes over, people become managers of the systems in their bodies. Unlike Nikolas Rose, in this radical critique Illich sees little benefit in forms of somatic individualism that turn people into self-regulating coping mechanisms, unable to either suffer or delight in the body.

The French philosopher Michel Foucault responded to Illich's arguments in *Medical Nemesis* in a lecture he gave in the 1970s that was not published in English until 2004.[7] He does not make a point-by-point critique of Illich but criticizes the nostalgic elements of Illich's analysis and his lack of historical perspective concerning how early forms of medicalization emerge and what the implications of its long history are. Yet both Foucault and Illich end at a similar point—medicine is not science but is a material practice embedded in the sociocultural context, systematically related to both economics and politics. They agree that medicine's iatrogenic effects are found not only in the context of its treatments and their dangers, but also in its enlarged sociocultural authority and its complex enactment of economic and political power. As a result, medicalization represents one aspect of the dangers with which modern medicine threatens modern people, but it is not the only danger. Iatrogenesis also resides within medicine, and threatens patients in the very context of treatment. Radical antimedicine stances move beyond the medicalization thesis to emphasize the problem of iatrogenesis as modern medicine's most significant overreach.

The People's Doctor

Robert Mendelsohn, MD, a self-described "medical heretic," popularized antimedicine arguments in the 1960s, 1970s, and 1980s in the United States, primarily through his syndicated newspaper column and newsletter, "The People's Doctor," and popular books like *Confessions of a Medical Heretic, Male Practice: How Doctors Manipulate Women,* and *How to Raise a Healthy Child in Spite of Your Doctor.*[8] Mendelsohn's arguments are rooted in an antimodern sensibility that accuses medicine of becoming a new religion. He included vaccines as dangerous technologies that are not necessary to the vast majority of children in the United States and relied on his clinical experience as a physician as well as experimental and anecdotal evidence for his arguments. Long a member of La Leche League's medical advisory board, he promoted home birth and breastfeeding and alerted readers to the dangers of routine use of X-rays (especially chest X-rays) and other technical procedures (such as nonreligious circumcision).[9] In these ways he argued against bureaucratic and technological trends in medicine that inhibited natural healing and supplanted traditional cultural institutions like the family that, in his view, support true health.

In *Confessions of a Medical Heretic,* Mendelson argued that the only real basis for people's trust in medicine is faith. He believed that this trust is misguided, as he portrayed doctors as not very reliable or knowledge-able. Nor did he believe that their practices led to actual health. It's un-clear why Mendelsohn had such low regard for his fellow physicians. He indicated that they are "only human" and therefore inclined to be narrow-minded, ignorant, uneducated, and (at times) boorish. His primary argu-ment is that, as the twentieth century wore on, doctors began to think of themselves as possessing magic powers and therefore like priests. Their quasi-magical powers resulted from new developments in surgery and the discovery of antibiotics, which allowed physicians to successfully treat conditions that previously were outside of medicine's capacity to cure. Ordinary people's faith in physicians as priests is dangerous because, he was quick to point out, they are only human. Their view of themselves as above others is what Mendelsohn thinks is dangerous, as he believed that physicians with such high opinions of themselves didn't scrutinize their own practices.

Like Illich, Mendelsohn believed that the practice of medicine had be-come less about healing than about the maintenance of medicine itself, and especially doctors' livelihoods. As a result, many medical treatments were self-perpetuating even though bad for people. A key passage toward the end of *Confessions of a Medical Heretic* demonstrates his point of view: "There is no way anyone can justify the billions of dollars we spend every year on 'health care.' We're not getting healthier as the bill gets higher, we're getting sicker. . . . Modern Medicine has succeeded in teach-ing us to equate *medical care* with *health*."[10]

Mendelsohn's arguments in *Confessions of a Medical Heretic* against vaccination detail the potential dangers of routinely administered vaccines in comparison to the risks to the population of epidemic diseases or to in-dividuals of illnesses. In 1980 those vaccines would have been polio, DTP, measles, mumps, rubella, and flu, although the latter was not as widely recommended as it is today. His discussion here includes vaccines as forms of preventative medicine that endanger healthy people, just like X-rays and other routine screening procedures. Here is a typical argument:

Any doctor who has had decades of experience with measles knows that while the incidence [of measles encephalitis] may be that high [one out of 1,000 cases] among children who live under poverty and malnutrition, among well-nourished middle and upper class children the incidence is one in 10,000 or even one in 100,000. Meanwhile, the vaccine itself is associated with encephalopathy in one case per million and more frequently with other neurologic and sometimes fatal conditions such as ataxia (discoordination), retardation, hyperactivity, aseptic meningitis, seizures, and hemiparesis (paralysis of one side of the body). (144)

He went on to argue that "numerous other factors such as nutrition, housing, and sanitation" determine whether an individual contracts a disease, implying that health could be supported through widespread public health efforts rather than by vaccination, which involved risks, however remote, to those vaccinated (144).

In his 1984 book *How to Raise a Healthy Child in Spite of Your Doctor*, Mendelsohn argued that "pediatricians are dangerous," primarily because they lead children into "a lifelong dependence on medical interventions," they are unlikely to "tell parents about the potential side effects of the drugs and treatments they prescribe," they "indoctrinate children . . . with the philosophy of 'a pill for every ill,'" they order unnecessary tests because of low pay, they fail to recognize real illness because they see so many well patients, they don't spend enough time with their patients, they "promot[e] and defend laws that force patients to use their services," they are against breastfeeding, and they "tacit[ly] support . . . obstetrical intervention that is damaging children."[11] His main concerns about vaccines focused on mass vaccination and the varied effects on individual children. He suggested that immunization clinics make it difficult to determine if immunization is contraindicated for a particular child, argued that long-term risks of "injecting foreign proteins into the body of your child" were unknown and not being researched, and mentioned the "growing suspicion that immunization against relatively harmless childhood disease may be responsible for the dramatic increase in autoimmune diseases since mass inoculations were introduced" (232). Mendelsohn discussed most routine childhood illnesses and presented arguments against vaccination for each one, including some illnesses (like scarlet fever and meningitis) for which there was no vaccine in the 1970s and 1980s. (In the case of scarlet fever, there still isn't.) His point in each case was similar—vaccinations are risky, and the illnesses at issue are not severe (at least not in children). In those cases for which the latter argument could not be made (such as polio), he suggested that the vaccine was not responsible for the reduction in disease prevalence.[12] This argument, heavily disputed by medical researchers and public health authorities, is nevertheless prevalent in some vaccine-skeptical communities today.

Whether Mendelsohn was right or wrong in his views on vaccination, they cohere with his overall belief that medicine had gone awry as a profession and become more like a religion intent on replicating itself and gaining adherents. Like Illich, Mendelsohn had a sense of the limits of medicine and was concerned about changes to human relationships that occurred as medicalization expanded medicine's social authority and replaced traditional experiences with medically managed ones. In 1987, he joined Illich in a statement for the School of Medicine at the University of Illinois, Chicago, against medical bioethics, which they argued was "irrelevant to the aliveness with which we intend to face pain and anguish, renunciation and death," in large part because, under the guise of bioethics, "medicine has ceased to look at the sufferings of a sick person: the object of care has become something called a human life."[13]

Yet Illich was more philosophically oriented in his objections to modern medicine than Robert Mendelsohn, who, I hasten to emphasize, was actually a physician. For Illich, a social critic and philosopher, the management of personhood through the proliferation of new concepts like "human life" was the problem. Such concepts became fetishes that the system subsequently protected and supported: "'A Life' is amenable to management, to improvement and to evaluation in terms of available resources in a way which is unthinkable when we speak of 'a person.'"[14] Mendelsohn's pronouncements are more firmly rooted in his experience as a doctor and his specific concerns about the practice of medicine. The two came together in warning against the inauguration of technocratic practices that supported medical care by substituting for actual healing, human experience, and the meaning of suffering in ordinary life.

For Robert Mendelsohn, medicine had left nature and consequently directed people's behaviors inappropriately. The example of breastfeeding is instructive here. Mendelsohn's promotion of breastfeeding was about the promotion of natural family organization and its corollary health practices. Today breastfeeding is another medicalized practice of maternity that is accommodated and documented in hospitalized birth and during well-baby visits. This is a fascinating historical development, especially because feeding with formula is a complex practice associated with a medicalized modernity. The promotion of breastfeeding in the 1950s, 1960s, and 1970s had a "back to nature" rationale and justification, against the medicalization of infant feeding that occurred with the takeover of infant feeding by formula in the first half of the twentieth century.[15] Yet breastfeeding itself, through its promotion within medicine, eventually became (bio)medicalized, although largely after Mendelsohn's death in 1988. But this development supports what Michel Foucault argues in his criticism of Illich, which is that positions that we want to take up against medicalization have already been medicalized or will eventually become medicalized. And it also suggests a limitation to Mendelsohn's influence in mainstream culture—his call to recognize the value of breastfeeding was ultimately followed, but only through its medicalization and thus its full integration into obstetrics and pediatrics, albeit unevenly. Mendelsohn's lasting influence in American culture is his steadfast opposition to vaccination, which means that, given how culturally accepted vaccinations have become, his influence is mostly evident in radical groups of vaccine skeptics.

Exposing Medicine's Overreach

The medical exposés discussed in this section touch upon and expand various elements of the medicalization and antimedicine arguments. In general, they highlight dangers that are the result of faulty research, purposeful deception, ethical conflicts in the process of scientific peer review, the desire of people to be healthy and free of pain, and the fact that most doctors find it difficult (if not impossible) to keep up with all of the relevant developments in their fields. Primary themes are overdiagnosis and overtreatment, as well as questionable research practices that range from worrisome to corrupt. In writing about these topics, the authors demonstrate how and why patients are complicit in specific instances of medicalization—why we, in other words, become enthusiastic adherents of treatment regimens that are questionable scientifically and clinically—and they explore how regulatory and research structures establish corrupt or deceptive practices at the heart of evidence-based medicine (EBM). The picture isn't pretty.

The titles of these texts are instructive: *Deadly Medicines and Organized Crime: How Big Pharma Has Corrupted Healthcare*; *Overdo$ed America: The Broken Promise of American Medicine*; *The Truth about Drug Companies: How They Deceive Us and What to Do about It*; *Prescribing by Numbers: Drugs and the Definition of Disease*; *Drugs for Life: How Pharmaceutical Companies Define Our Health*; *Overdiagnosed: Making People Sick in the Pursuit of Health*; *Better than Well: American Medicine Meets the American Dream*.[16] Providing a comprehensive discussion of each these books is beyond the scope of this chapter. In what follows, I pull out the significant themes and arguments that show the contours of the antimedicine argument as it is made in books written to expose varying levels of conflict of interest, endemic corruption, or criminality in medicine today. Taken together, these books provide ample fodder for significant and deep questioning of modern medicine and the negative impacts of medicalization—indeed, they suggest that neither medicine as a whole nor most doctors can be trusted to provide true information about the negative impacts of current medicines or treatments. They bolster Robert Mendelsohn's admonitions and provide a fertile context for vaccine skepticism.

H. Gilbert Welch, who wrote *Overdiagnosed* with his colleagues Lisa Schwartz and Steven Woloshin (all physicians), provides a persuasive argument about how the problem of overtreatment causes unnecessary medicalization and ill health among many people who aren't actually suffering from disease at all. Overtreatment is made possible by changing diagnostic features of diseases and so-called prediseases, by routine use of screening tests that find problems that don't produce symptoms or ill health, and by the rigid dictum that early detection saves lives. While Welch finds that pharmaceutical enticements are part of the problem of excessive diagnosis and, consequently, overtreatment, he also identifies a number of cultural factors, both within and external to medicine, that encourage the problem. His discussion does not emphasize the ethically suspect manipulations of pharmaceutical companies, although he does mention these sporadically. Instead, he focuses on the ways in which simple attention to the statistics of screening and treatment benefits versus the risks of overtreatment (or no treatment) demonstrates the evident problem—that our medical system is set up to encourage people to be treated for things that don't present as illnesses and will probably not kill them. This situation is *iatrogenic*, in that it leads to significant medicalization and dangerous modes of ill health through the seemingly healthful practices of screening, testing, and early detection. In this way, he highlights the systemic forces that lead to medicalization through overdiagnosis, rather than the particular actions of individuals or corporations.

Welch provides a clear assessment of the perils of excessive diagnosis. The specific medical practices that lead to increased and unnecessary diagnosis are (1) changing perceptions of disease markers that distinguish the sick from the well, absent symptoms of illness (for example, lower diastolic and systolic markers for hypertension, or lower total cholesterol numbers); (2) increased purposeful screening for disease, which is related to trying to find physical indications of illness before symptoms appear (such as mammography or routine chest X-rays, the latter of which was a particular pet peeve of Mendelsohn); and (3) increased discovery of abnormalities consequent to general screening or more specific screening for other reasons. These practices result from specific cultural tendencies and circumstances:

- pharmaceutical industry greed
- a market in which sellers, rather than consumers, create demand and "exploit buyers"[17]
- the widespread "true belief" that increases in diagnosis are "the path to better health for individuals and society" (157)
- researchers who rely on public grant funding to pursue research, which encourages them to identify topics *within* the current zeitgeist, rather than those that might challenge it
- a legal system that punishes potential undertreatment, which consequently encourages administrative requirements to order tests and promote screening as signs of quality health care
- physicians' desire to diagnose and treat rather than to live with uncertainty

Another systemic force is the self-reinforcing nature of testing: "To persuade you to be tested in the first place, someone . . . suggested that something might be wrong with you, something that could eventually have grave consequences, despite your current lack of symptoms. But now that your results have come back normal and that possibility is off the table, you feel good. You, and others like you in similar situations, become enthusiastic about screening" (176). He adds that this self-reinforcement is a psychological feedback loop: "Basically, the system that promotes early diagnosis induced a measure of anxiety and then took it away" (177). As a result, if you test positive for something and have treatment, then you assume that the treatment has extended your life, even though it is possible that you were simply overdiagnosed. Indeed, overtreated people are the most enthusiastic advocates for screening and early diagnosis:

> And what is most ironic is that the more overdiagnosis a screening program causes, the more popular it becomes. More overdiagnosis makes it increasingly likely that people will know others who have been diagnosed. This raises their personal sense of risk—so testing becomes all the more important. And an even more powerful reinforcement for screening is that more overdiagnosis also causes more people to believe that they owe their lives, or the lives of those they know, to screening. Remember, overdiagnosed patients tend to do extraordinarily well [because they are likely to be healthier already and their anomalies are likely to be benign], so it's easy to conclude that their lives were saved because their diseases were detected early. Once the cycle has begun, these influences will persist even if there are no other forces promoting screening (such as financial gain or true belief). This makes it difficult to back away from established tests, even when the medical community thinks it's the right thing to do. No matter what the experiences have been, the public tends to seek more testing. (178)

Jeremy A. Greene, in *Prescribing by Numbers*, provides the historical evidence for how the overdiagnosis described by Welch and his coauthors became a feature of contemporary medical practice, and Joseph Dumit, in *Drugs for Life*, corroborates these findings. Greene demonstrates how pharmaceutical companies came to play an "active role in the definition of these categories of illness," focusing primarily on hypertension medications, diabetes treatments, and cholesterol-lowering drugs in the second half of the twentieth century.[18] The upshot of these developments is medical practice that treat numbers and abstractions rather than the body and evident symptoms. (In other words, following Poovey, the numbers and abstractions come to stand in as facts for the body.) Greene highlights the close ties of marketing, research, and disease identification, showing how treatment is created through the development of pharmaceutical products and not the demand of clinicians and patients.

Like Welch, Greene does not focus on pharmaceutical scandal or bad behavior. Instead, his point is that it is the *normal* behavior of pharmaceutical companies that knit them to medical knowledge, medical research, and the dissemination of information about diseases: "The relationship between pharmaceutical companies and expert committees is not merely a question of conflict of interest, bribery, scandal, or bad science. Rather, this relationship is encoded in the very practice of 'good science' that is central to the circulation of medical knowledge. As a result, there is no organized opposition to the demonstration of benefit at more and more subtle levels of risk" (190). As a result, Greene can show that during the second half of the twentieth century, clinical trial became the mechanism that (1) makes sense of the disease state, (2) establishes efficacy of the drug, and (3) invents normal procedures for treating risk, all in the context of increased public attention to medical information. Dumit follows on these conclusions, analyzing what happens when pharmaceutical companies do their job, which is to increase profits and stock values for shareholders (not heal sick people): "I am talking about . . . what happens when companies do play by the rules and therefore use clinical trials to grow treatments. I have shown that if companies are allowed to design clinical trials, they end up shaping the very meaning of health, a health known only through those trials. . . . *Basically the only facts of health we have these days are about the value of more medicine.*"[19] In this way, Dumit, by focusing on how the pharmaceutical industry controls the production of medical facts, connects research results concerning specific drugs to an expanding idea of health. As a result, medications, nonhealth (or risk), and health all grow as a result of pharmaceutical clinical trials, and the latter (health) grows as a function of the growth in the former (medications) to treat the middle figure (risk).

Together, these exposés by Welch and colleagues, Greene, and Dumit show how treating people for asymptomatic conditions became normal. They also show how treating "by the numbers" rather than for symptomatic disease introduces problems that become culturally obscured, even though the evidence of overtreatment is all around us. The physicians John Abramson and Marcia Angell, in two books published in 2004 (*Overdo$ed America* and *The Truth about the Drug Companies*, respectively), work through much of the same territory as these authors. Angell is the former editor of the *New England Journal of Medicine*, so her concerns about research conflicts of interest are particularly troubling. The work of Abramson and Angell prepared the way for Peter Gøtzsche's *Deadly Medicines and Organized Crime*, published in 2013. Gøtzsche, a physician and scientist, is a founding member of the Nordic Cochrane Center (NCC). The NCC is part of the larger Cochrane Collaboration, a nongovernmental organization that conducts systematic reviews of medical research to check the safety and efficacy of approved treatments. These latter authors focus more specifically on research practices and corrupt relationships that lead to problems in medicalization.

Peter Gøtzsche makes four basic arguments in his book, *Deadly Medicine and Organized Crime*:

1. The statistical analyses used to demonstrate drug efficacy and safety are flawed.
2. There are corrupt relations between physicians and pharmaceutical companies.
3. There are corrupt relations between pharmaceutical companies and regulatory agencies like the Food and Drug Administration (FDA), as well as other regulatory deficiencies.
4. There is collusion between medical journals and the pharmaceutical industry in perpetuating false research outcomes that favor industry results.

To argue these points, Gøtzsche uses the tools of evidence-based medicine (EBM) against medicine itself, suggesting that we are not only overmedicated but endangering our health. (He also intersperses anecdotal evidence of corruption and worrisome research results throughout.) As a result, Gøtzsche provides a whistle-blower exposé of the corruption and questionable ethics involved in the development, research, and prescription of pharmaceutical products. (He doesn't delve into excess procedures, but he did that in a previous book, *Mammography Screening: Truth, Lies, and Controversy*; he also doesn't provide a social analysis of the phenomena he examines.)

Both Abramson and Angell are less enraged than Gøtzsche, but just as pointed in their criticisms. They claim that pharmaceutical companies

1. are deceptive with respect to their research interests,
2. use marketing as a form of education,

3. dominate clinical trial results such that bias is inevitable, and
4. remarket slightly new drugs in order to maintain patents and high
   profits.

Abramson and Angell also argue that the efficacy of many expensive drugs currently available is suspect, and that many patients would do better on older, less expensive formulations. Or they would do better with no treatment at all.

Angell is particularly eloquent about the role of medical journals in perpetuating what amounts to a form of academic fraud, having been the editor of the *New England Journal of Medicine* for two decades. Her book focuses on the pharmaceutical industry exclusively, demonstrating how Big Pharma keeps profits high without really contributing new medicines to improve health. Pharmaceutical companies come in for criticism in Abramson's *Overdo$ed America*, but, like Greene and Welch, he is interested in health care overall and how trends in medicine, including drug development, research, and usage, lead to overtreatment, excess expense, and iatrogenic illness. Abramson is particularly persuasive as he describes his efforts to determine if the evidence that he was reading in some journal articles actually matched the evidence of the clinical trials that is available on the FDA website (it didn't). Indeed, as a formerly practicing family physician, he describes how difficult it is to really know when newly developed treatments and drugs are helpful to his patients. Both Angell and Abramson end with advice about how to change the current iatrogenic circumstances of medicine.

Reading through contemporary antimedicine exposés, I am left with increasing cynicism and doubts about medicine in general and the pharmaceutical industry in particular. Remember that our vaccine advocates—Paul Offit, Seth Mnookin, Eula Biss, for example—have encouraged us to trust the science behind vaccines, and that one of the critics of science denial, Naomi Oreskes, did the same in encouraging trust in peer review of scientific findings. She appealed to readers to trust the real scientists rather than the corrupt ones. But these antimedicine critics have revealed some really corrupt scientists—or at least evidence that is created through systematically biased and corrupted practices. As a result, it is difficult to trust evidence produced in clinical trials of drugs that are funded by pharmaceutical companies, as almost all are. It is hard to believe that the information provided about these drugs—vaccines included—is trustworthy, because, according to these very persuasive books that I have read, the process itself invites and sustains bias. Jeremy Greene and Peter Gøtzsche are particularly convincing on this point—one needn't point a finger at individuals or corporations as specifically corrupted, because the process as a whole has led to a situation in which questionable or manipulated evidence of efficacy and safety can be used for licensure. In other words, normal operating procedure in the current system leads to inherent bias in results.

Joseph Dumit suggests that it is in the very construction of medical facts by pharmaceutical companies that the public's interest is neglected in favor of corporate interest. In chapter 6 I discussed the problem of the modern fact as an "epistemological unit"—while the latter is expressed numerically, and thus thought to have avoided the problem of interest or bias, facts are always situated in cultural contexts and thus beholden to those contexts for their meanings. Facts don't shed their circumstances of construction so easily. Dumit demonstrates, through a carefully argued account, that one problem with modern medical facts is that they are created in the context of the interests of pharmaceutical companies. Facts that doctors want to know—for example, when to *stop* giving a drug to patients—are not investigated because they are not in the companies' interests. As a result, the very notion of health that modern subjects currently operate under has been shaped by corporations whose main interest it is that we all take more medications and take them for life.[20]

Personally, my own sense that staying away from medicines is a healthy decision has been confirmed by my reading, but at the cost of becoming increasingly paranoid about the medical treatment of everyone in my extended family. Only significant self-restraint is keeping me from phoning all of my relations to warn them of the deceptions that have led them to trust their doctors and take their medications. To go back to the story about statins that I told in chapter 7, pharmaceutical companies' manipulations of data on statins and how well they prevent heart disease and stroke provide a cautionary tale. But should I pass on that cautionary tale? To do so is to suggest to my brothers, to my father, to other family members, to all my friends and acquaintances, that they shouldn't trust *their* doctors. Do I want to take on that responsibility? Do I feel confident enough in *my facts* to do so?[21]

My older brother was right—I resist particular medicines and therapeutic regimens because I am skeptical about the medical profession as
a whole. I am not skeptical that most doctors want to do well by their
patients, that they are in it for the right reasons, but I am suspicious about
the data used to support the highly intrusive, surveillant, and regulatory
nature of testing and treatment now considered completely normal for
insurance-protected Americans. I am suspicious that the reasons various
tests and treatments are recommended are influenced by structural problems that value profits over reasonable assessments of risk. To a certain
extent, I was primed for these positions and suspicions before I read these
particular books, because I have studied medicine critically for a number
of years and was already persuaded by the medicalization thesis. But reading these books has further convinced me about fundamental problems of
medicine in the modern world—its connections to profit-making enter-
prises like drug production, the increasingly blurry lines between health
and illness, and the normalization of "prevention" so that eradication of
all illness is the goal of medicine. This latter phenomenon is paradoxical,
as medicine's striving to rid the world of illness and suffering has occurred
simultaneously with (or caused?) more and more things being defined as
diseases or disorders and thus more and more people coming under treatment. Exposing the conflicts of interest, structural impediments to good
research, corruption, and seemingly unalterable trends toward overdiagnosis and overtreatment, these texts demonstrate that fixing this situation
will not be an easy matter, especially given how invested most of us are in
our own good health.

What is the relation of these exposés to vaccine skepticism in twenty-first-
century America? First, I find it interesting that vaccines are almost always
mentioned in all of these books as one of the surefire triumphs of medical
progress, even though they are made by pharmaceutical companies, their
clinical trials are conducted by those companies, and the results of those
trials are evaluated by the FDA—processes that are identified in these texts
as worrisome at the least. Mendelsohn is the outlier here, as he argues
that the iatrogenic effects of injecting foreign proteins into children's bodies are unknown and not a subject of significant research. I am not arguing that vaccines are not safe—nor am I arguing that they are safe. I am
arguing that these antimedicine jeremiads suggest that vaccines could be

dangerous, just like other pharmaceutical products. In other words, these books provide an argument that could be turned toward vaccines, as subject to the same kinds of criticism that these authors bestow upon drugs like Crestor and Zoloft.

And that leads to my second point. The antimedicine argument creates a context in which trust in medicine—both medical practitioners and medical treatments—is hard to justify and sustain. "Stay away except for emergencies" seems like pretty good advice. And that is precisely what my research group has seen in much of our interview data, which I will describe in more detail in chapter 10. Distrust is indeed promulgated by the arguments in these books, and for good reason. But if these authors are right—and, to my mind, they are really persuasive—then how does one make good decisions about medical care? Angell says that one question one should ask a doctor if he or she prescribes a new medication is "Has the evidence been published in a peer-reviewed medical journal?" even though she writes an entire chapter about problems in pharmaceutical-funded *published* research and links it to overmedication generally.[22] Abramson spends a significant amount of space in *Overdo$ed America* showing how medical journal articles spin research findings to make them appear to be significant, and Gøtzsche is practically apoplectic about the statistical manipulations to create significant findings in drug research. If the problem is as ingrained and foundational as Greene suggests, the entire system is based on the treatment of abstract risks, not real bodies or their symptoms. We are back, then, to Illich and the idea that systems-oriented knowledge and practice now substitute the manipulation of systems for the healing of people. In other words, medical understanding and practice are fundamentally alienating and lead to ill health because they "reduc[e] persons born for suffering and delight to provisionally self-sustaining information loops."[23]

Or should we believe that knowledge is power and understanding drug ingredients and efficacy are crucial to making good health care decisions? This is a pretty mainstream way of addressing the problems illuminated by the antimedicine critics, primarily because most of us are embedded in the system already and extracting ourselves completely is a tall order. Dumit's chapter 2, "Responding to Facts," traces the activity of "expert patients" who seek to inform themselves about treatments and medicines prescribed for them as a result of medical testing. Referring to a sociologist who represented his experience of seeking out medical facts after a prostate test, Dumit writes, "Having become suspicious of facts in the world, [Grove] nonetheless clings to truth, to the idea that with proper collection, assessment, and analysis of facts in the world he can come to the best decision for himself."[24] He might have been writing about many of us. We make ourselves feel more secure by conducting our own research—and the Internet has made this infinitely easier, at least for folks with broadband access. Indeed, one could argue that the rise in patients' Internet medical research is an attempt to counteract their growing sense that relying on their own doctors is not always a good idea. This trend is infinitely vexing to physicians and their national organizations, as they worry over the kind of information that people find, and want to ensure that it is scientifically reliable, although what that means given the exposés discussed above is anyone's guess. This trend is specifically difficult with respect to vaccine skepticism, as misinformation on the Internet is a favorite whipping boy of the vaccine promoters—all those gullible parents looking things up on the Internet and finding persuasive but misinformed pseudo-experts who tell them vaccines are poison!

Ivan Illich would see these kinds of information-seeking behaviors as part of a social field that demands management of the self as "a life" and repudiates the experiences of illness characterized by suffering and the challenges of being human. Michel Foucault would also see self-regulation at the base of these behaviors, but he would not emphasize the value of suffering or the meaning of being human. Instead, he would focus on the codification of information seeking as a mode of self-governance. He might also suggest that repudiation of such behavior is an apt resistance. The antimedicine physicians whose exposés are discussed in the final section of this chapter would see these activities as well worth the effort, as they arm individuals with knowledge that they can use to deliberate about their own health. Marcia Angell, remember, includes questions about medical research to address to one's own doctor. While none of the authors discussed here, except Robert Mendelsohn, specifically targets vaccines for criticism, all of them suggest that trusting medicine is an activity that must come with one's own information-seeking efforts. That is, since medicine is no longer trustworthy because of its entanglements with the pharmaceutical industry, its poor regulation by government agencies that are supposed to protect people from fraudulent, inadequate, or biased research, and the corruption of the scientific peer review process, people must rely on their own research to establish for themselves the right treatments and drugs to address illness, both symptomatic or imagined.

In this way seeking information about vaccines and making individual decisions about their advisability are fully in keeping with currents in antimedicine critique. The difference is that vaccines are not voluntary medicines, and in most states the mechanisms for exemption are limited to either medical contraindication or religious belief. Many parents, especially poor ones, might not be able to maneuver an exemption or feel that it is advisable to do so, even if they don't trust vaccinations. Thus, it is *completely understandable* that vaccinations would become specially contentious in the late twentieth and early twenty-first centuries, as antimedicine critiques proliferate and drug scandals seem routine. Vaccine skeptics are acting in a time-honored tradition (in the spirit of Robert Mendelsohn) as they hesitate to medicalize their children, or as they seek out independent information about vaccines and their ingredients, skeptical of the safety profile that is made available by both pharmaceutical companies and the federal government. They are practicing good biological citizenship in the twenty-first century.

9

VIRAL IMAGINATIONS

In fall 2010, the Vaccination Research Group conducted an online survey about attitudes toward the flu vaccine among local college students. We were surprised by two mentions of becoming a zombie after flu vaccination and four references to a Washington Redskins cheerleader who allegedly developed a rare neurological disorder from the H1N1 flu vaccine. Out of over 500 responses, these outliers stood out.

Initially we thought that these answers were just students fooling around, as college students are wont to do, but as we looked into them another possibility emerged. These responses signaled the power of urban legends and popular culture to shape perspectives on vaccines.[1] One respondent even mentioned *I Am Legend*, a 2007 movie in which a measles virus engineered for a cancer vaccine makes the entire US population vampiric zombies.[2]

This was my first experience thinking about zombies and vaccines. Doing more research revealed that zombies represent an outsized and deadly outcome of the very problems identified in the antimedicine critiques. One does not need to see a zombie as a real possibility of viral contamination, viral pandemic, or vaccines gone awry to understand what zombies represent—the possibility of system breakdown due to biotechnology run amok, bureaucratic procedures that cannot contain infections or experiments, dangerous linkages between medicine and the military-industrial complex, and the rapacious greed of pharmaceutical companies. And more than anything else, the zombie story tells us that in an outbreak, the government will agree to sacrifice some in order to save itself and civilization—a scenario that is eerily similar to allowing injury to a few in order to protect the health of the population as a whole, which is one way to understand the rationale for mass immunization.

Zombie apocalypse narratives are stories about the individual and the horde. Pandemic apocalypse narratives often involve mythic conflicts between good and evil. Often the two genres combine. In this chapter I explore how these types of stories articulate cultural concerns that resonate with vaccine skepticism. I do not argue that concern about vaccines makes people imagine that zombies could be real. Nor do I argue that mass media or popular novels create images that leach into people's minds and make them afraid of things that are perfectly safe, like vaccines. In other words, I am not trying to blame fiction and film for motivating vaccine resistance and refusal. Rather, in the spirit of science and technology studies, I suggest that these concerns and these stories are *cocreated*, in that they are part of embedded cultural processes in which we think about (and act on) the ways in which technological developments seem dangerous to us.

Novels and films are a classic way in which we express our concerns and also our beliefs, and they reveal ongoing worries about our collective capacity to control the unexpected outcomes of our prodigious efforts to improve human lives. They also recursively shape our conscious and unconscious responses to illness, health, disease, and medicine. We are not afraid of scientific and technical advancement in any simple way. Humans have always gnawed at the problem of how changes to society and culture affect our experience as living beings. Zombies represent this problem in particular ways.

We create our own monsters, and they represent not simply our fears or our social organization, but our sense of the future of humanity, our own capacity to imagine (or not) our survival, and our belief in the fundamental goodness and badness of humans. Soldiers fighting the zombie horde must decide if they are going to shoot people who are not sick yet but who may be infected. They must decide if they are going to simply follow orders or behave based on their own moral compass. Shades of Nazism are rife throughout the literature, especially in those stories in which the postapocalypse is imagined as a fight between egalitarian and totalitarian ideals. Importantly for my purposes here, a central question that is raised by the zombie infestation is how to save civilization from a horde that is incapable of any form of rational thinking and is motivated only by bloodlust, the desire to eat flesh.

A Brief Cultural History of Zombies and Vampires

In his book *Danse Macabre*, Stephen King argues that there are three archetypal monsters—the Werewolf, the Vampire, and the Thing That Has No Name. Zombies, he suggests, are variants of the vampire.[3] These figures, then, overlap somewhat, but King's distinctions are useful in understanding the importance of the zombie in the contemporary viral imagination. The zombie carries on a tradition of the vampire but also introduces specific distinctions that are noteworthy. Some of our most current zombie-like ghouls are really vampires.

The urtext of vampirism is, of course, Bram Stoker's *Dracula*. The general story is familiar enough, but in this case the specifics matter. *Dracula* follows a group of five men and one woman as they attempt to find and kill Count Dracula, who has moved to London in order to expand his territory of victims. Thanks to the diligence and skill of the one woman of the company, Mina Murray, the group is able to write up a record of vampire bites and deaths in the London area, and thereby both account for and track Dracula's movements. They eventually kill him, as well as three vampire women, at his castle back in Transylvania.

Dracula is the prototype of the undead vampire, rapacious and conniving, intent on spreading his evil, and seeking victims one by one. He is no match for the combined efforts of the vampire hunters who go after him. They are an odd lot, made up of the three suitors of Lucy Westenra (Mina's friend who is bitten by Dracula and turned into a vampire), as well as Mina's fiancé, Jonathan Harker, a famous doctor from the

Netherlands, Abraham Van Helsing, and Mina herself. What struck me reading the story is how isolated this group of vampire hunters is. They don't bring the police into their confidence; they don't alert the government or hospital officials to their suspicions; they go after Dracula on their own. They are independent and focused, and no one else knows what they are up to.

Mina is bitten by Dracula in London. He needs to be killed so she does not become undead. (Van Helsing deals with an undead Lucy with a stake through her heart and decapitation to ensure that she cannot come back as a vampire.) Fortunately, when Dracula is stabbed in the heart with a bowie knife (and also decapitated), his body disintegrates. As a result, Mina is saved. Of course, London is saved as well, but the story remains very individualized and narratively compact—it is focused on these few characters, on two basic settings, and on killing Dracula and his three close familiars.

How different from the representations of the individual versus the horde that characterize modern zombie narratives! In *Dracula* there is a sense of isolation, palpable in Transylvania where the count has alienated his countrymen with his weirdness and threatening manner, but also in London, where most of the action seems displaced from social context. This isolation may be an artifact of the construction of the novel from letters and diary fragments, collated by Mina Murray and ably typed by her. In *Dracula*, there is no horde, while contemporary zombification of the vampire introduces precisely this feature.

Roger Luckhurst, in *Zombies: A Cultural History*, locates the "zombie massification" phenomenon in the post–World War II period.[4] Prior to this time, the zombie was a lone character or "a gang of pitiful slaves under a single master" (109). In Luckhurst's view, the massification of zombies is partly a result of the discovery of the Nazi concentration camps, replete with masses of almost dead Jews, and the use of the atomic bomb over Japan, which also created a mass of people who could be termed the "living dead." He adds to these reasons other events and ideas that emerged during the 1950s, including the Korean War and the notion of a "human wave" of Asian soldiers, Red Scare anxieties, and concerns about an "other-directed" society—all of which, he argues, contributed to zombie massification.[5] In addition, mass culture contributed to the transformation of the zombie from individual to horde—at midcentury the zombie stood for "the abjected *form* of mass culture . . . becom[ing] a commentary on *massification itself*" (129, 109; emphasis in original).

Other events in the 1960s and 1970s influenced the idea of the "living dead." Luckhurst identifies the 1968 Harvard report on the definition of death in the instance of irreversible coma as a significant moment in the emergence of the contemporary undead.[6] The advent of the heart-lung machine necessitated a change in medically accepted categories of death, since the traditional understanding (cardiac death) did not apply to those whose cardiac function was taken over by a machine but did not have any neurological activity. According to Luckhurst, the so-called brain dead constituted an emerging category of the living dead, which contributed to the "boom in zombie narratives" (177). Arguing that on the individual level, changing technological capacities and definitions of death fed into the robust growth in zombie stories, he also points out that "the zombie *masses*, the ravening horde, also help figure another aspect of the contemporary medical imagination: the epidemic narrative" (179; emphasis in original). Not only have historical events created real-life zombie stories— such as the epidemic of "sleepy-sickness" in the 1920s—but the idea of the virus itself as a not-quite-alive particle that needs a host to reproduce itself "is the medicalized notion of the viral zombie in a nutshell" (181).[7] Thus viruses are zombies and also the cause of zombies, a staple element of the contemporary genre. The fact that ordinary infectious particles are understood to be the cause of zombiism, as opposed to a poison or witchcraft, represents something important about our particular cultural moment and what we think endangers us.

Luckhurst cautions that the figure of the zombie is complex and cannot be reduced "to a single explanation" or be thought of as "simply a metaphor" (196). In popular culture studies there is a tendency to see zombie fictions as critiques of capitalism, especially because George Romero's second zombie film, *Dawn of the Dead*, is located at a shopping mall and makes fun of consumer spending and desire.[8] (Romero was the director of the famous *Night of the Living Dead*, which was his first zombie film.)[9] It is also too easy to see zombie stories as articulating singular fears of viral contagion—scientific research gone haywire. Most of the zombie stories that I discuss in this chapter bring various features together, understanding the apocalypse to be caused by an intersection of greed, personality, basic human flaws, the structure of society and government, and individual (and sometimes collective) madness. Sarah Juliet Lauro, in *The Transatlantic Zombie: Slavery, Rebellion, and Living Death*, argues that zombie narratives since the mid-twentieth century have focused on misuse of science and technology, but that they have also been influenced by the development of weapons of mass destruction and advances in surgery and organ transplantation.[10] Likewise, in *Danse Macabre* Stephen King says that the superflu in *The Stand* is evidence that the "human race carries a kind of germ with it," but that it is "unleashed in a single technological misstep" (which he argues is not all that "farfetched").[11]

In other words, the apocalypse is always caused by one thing *and* another.

Zombie Hordes

Because zombies don't think and are motivated only by bloodlust, they engender a classic problem for those in charge: how to stop the horde and save civilization. The impulse of the government and military is to kill everyone who might be infected, even those who are healthy, in order to stop the outbreak. No one is an individual in a zombie apocalypse. Everyone is a potential member of the horde, and anyone can be sacrificed for the good of the group. This problem defines the zombie novel in the subgenre of apocalyptic fiction.

In addition to this generic problem, zombie novels reuse a similar cast of characters and set of issues. The characters include a doctor or scientist who wants to do good but is hampered by his or her own emotional limitations or investments, members of an ethically compromised military, rapacious mercenaries who don't care about human life, and an innocent but powerful figure who will save humankind. This last character is sometimes a not-so-innocent but good-hearted figure who needs to redeem him- or herself for past wrongs. The issues at stake include a desire for immortality and/or revenge against nature, the lack of control over the forces that are unleashed by medicoscientific experimentation, human error at the core of bureaucratic management (the glitch that unleashes the zombie apocalypse), and the too-easy corruptibility of medicine, in which doctors' core compassion and vulnerability are exploited for evil.

Dead of Night

In *Dead of Night*, the popular and prolific author Jonathan Maberry offers a pretty standard cast of characters for a zombie novel—a female Gulf War vet who is pretty (and buxom) now serving as a small-town Pennsylvania cop, her erstwhile boyfriend who runs a satellite TV news station, and an East German physician, recruited to the United States by the CIA, who now experiments on death-row inmates.[12] Zombification occurs when an executed killer wakes up at a funeral home. Developing a zombie version of a bioweapon, the doctor had injected the killer with a set of chemicals meant to paralyze him so that he would be maintained in a form of detached consciousness and experience himself being eaten alive by bioengineered wasp larvae: "Gibbon was supposed to be not only awake and aware in his coffin, it was my intention that he feel himself being consumed!" (169). Of course, the killer was supposed to be buried in a potter's field immediately after his supposed execution, but the doctor did not foresee his sole living relative requesting a decent burial for him. The larval parasites engender a zombie pandemic once they escape the sealed coffin at the undertaker's; they "were never intended to be allowed to enter the general biosphere" because they were "too unstable to use, even when deployed in remote spots" (170). Let loose in Stebbins, Pennsylvania, the zombies inevitably multiply.

The doctor, whose name is Volker, calls his superiors in the CIA, who inform the president. Thus, the highest level of government is involved. The area around the outbreak is locked down, and the National Guard brought in. Soldiers are told to shoot on sight, with the idea that everyone in the area is infected or potentially so. In the final pages of the book, with the uninfected squirreled away in the local elementary school, the police officer, Dez, and her sometime boyfriend broker an agreement with the feds, moments before a squadron of air force jets is scheduled to bomb the facility. They agree to be quarantined in the school for an indefinite period of time, with food and weapons airdropped in as needed. Their bargaining chip was a satellite feed to a reporter in the next town over, who put up streaming videos from inside the school. As their situation was played out over social media, the school inmates were able to garner sympathy from the rest of the country and turn the government away from its initial strategy to kill everyone within Stebbins and the immediately surrounding area. (Of course, the last scene of the book is of the convicted killer zombie Homer Gibbons showing up at the Starbucks where the satellite feeds are being uploaded to the Web. On to the sequel.)

Dead of Night thus offers the basic ingredients of zombie fiction—the foreign doctor who works for the CIA but whose sister was tortured and killed (thus making him liable to poor judgment as well as emotionally attached to his bioweapons research), a government-sponsored bioweapons program that uses convicted killers as research subjects, a zombie outbreak that spreads before anyone understands what is going on, and a government decision to sacrifice everyone in a small town as a method of containment. (This last element should remind readers of the movie *Outbreak*, in which a similar action was going to be taken, even though the antidote to the contagion was ready.)[13] In other words, we have misguided people who serve evil ends, innocent victims, calculating government officials, and resourceful and honorable heroes. The origin of the zombification, Dr. Volker, serves as the well-meaning servant of evil, but, as in Stephen King's *The Stand*, the origin of the outbreak is a bureaucratic glitch that he did not foresee.

World War Z

The novel that showed me how important the zombie narrative is in articulating certain kinds of vaccination concerns is *World War Z*, which chronicles a global zombie apocalypse through the oral history of a United Nations professional who interviews folks from all over the world in the aftermath of the disaster and recovery.[14] In *World War Z*, the strategy developed to counter the zombie apocalypse and save civilization is known as the Redeker plan. Paul Redeker is the name of a fictional Afrikaner apartheid architect who developed the plan that would prove successful against the zombie hordes. The Redeker plan is based on an also fictional "Plan Orange" that was designed to protect the white minority in the event of "an all-out uprising of its indigenous African population" (106).

Under the Redeker plan, the first thing governments had to accept was that it was not going to be possible to save everyone by the time a zombie outbreak was recognized, both locally and nationally (except in Israel, which presciently entered into a voluntary quarantine before everyone else). The plan thus involved pulling the military back to a semiquarantine zone that could be defended. That was the first step. The second step involved evacuating some citizens to the safe zone, as well as, far more controversially, the establishment of "special isolated zones" where human communities were sustained as "human bait," so as to protect the safe zone from a full-out onslaught of zombies (109). As zombies are drawn to living people, there needed to be enough living people among the zombies in the war zones that the military in the safe zone were not always on the defensive.

World War Z strongly suggests that all countries had to adopt a version of the Redeker plan, however seemingly humanitarian those versions were. That the successful strategy against the zombies was created by a proponent of apartheid is significant. This fact links the solution to the zombie apocalypse to a hated form of institutionalized discrimination, much like the link in *Dead of Night* of the cause of the zombies' emergence to biochemical warfare research behind the Iron Curtain. In both cases, there is a connection to selective survival and the forces of evil that condone such behavior. In *World War Z*, a figure meant to represent Nelson Mandela embraces Paul Redeker and enables the implementation of his plan in the face of political opposition, a feature that does not erase the implicit critique of Redeker's links to apartheid. Instead, this feature demonstrates that in the context of a zombie apocalypse, survival is not a humanitarian endeavor but the result of strategic action. The person who was willing to create a plan to save the Afrikaners from an uprising of the majority black population is exactly the right person to imagine a solution to the zombie horde, because that person is already trained to consider some lives eminently expendable without sentimental or moral hesitation.

Because of its unusual generic framing, *World War Z* does not utilize the familiar cast of characters of popular zombie fiction, but its issues are certainly similar. For example, the zombie apocalypse was not recognized initially because bureaucratically minded government officials had other things on their minds, or were snookered by the Chinese, who knew there

was an emergent infection going out of control but managed to fool outsiders by starting a war with Taiwan. The message here is that bureaucrats cannot be trusted—their allegiance to higher-ups, their adherence
to norms, and their lack of independent judgment make them unreliable.
They also simply cannot know everything that they need to know in order
to maintain citizen safety from the zombie horde.

The Passage Trilogy

In Justin Cronin's *The Passage*, as in *Dead of Night*, the initial expendable lives are incarcerated inmates awaiting execution.[15] In zombie fiction,
considerable effort is expended to contain the experiments to the chosen
individuals, those destined for execution, but the effort is never fully successful. It is here, in part, that the story criticizes bureaucratic control—no
one, it seems, is able to adequately protect against the escape of zombies
or, in the case of *The Passage*, zombie vampires.

   The Passage begins a story of apocalypse that tracks between the situation that initiates the outbreak—a USAMRIID (United States Army
Medical Research Institute on Infectious Disease) project to create
human bioweapons—and the postapocalyptic society almost a hundred
years in the future, where isolated human communities across the United
States are organized in response to the ever-present threat of viral hordes
intent on killing all living mammals. The human bioweapons, called
virals, were created by a doctor who went to the Amazon to find a virus
that was thought to extend life. Most of the research team was killed in
South America by vampire bats, but those who survived showed rejuve-
nation of the thymus gland in addition to less desirable qualities.[16] The
initial involvement of USAMRIID in the research project is unclear, but
by the time the researchers are in South America, the army is running the
show. After the survivors are evacuated, research continues at a secret
facility in Telluride, Colorado, and death-row inmates are recruited as
experimental subjects. The original doctor, Jonas Lear, is working on the
virus ("refining" it) to see if it can be injected without turning people
into vampires. When the officials in charge are about ready to move the
thirteen virals to another facility to begin training them as humanoid
bioweapons, the virals themselves break out by telepathically influencing
their keepers to free them. They escape and infect the entire continent.

At the same time a six-year-old girl who has been injected with the attenuated virus also escapes. She retains her form as a human and can communicate with the virals, but is not fully one of them, although she does age very slowly.

We have, then, the familiar cast of characters—a curious and emotionally lost doctor who is manipulated by the military, ethically compromised military officials, rapacious mercenaries who don't care how many people die to protect the project, and an innocent but powerful girl who is going to save humankind.[17] With respect to the girl, Lear, the doctor, says, "Once I *saw*, once I *knew* what they were planning, how it would all end, I wanted there to be at least one," meaning that he wanted to see if his own goal, to use the virus to extend life without making a vampire, could be achieved (228). This desire to live as long as possible, which is clearly considered normative within medicine today, was co-opted by a military that imagined the virals could be bioweapons of an unparalleled capacity. And, of course, the attempts to control and contain them are inadequate—in the zombie apocalypse narrative the force is always unleashed, usually because there is a moment of human error, an inability to maintain the necessary control at all times. In *The Passage*, the forces nominally in control experienced the dreams that were the effects of the virals' telepathy, but tried to ignore them. It didn't end well.

The figure of the doctor who is so overcome by his own grief that he is easily manipulated by the military is reminiscent of Dr. Volker in *Dead of Night*. The message here is that medicine is easily corruptible—even the benevolent dreams of medicine can be manipulated to evil ends. The military, of course, is always already corrupted, filled with people of questionable ethics whose job it is to make people disappear, no matter what the cost, or who are simply willing to bend all rules in order to get the job done. All of the functionaries in *The Passage* are compromised individuals, and the crisis of the virals' escape offers them the opportunity to be heroes, to sacrifice themselves or be sacrificed, or to take advantage. Cronin offers us examples of all three types, taking the story into *The Twelve*, in which the action is all in the postapocalyptic future and the showdown with the virals figures as the climax of the novel.[18]

The third book, *The City of Mirrors*, reaches back like *The Passage* into the pre-apocalypse to offer a closer portrait of the original viral, Zero, painting him more as a classic vampire individually bent on killing his rivals. It also chronicles the discovery of Amy, 1,000 years in the future, as the sole humanoid survivor of the North American continent. Zero is Tim Fanning, a researcher infected on the original trip to Bolivia, but he is also, like eleven of the other original virals, a murderer, although no one but himself knows it. (The one original viral who was on death row but wrongly convicted, Anthony Carter, becomes a hero in *The City of Mirrors* as he helps Amy fight back against Fanning's viral minions.) Fanning's backstory is a focus of *The City of Mirrors*, and its telling, as well as other elements of the story's wrap-up, makes it a moral tale. The evil characters get what they deserve, even if many innocents have to die in the meantime. And Fanning's evil nature—developed initially through his unrequited love for his best friend's wife, and then honed by a century of waiting and planning the demise of the humans who believe, after the massacre of the Twelve at the Homeland, that the virals have been vanquished—makes his vampirism an outgrowth of his evil nature, rather than just the effect of being bitten by the bats in South America. He is a postmodern Dracula, a figure who reigns over a dead city, waiting for his victims to enter at their peril. He also makes a critical, fatal, mistake, allowing himself to be strangled by Amy while on a wildly undulating crane above a city breaking apart.

Because Cronin's virals are zombie-like vampires, their activity is somewhat different from the completely mindless hordes of *World War Z* or *Dead of Night*. They are able to be controlled by more human-like vampires, such as the Director and Lila, who use their power to capture others to serve as laborers in the Homeland (set in Iowa City, where the author and I went to graduate school). They are also controlled, in *The City of Mirrors*, by their progenitors, the original virals that escaped from the USAMRIID facility in Telluride. The virals can be on their own, although they are more likely to appear in pods of several. Nevertheless, the virals mostly act through bloodlust, and there are so many of them and they are so consistently dangerous that they represent a horde, especially when massed. In *The Twelve* they are "clustering," in part because there are so few humans left. And Cronin's virals are like other fast twenty-first-century zombies, not the ponderous slow-moving hordes of the earlier twentieth century. James Thompson, in a chapter of a book titled . . . *But If a Zombie Apocalypse* Did *Occur,* suggests that these "fast-moving and feral" zombies are "usually the victims of science gone astray, and not necessarily a risen corpse, but rather a transformed human monster."[19] Bingo.

Cronin's trilogy treads much of the same territory as classic pandemic apocalypse novels, where the purpose is to show how new societies form in the wake of widespread social collapse. His story about the ongoing confrontation with a zombie apocalypse reaches a climax a century after the initial release of the horde. What is striking about the postapocalyptic society is that there appears to be no attempt to manipulate the virals' blood, to continue the "refinement" that has led to the girl's (Amy's) existence as a nonviral who nevertheless is of their kind. This sort of lack of technical sophistication is typical of many dystopian apocalypses, such as *Station Eleven*, *The Stand*, and even *Oryx and Crake*, where the apocalypse has not only stopped technological progress but actually forced the human population into a situation of far more primitive technical capacity.[20] Usually the enforced primitiveness is a result of a loss of electricity and other forms of energy, as well as the death of most of the professional and educated classes, but it is also a way of criticizing that very technical prowess. Technical sophistication is partly what gets us into the mess, and the punishment of the apocalypse is to put humans back into a time when we are unable to use these same methods to threaten our existence. Of course, the postapocalyptic societies have other threatening activities, as many more basic forms of violence and aggression endanger the lives of those who survive. Significantly, the primary threat to human existence in *The Passage* and *The Twelve* is the rise of leaders willing to sacrifice the lives of some humans in order to save the group (this is the story of the Homestead in *The Passage*) or to sustain an authoritarian society and therefore save the elite (this is the story of the Homeland in *The Twelve*).

Notably, in none of Cronin's stories is a general argument made for sacrificing the few to save the many, except in the instances just noted where the sacrifice is *required* by those who demand human blood in return for keeping some people alive, or in the context of the hero-like sacrifice of an individual who volunteers to fight against impossible odds. The sacrifice is not made so that civilization as we know it can be saved, but (in the negative sense) so that the evil forces can retain their power or (in the positive heroic sense) in a desperate kamikaze move to take the other out. It is not sacrifice for the human race but execution demanded by the virals or their familiars, or it is self-sacrifice. That the self-sacrifice is meant to save humankind, or at least the known survivors, does not make it like the mandatory sacrifice of *others* that characterizes the management of zombie hordes. In this sense Cronin's trilogy is more like vampire than zombie fiction, as it retains enough of the individual's ethical sensibility and turmoil to refrain from violence, especially characters like Alicia who have been bitten but also saved by injection with remaining virus (i.e., partially vaccinated), or Anthony Carter, the last of the original virals, who struggles throughout the story to understand why his former employer used him to kill herself. The trilogy is also, in a very significant sense, about blood, which makes it more like *Dracula* than *Dead of Night*. It matches the zombie narrative most closely in the initial events that set the apocalypse in motion and in its implicit criticism of the medical experimentation that leads to it.

Cronin's trilogy never attempts a medical solution to the problem of virals, which distinguishes it from the movies I'll discuss next. It gets close when Amy tries to save Peter, who has been bitten by Fanning and has "turned," by mixing their blood (thus mimicking the transfusions in *Dracula* meant to save Lucy). It appears that this action does keep him alive, although not as long as Amy, and it does not prevent him from being a viral. But this is a low-tech solution. Also, in *The Passage*, Peter uses one vial of the attenuated virus that was injected into Amy to save Alicia from becoming fully viral. It works, but then Amy destroys the rest of the vials to prevent any of the others from becoming like her. Symbolically, this means that the solution to the problem of the virals is not medicine or technology, but good conquering evil in the form of a knock-down, drag-out fight that is the staple of modern morality tales. None of the volumes in the trilogy disappoints on this count.

In *The City of Mirrors* we find out that the virus that escapes the USAMRIID research facility in Telluride mutates later, after a worldwide quarantine of North America. It mixes with an avian virus and becomes both airborne and lethal, killing those it infects within thirty-six hours, before they can "turn" and become virals. One of the characters comments that the quarantine of North America is precisely what saves the human race, as there are no other human survivors in the world. Within the quarantine, what saves the human race is good old American ingenuity, technical smarts, lots of luck, grit, good leadership, and knowing when it is time to take a stand. Not everyone survives, not by a long shot, but enough do, eventually seeding a new human civilization halfway around the world.

Earlier in the novel we found out that those communities where individual integrity and self-confidence did not survive are doomed: their inhabitants cannot rule themselves effectively, epidemic illness takes hold, and no one knows how to make a community run. That is, in places where not enough people with grit, ingenuity, and good leadership survive, everyone is vulnerable to the predations of the virals. The eventual survivors from North America all come from the well-functioning community of Kerrville, Texas, from whence they escape to a refurbished boat on the Gulf of Mexico and sail east past the Horn of Africa to an uninhabited tropical island. The successful response to the vampire apocalypse is to get the hell out of Dodge.

Filming the Zombie Apocalypse

To a certain extent, the melding of zombies with vampires, the creation of what amounts to a vampire horde, allows for a more complex plot, as the vampire horde involves more intentionality and thus necessitates more cunning on the part of the humans fighting it. This is clearly the case of the movie version of *I Am Legend*, a zombie apocalypse film that has almost nothing in common with its vampire novel origin. In the original 1954 story, it is a bacterial pandemic that creates vampires who gather nightly outside of Robert Neville's home and chant his name, egging him to come out to be bitten.[21] In the movie, the mutants are vampire-like creatures who resemble zombies in their horde-like fixation on biting, the result of an engineered measles virus used to create a cancer vaccine. It represents a clear case of humans inadvertently creating the circumstances for their own demise.

The film *I Am Legend* is notable because for most of the movie there appears to be only one human survivor, Lieutenant Colonel Dr. Robert Neville, and his dog, Samantha. Neville's implicit sacrifice—when he enables the escape of the two other humans, a mother and son, who will take the vaccine to a mythical colony of the immune in Vermont—is a personal sacrifice meant to save humankind. But Neville does not stay as bait, drawing the mutants toward him so that the other two can escape.

He closes the door of the chute and then pulls out a grenade that will blow up his lab and the mutants in it. He becomes a legend with his sacrifice—this is what he is "supposed to do," as he puts it. The fact that he has discovered a cure for KV (which stands for the Krippen virus, named for the doctor who genetically engineered the measles virus as a putative cure for cancer) is what makes him a legend and allows his sacrifice to have meaning. In the end, he makes things right, which has been his tragic goal throughout the whole film, implicitly to make up for the death of his wife and daughter as they try to leave New York City on one of the last military transports out before the city is officially quarantined. His sacrifice is the usual one for a hero of this sort, not the staged and involuntary sacrifice of those who are willingly killed by others in order to save civilization for the rest of us.

The movie version of *World War Z*, like *I Am Legend*, diverges significantly from its novelistic origin.[22] Instead of focusing on the strategic maneuvers to beat the zombies at their own game, the movie version creates a biotechnical solution. Because the zombies do not recognize the existence of the sick, the protagonist, played by Brad Pitt, is able to save himself from zombies in a WHO medical facility by infecting himself with a known virus. This potentially self-sacrificing action leads to the invention and dissemination of a vaccine that mimics the signs of illness and saves humankind from the zombie hordes. Interestingly, the movie shows that Israel's early voluntary quarantine does not hold (going directly against the book's narrative), suggesting that medicine, not governments or military action, can be the savior of humankind. In this way the movie's message about zombies is exactly the opposite of the book's, although it aligns with *I Am Legend* in proposing a medicalized solution.

I Am Legend brings us back to where I started the chapter—with vaccines and the fear of becoming a zombie. I don't really think people have that explicit fear, but there is certainly a festering uncertainty about the engineering of viruses that the film expresses and also shapes. Many vaccines today are created through engineering of the germs that cause disease. Such manipulation is supposed to make vaccines safer, as they use only enough of the microbe to create an immune response to the appropriate antigens. As a result, the vaccines cannot cause true infection, and they include fewer antigens than older vaccines. But the concern represented in *I Am Legend* suggests that there is some discomfort about all this monkeying around with dangerous microbes. In these fictional dystopias, there are always unforeseen consequences. We are always playing with fire.

It is tempting to try to wrap up this chapter in a neat argument about how fiction and film express anxieties about contemporary medical technology and the military-medical complex that, behind the scenes, creates humanoid bioweapons without being able to control them. As I have shown, this is a strong theme in the genre, set alongside the repeated idea that bureaucratic organizations and government officials are inadequate to their securitizing responsibilities. But zombie novels and films, and their vampire horde cousins, articulate a deeper set of concerns about the implicit trade-offs that we seem to have already accepted with respect to individual and population health. Do we really, they ask, believe that it is moral to sacrifice some citizens in order to save the country—or civilization—itself? Is injury to some acceptable in the overall scheme of things? These are questions that are raised by the zombie horde, and echoed in contemporary vaccination controversy, where many vaccine skeptics use injury narratives to raise questions about vaccine safety. Whether or not the specific injuries claimed are real is immaterial to the argument, because everyone who is party to the controversy acknowledges that no vaccine is 100 percent safe for every person all of the time. Some people are injured by vaccines every year, and very little is known ahead of time about who those individuals will be (beyond the ordinary contraindications of allergy to vaccine ingredients or previous adverse reaction to the vaccine). Stories about the zombie horde emphasize this central question about the value of the individual in relation to the group and the ethics of population health. They represent our collective worry about who will save us when the next mistake happens, and whether we will be able to recognize the mistake before it overcomes us all.

Mass immunization is one way to imagine the creation of a zombie horde. Another is using vaccines for something honorable and monumental— curing cancer!—as in the movie *I Am Legend*. In pandemic apocalypse stories, such as the movie *Contagion*, the vaccine is what saves civilization.[23] Yet the notion that populations can be sacrificed for the health of others also circulates in these stories, notably in a Korean movie simply called *Flu*.[24] In *Contagion*, state governments set up hard borders to keep the virus from spreading across state lines, and in the movie *Outbreak*, the military is ready to bomb a town where the infected are sent. In *Oryx and Crake*, the first novel in Margaret Atwood's *Madaddam* trilogy, evil genius Crake seeds the entire world with a pandemic virus in order to wipe the slate clean for the genetically superior humanoids that he creates—this is the ultimate sacrifice of some humans for the sake of the survival of others. While it is true that the "Crakers" survive and begin to procreate, some humans also survive, and it is uncertain whether demolishing the old, corrupt society has cleared the way for a different kind of civilization to be born. (The problem in both *The Stand* and *Oryx and Crake* is that enough of the old society survives to recreate violence and the forms of inequality that led to the corruption in the first place.) In *Oryx and Crake*, vaccination saves the protagonist Jimmy, as Crake wants him to survive to protect his invented humanoids. But the overall destruction and his own personal desolation leave Jimmy in no position to do much besides save himself, and even there he is not altogether successful.

Modern writers have worried about scientific developments and playing God since Nathaniel Hawthorne wrote about the unfortunate consequences of altering nature in the story "The Birth Mark." *Frankenstein* by Mary Shelley is an obvious example as well. Altering nature is dangerous. One incurs the wrath of God, or of Nature, in tinkering with what is given. Our uneasiness about medicine reflects a long-standing concern about how manipulating nature changes our relationship to God and to the natural world. Zombies and vampires are one way to figure that concern, as they are humanoid creatures who seek to kill us. Vampires, especially, represent the human cost of our desire for longer life or escape from death. It only makes sense, then, that one of the most heralded medical triumphs of the twentieth century, vaccination, would share the viral imagination with zombies and vampires. Cheat death, and this is what you get.

But more significantly these fictions warn us that we cannot trust those who mean well and hope to secure our health and safety. Accidents happen, and dangers lurk. The question is what and whom we trust to create and sustain our health. How can we secure our own futures, ensuring that we are not the ones who are sacrificed when the procedures break down, the germ escapes the lab, or the wrong people gain control of the bioweapons? Given that good people can be manipulated for bad ends, how do we know that the professionals we trust with our lives are telling us the truth? That is a strong message across zombie and pandemic apocalyptic fictions, and it reflects the fractured contexts of contemporary modernity, in which we seek the truth ourselves, wary of relying on governments and groups that have failed us again and again. Recognizing that there is a limit to how much we can trust those who are ostensibly responsible for our health, many of us use the reflexive knowledge practices characteristic of modernity, and the new tools available to us (like the Internet), to make decisions on our own. And in the United States, where common cause has been eroded for decades by a sense that individuals matter more than the collective good, the notion that some people should be willing to sacrifice for the benefit of others is not necessarily widespread. One might say that it is an ideal honored more often in the breach.

10

ANTI/VAX

This chapter discusses interviews about vaccination and health beliefs that have been conducted by members of the Vaccination Research Group (VRG) for over six years.[1] The interviews were part of three small studies.[2] The oldest study looked at H1N1 flu vaccine uptake in far southwestern Virginia public school vaccination clinics, while the more recent projects investigate a small community with cyclical pertussis outbreaks as well as more general health beliefs and vaccination practices across a broader region. None of the findings from these studies are generalizable, which means that our interpretations are specific to the participants we interviewed. Yet our work confirms other studies published by social scientists, most notably the anthropologists Melissa Leach and James Fairhead of the United Kingdom in *Vaccine Anxieties*, and we believe that our methods deserve to be used more widely. Simply put, asking people about their vaccination practices in the context of their health beliefs provides a wealth of information about vaccine skepticism that challenges popular opinions about the motivations and ideas behind vaccine refusal.

I didn't start the VRG thinking that we would conduct interview studies—I am not trained in this type of research method. I started the VRG because I wanted to learn more about why people refused vaccination and what the controversy involved. In 2011, however, I was asked to collaborate with faculty in public health to conduct the H1N1 study, which was funded by federal stimulus funds funneled through state public health programs. I pulled in a linguist colleague who routinely goes into people's homes to talk to them about all manner of things, and she wanted to do interviews. Then a few years later a local public health district office asked us to partner with them to improve communication between public health employees and members of a community with multiple pertussis outbreaks. A graduate student in science and technology studies wanted to study vaccination controversy with me and started up the third study. Before I could turn around, it seemed, I was directing three interview studies that try to make sense of people's vaccination practices and beliefs. We are still in the middle of interpreting the results.

The questions we ask in what are called *semistructured interviews* allow participants to tell their own stories. This approach allows us to interview people who might otherwise be unlikely to participate in research studies about vaccine skepticism, and it is crucial to revealing beliefs about vaccination and health that are obscured by the current media obsessions with celebrity vaccine refusers and erroneous information on the Internet. We have found that the people we interview make deliberative, intentional decisions in the context of their lived experience and social networks. They seek information appropriate to their worldviews and experiences with illness and medicine. Indeed, we think that vaccine-skeptical parents make decisions in much the same way that other parents make decisions, and often consider similar issues and experiences.

In our research, a number of factors appear to distinguish vaccine skeptics from wholehearted vaccinators, including alternative views of health and illness, valuing illness as crucial to good health, and accepting the uncertainties of illness over the uncertainties of medication or preventative treatment. We find as well a belief in the body's capacity to be ill and recover, a suspicion of pharmaceutical companies and medicine as a business, and highly personalized ways of understanding and experiencing oneself as a responsible and health-conscious community member. Our participants who don't vaccinate or only partially vaccinate do not like to be "bullied" (their words) by medical providers to comply with standard directives, and they often had negative experiences with physicians or other mainstream health care providers. These factors, as well as the fact that many participants are somewhat isolated geographically, contribute to their beliefs and practices about vaccinations.

But we do not believe that any particular belief or practice will automatically identify a person as a vaccine skeptic or refuser. Indeed, we think that people's health decisions generally, and vaccination decisions in particular, are characterized by complexity—of experience, belief, and practice—which makes identifying a particular thing that can be changed to make vaccine skeptics accept vaccination a nonstarter.

What We Have Learned

What are the assumptions that people bring to vaccination? How does vaccination fit into the rest of people's lives, especially with respect to views of medicine, health, and illness? In what ways do parents and others make sense of vaccination as a practice, and in what ways does it not make sense to certain individuals, given their belief systems and worldviews? How do people make health care decisions generally, and how do their decisions about vaccination fit into this pattern? How do external events and representations (especially media reporting) affect people's decisions about vaccination and their experiences with health care providers?

These are the questions that have guided our studies on health beliefs and vaccination. The interview transcripts are lengthy, nuanced, and fascinating—people discuss birth experiences, family relationships, illnesses and treatments, and employment decisions as all contributing to their ideas about health and their vaccination practices. In this chapter I cannot possibly do justice to the complexity of the data, which, in any case, will be more formally analyzed by the research team for article and thesis publications. Here I present two ways of framing their responses: (1) listing reasons for vaccine skepticism or refusal that we have extracted from the data, and (2) discussing the complexity of their interrelation, in order to show how embedded vaccination decisions are in the fabric of people's lives.

What Bothers People about Vaccines?

The following list offers some reasons that our participants provide to explain why some people are skeptical about or resist vaccinations:

- belief in the value of natural illness
- desire to avoid unnecessary medicine and treatment
- belief in nutrition as the first defense against illness and as essential to basic health, often including specific, and nonmainstream, dietary advice
- enmeshment of ideas about health and the body with spiritual and religious practices
- alternative views about health and medicine, including holistic, herbalist, oriental, integrative, naturopathic, and chiropractic medical systems
- lived experience with illness, especially with illness that is not effectively treated by mainstream medicine
- protection of the body and control over what goes into the body
- experience with perceived vaccine injury
- distrust of mainstream scientific studies of vaccine safety
- distrust of medicine's entanglement with big business (especially "Big Pharma") and government
- rejection of the idea that vaccinations are necessary to health
- perception that too many vaccines are given routinely to children
- perception that vaccine mandates do not distinguish between less severe and more severe illnesses
- rejection of one-size-fits-all prescription of vaccine mandates
- belief that parental responsibility for child health involves deliberative decision-making about vaccination
- concerns about toxins in the environment, food, medicine, and household goods
- experience of being bullied by mainstream health care providers, primarily in birth experiences but also in pediatric care
- responsibility to the community that involves not going out when sick
- global worries about how vaccination may change the world and children's futures
- perception of children as persons with rights over their bodies

In this chapter I do not have the space to discuss at length all of these cumulative concerns. It is clear that participants in our studies echo some of the concerns that I have discussed in previous chapters, such as the distrust of government officials and mainstream medical professionals concerning the safety and efficacy of vaccines, the role of pharmaceutical companies in conducting safety and efficacy research, and the way in which current medical perspectives on individuals and genetics makes one-size-fits-all approaches to preventative health care suspect to some people. Asking our participants how they get their information and whom they trust led to varied responses about social networks, Internet sites, and scientific research. The complexity of our participants' narratives about their ideas about health and their practices in the face of illness is the subject of the next section, but it is an integral element of teasing apart the significance of the list of concerns above—the list comprises discrete items, but the participants did not relate them as bullet points. Instead, they are integrated within holistic approaches to health and well-being.

To flesh out this list of vaccine concerns, I will focus on three topics: nutrition, illness, and responsibility. The first two topics allow me to explore the alternative health beliefs of our study participants, in a way that shows how they approach vaccination from within their own worldviews. The final topic, responsibility, lets me bring the conversation back to a concern of an earlier chapter about the responsibility of parents to vaccinate their children for the good of the community.

Nutrition   Most of our participants mentioned nutrition and diet at one point or another during their interviews, and many of our vaccine-skeptical participants subscribed to very specific, and culturally anomalous, diets, at least in comparison to the mainstream American diet or even the typical medically advised diet (low fat and high fiber). In response to the question "What does being healthy mean to you?" one study participant discussed her family's dietary practices in detail:

> Okay. Um, for us, being healthy is all about diet and lifestyle. So we've chosen to, um . . . well, a lot of the reason we've been farmers has been to raise healthy food for our family and our community and we're passionate about keeping our family healthy through the food that they eat and so we're very focused on making sure they always have nutrient dense food, very few empty calories, very little, um, well, very little if none processed food, very little sugar, and certainly no artificial sugars. Not to say that they don't get

to indulge in the wonderful things of life like, you know, sweets that are homemade, or, or, if we feel okay about.[3]

When the interviewer followed up with a specific question asking for clarification of her beliefs around food, this participant responded:

Yeah, we focus primarily on the Weston A. Price, um, diet. So, animal products, animal fats, um, also other good fats like coconut oil and, um, lots of raw milk. We used to raise raw milk. Um. And. Our kids eat tons of veggies, fresh veggies. Um, very little in the way of carbohydrates and grains. I personally have recently needed to go gluten-free for my own autoimmune issue that came out of Lyme disease, but for the most part I don't have to worry about that with the kids. But we still just don't eat a lot of gluten-rich products. Um. And. Um. You know, making sure the kids are, are interested in bitter foods and sour foods. We eat a lot of fermented vegetables. A lot of sauerkraut and things like that and the kids love it. Um, so making sure they have a broad range of what they're willing to accept and enjoy. A lot of bone broth.[4]

Another interviewee responded, in part, "Hygiene and food as medicine and prevention" to the question about what it means to be healthy. When the interviewer followed up for clarification with the question "What do those choices mean for you for healthy food?" she responded:

Meat that I know where it came from, that doesn't contain hormones or antibiotics and hopefully that's grass-fed and raised right around here. Um, or, you know, at least organic if not local. Um, and then vegetables also that are organic. We just, we really try not to have any pesticide residues on our food if we can help it. Except for when we eat out and you don't really, you know, we do choose to eat out sometimes and you don't have a choice in that matter. But, um, but, yeah, we just, and we do choose to drink raw milk because we feel that it's healthier and that it had a lot of, a lot of things in it that are health enhancing. Also raw butter and um, and um, eggs, um, I feel are very very healthy. Very healthy food. We also do take cod liver oil because the vitamins A and D are really important. And in combination with the raw milk, I feel like we're getting a lot of protection from those foods.[5]

Another interviewee responded to a question about what the family does when someone gets sick: "Um, we eat . . . well, you talked about diet,

I didn't really think about this, but we eat foods that are known to be immune boosting. Things like garlic and, um, bone broth and, uh, ginger and lemon juice and . . . you know, I mean, all of the things."[6]

Our more mainstream interviewees also mentioned nutrition. One answered a question about what being healthy means with the following comment: "So I think happiness is the most important, and I think eating a good diet is second. And a good diet to me is a lot of vegetables, a lot of food without added chemicals, unprocessed, um, you know, you, you know how it's produced. It's produced in fertile soil and not in soil that just had a lot of chemicals dumped on it [*sighs*]. Um, same goes for meat."[7] Another participant responded to a question about health responsibility for herself, her family, and for others by referring to nutrition: "I think that, um, my responsibility to be healthy is to do everything I can to ensure that my kids are healthy and also safe [*laughs*] and, um, like I mentioned, I, I've done that through breastfeeding my babies and providing them healthy food."[8] One couple discussed their frustrations with a teenage son who didn't eat as healthfully as they would have liked: "My oldest son eats crap. Um, I mean, just, uh, he just eats the shittiest food, and we're, you know, we're so careful about, like, you know, health, you know, buy organic food and cook, cook dinner every night and all this sort of stuff, and then he gets his, you know, frozen, um . . . Hot Pockets."[9]

Nutrition and eating habits were thus frequently mentioned in respondents' comments about how to be healthy. (No one that we talked to mentioned medications or vaccines as a primary way to be healthy.) In the Pertussis and Health Beliefs Study, participants who espoused alternative health ideas implied that poor eating habits led to susceptibility to illness, and they linked those habits to mainstream medicine. One participant, for example, criticized the practice of giving Jell-O to people recovering from surgery:

> I would not consider 80 percent of the people that walk into a doctor's office and the doctor tells them that they're healthy and fine, I probably would not agree, with them, you know. But, most physicians don't have any problem with the standard American diet either. You know, they don't have a problem with feeding, you know, a person who just got out of surgery, high fructose corn syrup Jell-O. . . . You know, like wait a minute. You've got someone who is trying to *heal* from *surgery*, and you're going to give them a bowl full of sugar? You know, to me, that is completely contraindicating

the health and balance of the body. You know, why aren't you giving them a bone broth soup? Like that gives them everything.[10]

She also mentioned that her children ate corn chips with salsa, but not "Doritos."[11]

Illness as Natural and Beneficial to Health   The World Health Organization's constitution defines health as "a state of complete physical, mental and social well-being and not merely the absence of disease or infirmity."[12] None of the participants in our studies has given us a definition even close to this one. What they articulate is usually closer to what one participant offered: "a body that supports you in the life you want to live." When asked further about sickness in relation to health, she responded:

> I think sickness is a part of life. I, um, think that some sickness can be a good thing. I haven't looked into this extensively but have recently been interested in the idea that experiencing childhood illness can kick the, uh, certain period of development into action when it needs to be. . . .
>
> And, yeah, I don't think there's really anything wrong with sickness. I, it's one of the big reasons that I wanted to be at home. I used to work in a day-care center. And I saw all parents, you know, lying about giving their children medication so that they could go to work. And it, I just, I saw miserable kids who wanted to be with the people that they loved, where they felt safe, when they, you know, maybe weren't so sick as to have a high fever but were sick enough that they needed to just be resting. . . .
>
> And, and be comforted and I think that's part of childhood, I think that's part of life. You know, hopefully when we're adults we've built healthy immune systems, and it doesn't happen to us often. That's been my experience. But, um, but, yeah, I don't think it's something that really can or should be eradicated completely.[13]

Other participants responded similarly: "If I'm sick, I don't go to the doctor. There's not a point in that; I just let my body cook until it's done cooking, and then, you know, I'm okay, but I honestly get sick very, very, very rarely."[14] "You know, it's like muscles. If you don't lose, use them, you lose them. And with some illnesses and childhood illnesses, they actually make your immune system stronger. I have a lot of, uh, stories, uh, with, um, people who survived, you know, in their childhood, you know, some, some kind of more serious and prolonged flus and colds or measles or whatever, and then, you know, they're ninety and they never went to a doctor."[15]

Our vaccine-accepting interviewees are more liable to have negative views of illness than our vaccine-skeptical participants. Among the vaccine skeptics, we had strong indications of positive approaches to illness and its benefits for health. One participant had a lot to say about the relation of illness to health:

> But, illness comes into play, our family gets the flu and it's four days, maybe a lingering cough for, you know, the fifth or sixth day. But then we're fine, and we bounce back and we're healthy and we're strong and we can keep moving with our day. It's not, you know, the flu that everybody got last January, um, our family was one of the only families that bounced back like that. You know, everybody else, I mean people had that cough for *three months*, you know, and to me, that is where, um, someone's picture of health begins to degrade, and that wellness is no longer there. . . . [But] everyone's going to get sick. How you process that illness in your body is I think a big, a big part of it. . . . And so I think that those basic hygiene, basic nutritional stuff, our society's gotten really soft about. And we don't remember that those are key components to how much health and wellness we actually have.[16]

Another nonvaccinating mother put it this way:

> I think if you're healthy, you probably won't get sick as often, but you're able to handle it. And, I think, specifically with children, getting sick is an important part of being a ch—, being a child. It's part of, it's kind of like use it or lose it with your immune system. And I think the, um, how people won't let their kids be ill, um, is, causing a lot of the, the chronic, the chronic illness epidemic that's happening. People's immune system, it's kind of like your muscles, if you don't use them, they're just going to become noodles, and I think your immune system's the same way.[17]

This mother in particular was very concerned about children who are simply given antibiotics when ill:

> But I, you know, I see, the other people, the people who did the antibiotics [during the pertussis outbreak], for their kids they just gave them antibiotics. And they say you're good after that week. And then they just send them

back to school, and they're like coughing all over. They're sick! They're not, they didn't give them any other support, to help them. And the kids like that, might have chronic lung issues, their whole life, probably will. I think there's a good chance they will, because you're not giving them any support. You just give them antibiotics and then they're not even getting their rest or the care or anything, and I thought that was kind of brutal in a way.[18]

Another mother spoke of the experience of fever in a way that demonstrates her positive attitude toward illness: "Well actually, I can give my kid some feverfew tea, and some yarrow tea and 90 percent of the time their fevers go down to a healthy, you know 100 degree fever that then helps their body kick out what's going on."[19]

A few of the vaccinating participants commented on the issue of sending children to school while sick. One put it this way:

> I mean, again we have the luxury now because we have all these over-the-counter medicines that make us feel better in a, in a moment, of, like, continuing to work and just push through and do all those things, and so people just; we just have such a weird view of health right now. It's a strange time regarding that. Um, like, I think that people before, when we felt more vulnerable because there weren't vaccines available and these over-the-counter medications weren't available, and things like that, I *wonder* if people maybe were more, like, cognizant of not going out, and being in public, when they were coughing or hacking all over everyone.[20]

Another ruefully explained sending her kids to school when they were sick and she was working: "So hard when I was working 'cause I would send them to school . . . and then I felt so bad about it because what I would do is, if they were sick they'd stay home because if you stay home your s—, illness will last three days. If you go to school, it's gonna last a week or two, but they were good, they did it, they went not with fevers 'cause you can't send them with a fever, right? But . . . I always felt bad about that."[21]

Responsibility to Community   I have already shown that a number of our participants argue that people should stay at home while ill. The more radical of these arguments suggest that modern society has created a demand for medicines and vaccines so that people can go out in the world when ill, even to the eventual detriment of their health.

The nonvaccinating families created contexts in which the parents could stay at home with their children or spouses when ill, allowing family members to rest and "be supported" through illness. They tended to be very defensive about perceived accusations that they were not responsible community members. For example, one participant said the following, as if responding to a physician who claimed she was being irresponsible:

> Well, when I answered him I was just, like, "Actually, I'm very responsible because I'm proactive in learning about these issues." Um, it, I mean he doesn't know me. . . . But, . . . I didn't give up ten years, eleven years of . . . You know I made a choice to be with my children and I drive a tiny little car [*laughs*] that has about a million miles on it, as does my husband. So don't tell me. You don't know me. . . . And I don't appreciate your judging me and I think what the issue is, is that you don't like the fact that I'm questioning you, and you're not used to that. So actually, I'm very responsible because I can think for myself. Um, and I'm being responsible to my children, because I'm protecting their health from what I understand and believe. . . . And I'm also teaching them to think for themselves.[22]

Previously in the interview she described an interaction with her brother over her responsibility to other children who were immunocompromised as a result of chemotherapy:

> If, if, if a child were undergoing chemotherapy and my child had a, one of these other things they don't vaccinate for that they can catch at school, the child having chemother—, chemotherapy could be compromised. I certainly would not send my children to school sick, and I would like to think that the parents of the children who's undergoing chemotherapy would be mindful of taking precautions to make sure their child was safe. Nobody wants to take responsibility for their own health. . . . So that w—, and then it was interesting, I said to him something to the effect of my children going to school and people sending their kids to school sick all the time, and he says, "Well, parents can't help it. They have to send their kids to school sick because their, um, they can't get off work." . . . My kids last month had, uh, Fifth's disease that was going around their school . . . I talked to the school nurse. She's, like, "It's, it's not bad. It's not . . . they're probably not contagious."[23]

The nonvaccinating participants all responded to questions about responsibility with comments either about their responsibility to their own children's individual bodies and health or about their actions that demonstrated their responsibility to their communities, or both. In the Pertussis and Health Beliefs Study, all community participants were angry that some local health care providers refused to test for pertussis, even after the health department had identified an outbreak in the community. Several participants suggested that this was the most irresponsible behavior, which allowed the outbreak to spread unnecessarily. It is important to point out that even people who practice alternative medicine need the diagnostic tools of mainstream health care for proper diagnosis; often their alternative regimens depend on specific and accurate diagnosis made possible through physician testing. And one nonvaccinating participant in the Health Beliefs and Vaccination Study mentioned that she did vaccinate her children against pertussis when they were interacting with a family with a newborn who was too young to be vaccinated for it, demonstrating considerable flexibility in her own practices in order to protect others in her community.

Complexity and Vaccination Practices

Complex relationships and networks of meaning are pervasive in the way people think about vaccines. It is impossible to read these interview transcripts and say, "These people don't vaccinate because of X." Instead, we have found that people's approaches to vaccination are deeply embedded in personal experiences that are hard to generalize. It's impossible to know why people come to certain kinds of decisions about vaccines unless you *ask them* in a way that is respectful of those decisions and tries to address, rather than bracket off, their complexity.

The focus on nutrition and its importance to health is illustrative. In the United States at this time, it is completely normal to believe that eating well contributes to good health. In 2016 I collected all the articles that the "YouDocs" (Mehmet Oz and Michael Roizen) published as a weekly syndicated column in the *Roanoke Times*. The most common topic that they discussed in their columns was disease, with nutrition and diet second. The YouDocs follow the mostly mainstream low fat/high fiber diet dicta, but they are slightly more radical than the mainstream. For example, they suggest that red meat is not good for you in any amount, rather than advising that it can be eaten in moderation as the USDA suggests.

Some of our study participants have very unorthodox nutrition beliefs, but their investment in the power of food to prevent illness is not unusual. A nutritional approach to health is a functional approach, one that emphasizes personal control and a cause-effect mind-set. When the mother of one of my colleagues had a stroke, the person who informed me mentioned that "she was really healthy, eating right and exercising into her eighties," implying that her good diet and exercise habits should have prevented cardiovascular disease. Because we feel this way—either intuitively or as a result of reading the ubiquitous and ever-changing news reports on health and nutrition—control of diet is seen and experienced as a primary way to ensure good health in families that are focused on health. And, in another register, many of us have fond memories of the kinds of foods that we got to eat when sick—saltines and ginger ale when home with the flu, for example, or chicken soup for a bad cold. Food, health, and illness are intertwined, although dependent on a family's nutritional disposition, belief system, socioeconomic status, and access to grocery stores or other places to purchase desired items.

For some of our study participants, nutrition is a value system and way of life. This is so, in part, because their nutritional beliefs put them at odds with mainstream US culture, so much so that some mention whether or not they violate their own rules when eating out or when their children go to parties or playdates. The isolation that some participants created when their families were ill extended more generally to their nutritional choices. One participant talked about how she and her family were creating thoughtful cold lunches because her children were attending a school—this constituted a change to their regular hot lunches when the children were being homeschooled. Other families came to their nutritional choices because of specific medical problems that they or their children experienced, such as chronic constipation, celiac disease, or Lyme disease. As seen above, one couple lamented their teenage son's food choices, but were unwilling to police his habits, preferring to simply offer healthier choices at dinner and hoping that he would conform to family practices eventually—a disposition that many families can relate to.

The focus on nutrition and many participants' adherence to nonmainstream diets reveal their confidence in the familial management of health. This confidence extends to their approach to illness, which for many of our participants is perceived and experienced as a normal aspect of life and one that contributes to or demonstrates good health. Illness always represents an uncertainty, but our participants by and large felt that illness functioned as a reminder that something might be wrong but also that what was wrong could be ameliorated. Illness was seen as a challenge to one's immune system that would, through supported recovery, make an individual stronger. Medications, in relation to this way of thinking about illness, are equivocal. They mask true illness and the body's needs, are potentially harmful to long-term health, and allow people to participate in social life (work, school) in ways that threaten both the individual's and the community's health. Illness requires adjustment—renewed focus on healthy foods, support for the body's unique needs, and recognition of the body's response (fever, for example).

Participants' approaches to social responsibility also expressed confidence that illness could be contained and managed so that infectious outbreaks would not result from individual experiences. As explored above, our most ardent vaccine-skeptical parents reported that they did not think sending children to school while ill was appropriate, and they reported that they had set up their lives in such a way that managing illness at home was workable. Some of the families living on remote farms were able to completely isolate themselves during the pertussis outbreaks in their community.

Responsibility to one's family and community through vaccination is a prominent element of public health messaging about vaccines. Public health authorities imply or state outright that nonvaccinating parents are irresponsible, especially with respect to others in their communities who cannot vaccinate or are especially susceptible to infectious disease. Pro-vaccine writers, reporters, and scholars repeat these sentiments, contributing to the public perception that vaccine skeptics are selfish and inflaming public debate about voluntary nonvaccination.

Yet our research participants spoke of a different kind of responsibility—to the body, the earth, and the future. Some of our participants feared that manipulation of viruses and bacteria through vaccine development would fuel the creation of superbugs, for example. Other concerns focused on the body's capacity to fight off illnesses on its own, and the overuse of medications generally that vaccines were seen to be a part of. And participants expressed a range of concerns about changes to children's futures through vaccination. One participant was quite eloquent on this

particular point, speaking "of the risk that is there that we have not un-
covered because the research hasn't been done. And so I just, I'm, I'm
really worried that we are changing our children in ways that we can't
even predict. And that we will never know who these little people would
have been if they had not been injected time and time and time again,
with diseases and foreign substances throughout their childhood."[24] Here
uncertainty is not attached to illness but to medications in the form of
childhood vaccines.

The standard public health approach, to counter the uncertainty of
illness with the certainty and control of vaccination, would not persuade
many of our participants. The people we spoke to are likely to rely on
domestic practices as dependable approaches to illness. For them, vaccines
are things that may bring uncertainty to their children's futures, rather
than control and health. Responsibility in this context is different from a
straightforward obligation to keep oneself from becoming ill in order to
protect others. When people feel that they can control their own exposures and potential exposures to others, and when the experience of illness
itself is valued, other kinds of uncertainty are more influential in guiding
behavior.

Acknowledging these complex perspectives on health, illness, social responsibility, and vaccination does not lead to a quick fix to the problem of
voluntary nonvaccination. Where one sees uncertainty and how one en-
acts control or management are effects of one's worldview. Many of the
families that we spoke with reported significant independent research and
deliberation about whether vaccines were right for their children, as they
tested their own sensibilities by consulting external sources and trusted
members of their social networks. Their research did not simply shore
up preexisting views; it helped to shape those views with information, reported experience, and affective identifications. Our participants did not
simply adopt other people's ideas, nor were they swayed by celebrity en-
dorsements. Instead, their approaches to vaccination were part of larger,
complex worldviews in which illness, responsibility, and bodily experience each played a significant and interacting role.

Portraying these participants' worldviews as *wrong* is not an anthro-
pologically sound way to understand why people believe certain things
and not others. More significant for public health, it isn't an effective way

to have a conversation with people whose behavior one needs to guide in the context of an outbreak of infectious disease. The typical public health presentation of vaccine recommendations and mandates provides cost-benefit comparisons and evaluations of the burden of disease on families, communities, and the state. Yet the alternative perspectives that our non-vaccinating study participants revealed to us rely on a different calculus. If disease is functional and produces improved immunity, then the cost of illness cannot be measured only in dollars and cents. If health is a product of support through illness and demonstrated by recovery, the uncertainties of illness are not feared but embraced. If medicines allow one to live in a kind of fake health, then they are to be avoided. And those who promote them cannot be fully trusted.

The most radical of our study participants are making a kind of argument against modernity and its reliance on the circulation of people, goods, and money in modern economies. Clearly, they are reiterating concerns that we saw expressed by the antimedicine advocates, especially Robert Mendelsohn and, to a certain extent, Ivan Illich. Significantly, their interviews demonstrate that the problem of trust—discussed throughout this book—remains at the center of vaccination controversy. For a person who thinks that Jell-O is a ludicrous food choice for someone recovering from surgery, trusting mainstream medical advice about vaccines may be a stretch. That is, for such an individual, criticism of medicine *as a system* makes sense. She sees medicine as being overly reliant on industrial food and medicines, not acknowledging basic truths about nutrition and its fundamental role in health, and too readily treating all patients the same. For a person whose fundamental approach to health is framed by a disposition to criticize medicine in these ways, being skeptical of vaccination makes sense. Such a person cannot trust information about health, safety, and efficacy broadcast by an institution that considers Jell-O a healthful food.[25]

The discussion in this chapter shows that there is no magic bullet of knowledge that can reveal why some people reject vaccination and others (the vast majority of US citizens and residents) embrace it. The studies reported on here show that there is a grave need for more such qualitative research, and on a larger scale. More significantly, we need something of a moratorium on those limited research studies that try to determine how to manage, with the least amount of effort, parents' questions about vaccines, or how to regulate, again with minimal effort, patient populations into compliant behaviors. Instead, we need to pay attention to complexity in the context of rich and exuberant perspectives on health and illness. And we need to consider why vaccination controversy emerges so forcefully now—not simply as an effect of the historical forces discussed in chapter 1, but as an exemplar of the kinds of challenges that modern social systems grapple with: the promise of technologies to manage problems of embodiment, the meaning of illness and bodily vulnerability in modern economies, and the public role of social resisters in a bureaucratic democracy. It is to these topics that I turn in the conclusion to this book.

CONCLUSION

What Vaccination Controversy Can Teach Us about Medicine and Modernity

Modern science aims to understand, and thereby control, nature. Modern medicine, insofar as it depends on, and touts itself as an example of, modern science, shares that dream. At mid-twentieth century, because of the successes of vaccination and antibiotics, control of infectious disease looked possible. But in the last quarter of the twentieth century, nature came roaring back—in the form of antibiotic resistance, multi-drug-resistant tuberculosis, HIV/AIDS, and other dangerous viral diseases like Ebola. Even though smallpox was declared eradicated worldwide in 1980, these emergent and returning illnesses came to demonstrate the limits of medicine and science in ridding the world of infectious disease.

In the twenty-first century, controversies about global warming, genetically modified organisms (GMOs), vaccination, and HIV/AIDS—often characterized as *science denial*—are examples of uncertainties promulgated by science's own successes. They demonstrate, perhaps, the limits of modern dreams about the control of nature. Vaccination skepticism in particular may be a special example demonstrating the limits of modern confidence in interventionist approaches to disease prevention, at least for some people who see in conformity to technocratic regulations a capitulation to a worldview and a theory of bodily health that does not make sense.

In this book, I have tried to show that doubling down on the side of science does not address—or even acknowledge—the beliefs and concerns of those who question the triumphal vaccine narrative.[1] If the goal is to reorient public stalemates about vaccination controversy, then heralding "science as truth" is a failure, especially when mainstream science, or mainstream interpretations of scientific data, are the only accepted positions. What needs to happen is much messier and more unclear. Understanding must take place without the goal of control, given that what motivates vaccine skepticism are some fundamental concerns about modernity and human thriving.

Vaccination controversy offers us a chance to consider three important and philosophically challenging propositions of modern societies—the promise of technologies to manage social problems, the eradication of illness as a sign of social progress, and the capacity of bureaucratic democracies to manage social welfare and human well-being. My framing of these propositions demonstrates my strong sense that we must move the conversation away from an adjudication of the rightness or wrongness of people's viewpoints with respect to scientific data. What we do to our bodies in the service of health is never only an effect of data and scientific considerations. This framing allows us to see that vaccination controversy stages another conversation altogether—a consideration of modernity, its promises, and its assumptions.

Biomedicine and scientific research provide particular ways of framing health, and the government uses scientific and biomedical research data to create a *technocratic frame* in which science is put to bureaucratic uses. Technocratic framing often makes sense to people educated in this worldview, especially those whose professional identities are linked to it, or to people who are convinced that bureaucratic processes and scientific evidence are generally beneficent. But daily life provides a powerful set of experiences that frame alternative worldviews that may or may not align with the technocratic framing of data. In addition, societies develop and sustain diverse symbolizations that contribute to culturally typical frames for health, well-being, and medicine—and these may or may not match how vaccination is framed by health care workers in any given community.

The anthropologists Melissa Leach and James Fairhead, authors of *Vaccine Anxieties*, suggest that the framing of vaccination as a public triumph of technoscientific achievement lends credence to the perception that those who do not believe in vaccination are ignorant or willfully misled by celebrity deceivers. In their view, the framing of the problem in terms that are accepted and valued by biomedical scientists and public health officials creates the notion of the ignorant or gullible parent as the cause of vaccination resistance. Typical frames, then, that blame rumor or ignorance for vaccine refusal reflect technocratic, not parental, perspectives.

The public controversy over vaccination in the United States has created two different narratives about vaccination: (1) that vaccination is safe and effective and poses almost no risk to individuals, and (2) that vaccination is dangerous to some or all citizens and is only marginally—if at all—effective. It is not clear that people who subscribe fully to the second position can be persuaded of the first one, although people who fully believe that all vaccines are dangerous appear to be very rare in the population as a whole.[2] Furthermore, a sense of urgency is created by the public nature of the controversy itself, which inflames mechanisms of blame. Earlier in the book I discussed the increasingly inflammatory news reporting on vaccination controversy. This reporting context distorts our idea of what the problem is.

Faith in technological solutions to social issues obscures historically long-standing resistance to state-mandated vaccination, making it seem like there is a quick-fix solution to force people to accept medicine's truth that vaccines save lives. Historical reframing can remind us that there have always been people who have refused, resisted, or been skeptical about vaccination, and that exemptions have been used as a way to manage dissent politically. The historical literature reveals that there have always been attempts to discredit the beliefs of vaccine skeptics—to suggest that they are against medical progress, that they subscribe to dangerous ideas about health and the body, that they believe in "quacks." Discrediting vaccine skeptics is one mechanism for shoring up support for vaccination as a valid and valuable public health effort in the context of an outbreak of infectious disease, and it was used frequently during smallpox outbreaks when vaccination was a primary method to stop ongoing epidemics. Leach and Fairhead remind us that discrediting vaccine skeptics in this way demonstrates the power of technocratic frames in understanding vaccination controversy—the dominant public framing is that of the government and its allies in public health, which delegitimizes the experience and perspectives of those who disagree with it, in order to further their own agendas. At least, this is what such framing looks like from the perspective of those who don't share it.

When we reframe vaccination controversy as a clash between worldviews, the question "Do children receive too many vaccines?" is not only a question about the capacity of small bodies to tolerate multiple shots and numerous foreign proteins. It is a question about the dream of disease eradication and the future of human life without infectious disease. It is a question about the modern body and our expectations of its performance, and it lodges an implicit criticism about what it means to have a childhood free from illness. Our answers to this question must address these embedded questions, which are not amenable to what goes by the name of scientific reasoning. While many of us may not subscribe to the notion that saving lives with medicine is a dangerous way of "playing God," we may still have lingering doubts about the extent to which we can transform human experience to do away with the burden of infectious disease for everyone. We may still think that days spent at home with a cold or the flu are valuable in the calculus of human immunity, survival, and thriving.

In her evocative essay "On Being Ill," Virginia Woolf points out that being ill reorients one's perspective; while lying prone, one looks up: "Now, lying recumbent, staring straight up, the sky is discovered to be something so different . . . that it is a little shocking. This then has been going on all the time without our knowing it!—this incessant making up of shapes and casting them down, this buffeting of clouds together, and drawing vast trains of ships and wagons from North to South, this incessant ringing up and down of curtains of light and shade, this interminable experiment with gold shafts and blue shadows, with veiling the sun and unveiling it, with making rock ramparts and wafting them away—this endless activity."[3] Being ill also changes one's disposition—for Woolf this meant an appetite for poetry, rather than prose, and for the predictable biographies of ordinary women. One could be sympathetic to these women, while ill, as illness creates a kind of sensitivity to others that, ordinarily, people lack. Being ill, for Virginia Woolf, was a generative state, even though it brought one uncomfortably close to one's mortality. That, of course, was part of the point.

"On Being Ill" was published originally in 1930, by one of the foremost modernist authors of the twentieth century, someone who explicitly addressed the changes of sensibility and disposition that modern perspectives created. A chronicler of modernity's effects on women and the novel, Woolf wrote in *A Room of One's Own* about how modern writers could no longer rely on the cadences and words of their Victorian forebears: "When the guns fired in August 1914, did the faces of men and women show so plain in each other's eyes that romance was killed? . . . The illusion which inspired Tennyson and Christina Rossetti to sing so passionately about the coming of their loves is far rarer now than then."[4] Indeed, "the living poets express a feeling that is actually being made and torn out of us at the moment. One does not recognize it in the first place; often for some reason one fears it; one watches it with keenness and compares it jealously and suspiciously with the old feeling that one knew" (14). Thus it is not without significance that she wrote similarly about the meaning of being ill in modern times—it makes one long after that "old feeling" through reading poetry, it makes one sympathize with others in the old way. Illness itself is nonmodern, or so, at least, modernity would have us think.

And yet chronic illness and disability are, arguably, more prevalent now than previously. Perhaps they come to the fore of experience as infectious disease is more handily prevented and treated, and as people live longer. Affluence is clearly a cause of some chronic illness—diabetes is a prime example, and cancer may be another. We now manage disability and chronic illness with laws, regulations, and technologies, and those who are physically disabled are not locked away or hidden, even as they struggle in a society created and sustained for the able-bodied.

Moreover, the widespread use of medication for disease prevention turns all of us into the pre-ill, medicalizing our existence in an attempt to forestall illness. Does that make us healthy or sick? When we prescribe "by numbers," are we maintaining our health or succumbing to disease? While seeking after cures is an age-old practice, there is something particularly modern in our pill-oriented lifestyle, when catching up with old friends means learning about their children's multiple diagnoses and medication regimens.[5] These medications keep us vital and strong, able to circulate publicly without embarrassing skin lesions or crippling anxiety, or they give us the few more months with our families that we crave. At least, that's what we are led to believe.

The counterargument that we saw in the antimedicine critiques is that there is no way to know who really benefits from all of this preventative treatment—the sense that prevention is good is so ingrained in us that we don't pay attention to how the numbers don't always add up. But the deeper questions have to do with how our relationships with medicines and preventative regimens are markers of our modernness—they define a particular relation to disease that is characteristic of our era. That is why so many vaccine promoters criticize vaccine skeptics for wanting to "go back in time" to periods when thousands of children were sickened by infectious disease, and many died. Vaccination is itself a product of modernity—the emblematic medical practice of the germ theory of disease, it represents modernity's promise of personal and population health with the tools of science. Vaccination is one medical practice among many that knits us into a particular relation to modern medicine and its requirements, and that's one reason why Robert Mendelsohn was so against it, because it trained children to be reliant on their doctors and to experience themselves as medicalized subjects.

Virginia Woolf, whose own physical and mental vulnerabilities were significant, reminds us that illness is a human experience with meaning, a sentiment that is repeated in the interviews with vaccine skeptics that my research team has collected. Her political writing, especially *Three Guineas*, stakes a claim for the role of an "outsider society" that resists norms and mainstream positions, especially those that are supported by tradition and institutions.[6] Vaccination controversy, including the decisions of radical vaccine refusers, raises questions about the public role of resisters in a bureaucratic democracy, allowing another interesting link to this icon of modern literature. Those who fashion themselves as vaccine safety advocates argue that they are acting as whistle-blowers, revealing significant deficiencies in the licensing, recommending, and mandating of vaccines by federal and state bodies. Most of the vaccine skeptics that my research team has interviewed simply opt out of the system, either formally or informally, using their actions to articulate disagreement with immunization laws.

How are public health decisions made in a bureaucratic democracy? The distrust apparent in our interview data as well as published work on vaccination demonstrates that the existing system does not engender trust in some people. As I have argued above, promoting science and its data in favor of vaccination does not create trusting vaccinators out of skeptics, at least not the ones that we have spoken to, even though most of the people we have interviewed are not full-on vaccine refusers. The distance of most ordinary people from the agencies and committees that deliberate about vaccine licensure and approve vaccination recommendations is one way to characterize the problem. While the lengthy research protocols and licensing approval process are meant to ensure trust in the system, the obscured bureaucratic processes seem to make many people less trusting, especially when exposés show that many of those involved in decision-making are also insiders, either vaccine inventors or industry experts.

In other words, the way that large modern democracies work—through legislative and bureaucratic mechanisms, both of which are often seen to be influenced improperly—is an obstacle to creating more trust in vaccines and vaccination recommendations. In the United States, at this writing, there is not a lot of trust in government. It is not only political partisanship that is the problem, although partisanship contributes significantly to this lack of trust. It is that ordinary people do not see how their experiences and their views are represented in government decision-making, which is perceived to be dominated by elites. And this problem raises the question of how decisions about issues of public health, which are dependent on scientific evidence, are to be made in ways that the public accedes to. It is one thing to mandate clean water for all residents of a city and to clean up reservoirs and create sewers; it is quite another to demand that all citizens be given shots to keep them well. To what extent are citizens able to make a case for their points of view when their bodies are on the line?

These questions go to the heart of modern forms of government and their promises to promote the welfare of their populations. Michel Foucault's later career was dedicated to understanding the origins of these problems in the eighteenth and nineteenth centuries. Current public contestations over vaccination represent one way that these questions and the problems they point to are made manifest. They reveal the nodes that draw together democracies and modernity in dreams of self-government, independence, and triumph over nature. They demonstrate that techno-scientific modernity and democratic decision-making do not necessarily go together, especially when people feel that technoscience is aligned with big business and profit making and not dedicated to the real well-being of ordinary citizens.

Stories of viral pandemics and the zombie apocalypse alert us to concerns that go beyond predictable worries about meddling with dangerous microbes. They expose more basic anxieties about whom we can trust when the chips are down. Bureaucrats do not come off well in these depictions of the end of the world as we know it. Instead, the heroic actions of the few who are willing to buck the system usually save the day. Going rogue is a valued tradition in American culture. It is not unusual that some individuals choose to do so by avoiding or actively resisting state compulsion to vaccinate.

At this point, I feel compelled to take a stand about science, a stand that I have resisted throughout the entire text. At various points in this book, I have wriggled out of this felt requirement by arguing that our relation to science is affective, mired in circumstance, and influenced by mechanisms of trust that are not fully rational. I have discussed at length how scientific facts continue to carry with them problems of interest. I have demonstrated how to think about scientific facts as both cultural constructions and renditions of an objectively real world. I have suggested, throughout, that people believe different things, even when faced with similar facts. Indeed, I have argued that the abstraction and expertise that are the hallmarks of modern systems of bureaucratic science and governance can be alienating and provoke resistance among the very individuals that they are meant to persuade.

Writing this book has demanded of me a radical alienation from claims about scientific reasoning and scientific truth. Just as my research group has developed a neutral stance toward vaccination in order to solicit research participants and more effectively understand the concerns of vaccine resisters, I have had to bracket my own commitments to medical science and vaccination to draw out the arguments that make up this book's primary contributions to public debate. As I noted in the introduction, researching vaccination has made me more of a skeptic than I used to be. And yet I still get my tetanus shot every decade.

So why do I feel as if I need to take a stand about science, for science? I worry that my comments here will be taken to mean that I don't respect science, that I don't believe in science, when all around me the negative consequences of the social repudiation of scientific evidence (global warming, polluted air and water, environmental contamination) pile up. In the polarized political context in which we find ourselves in 2018, will the kind of stance I have taken in this book become evidence for being on the wrong side of history?

And yet, I believe wholeheartedly, now more than ever, that the problem of vaccination skepticism is not a scientific problem so much as it is a social one. Medical controversies in the public sphere are inevitably social controversies, and as such they demand social solutions. My almost three decades of research on these issues have convinced me that public debates about them are always also conversations about *something else*—questions about what it means to be a person, to be a member of a community, to be a human being living in consonance with other kinds of beings and bodies. To get at the *something else*, we have to be willing to bracket science and its contribution to understanding the problem. This is not to say that scientific perspectives are unimportant. But we must recognize that when we allow science and its conclusions to dominate our responses to medical controversies in the public sphere, we limit our understanding of what motivates those controversies and how we might solve them.

The answer is science *and something else*. The answer is not communicating science better, as if the problem is a lack of clarity or the complexity of scientific practice or results. Sometimes that is part of the problem, but in the tangle of issues that I have discussed in *Anti/Vax*, identifying better science communication as a primary solution only promotes the popular, and damaging, idea that vaccine skeptics are scientifically illiterate, confirming the deficit model of the public understanding of science. The *something else* has to do with understanding in a deep way the cultural mechanisms and beliefs that support our lives and make them meaningful. The *something else* is how vaccination controversies point toward fundamental questions about human flourishing and the meaning of illness in healthy lives.

Science is not sufficient to address vaccination controversy and the problems that it can present to public health efforts to prevent and contain infectious disease. In an earlier version of this conclusion, my parting line was "The social response to vaccine skepticism is not science, it's democracy." While I still believe that we must attend to the challenges of modern bureaucratic democracies in understanding and addressing public contestation of vaccines and vaccination mandates, I now think that a better way to frame the problem is through the forms of knowledge that we use to understand it. Epistemologically, science does not offer us a lot of help in identifying and explaining the various threads that are woven through vaccination controversy. My analysis has shown that existing scientific approaches are limited. Scientific efforts are too disembedding—they require that we bracket idiosyncratic influences, those things that make us singular and distinct. They demand generalizability and quantification. Instead, close reading and cultural interpretation demonstrate how a number of social trends coalesce to enable a robust skepticism of vaccines in contemporary culture. Attention to rhetoric, argument, and language use illuminates patterns and meanings that are otherwise obscure to most of us. Telling and interpreting stories reveal concerns that we did not know we had.

In other words, the humanities and their characteristic hermeneutic approach offer insights unavailable to scientific reasoning. In medical education, narrative medicine and the health humanities have responded to a felt need for more human-centered approaches to healing after the technological advancements of the last half century. Illness memoirs dominate best-seller lists, demonstrating significant public interest in the experience and ontological significance of being ill. But in public debates about vaccination, climate change, and genetically modified organisms, simplistic renditions of science and its truths dominate the discourse.

The humanities—emphasizing multiple interpretations, linguistic complexity, and subjectivity—can help us rethink the way we use evidence and how we might talk to one another as fellow citizens committed to culturally relevant solutions. Invested in both pluralism and painstakingly acquired evidence, humanistic modes of inquiry and analysis model a conversational and democratic epistemology. They represent the *something else* that must be engaged if we are to productively reframe vaccination controversy today.

NOTES

Introduction

1. Lloyd Bitzer, "The Rhetorical Situation," *Philosophy & Rhetoric* 1, no. 1 (January 1968): 1–14.

2. Nadja Durbach, *Bodily Matters: The Anti-vaccination Movement in England, 1853–1907* (Durham, NC: Duke University Press, 2005), 4.

3. Measles has not been eradicated. The most infectious disease known to humankind, it has been eliminated in the United States, which means that there are no known endemic infections in the United States. All new outbreaks in the United States are traced to foreign sources.

4. Vaccination Education Center, Children's Hospital of Philadelphia, "A Look at Each Vaccine: Rotavirus Vaccine," CHOP.edu, accessed October 1, 2017, http://www.chop.edu/centers-programs/vaccine-education-center/vaccine-details/rotavirus-vaccine.

5. I don't spend much time on two signature topics in current reporting on vaccination controversy: Jenny McCarthy and the MMR-autism connection. Each has become a proverbial whipping boy of the vaccination debate, and since the purpose of this book is to understand "why this controversy and why now?" neither Jenny McCarthy nor the MMR-autism connection will be targeted as examples of what is wrong with the thinking of "those people" or as emblems of the controversy overall. In many studies, the prominence of McCarthy and the MMR-autism connection in vaccination controversy demonstrates how certain popular ways to understand the debate obscure the complexity of what is really happening in the

heterogeneous contexts of people's lives and individual decision-making. As a result, I don't preoccupy myself with these ways of conceptualizing vaccine skepticism.

1. So What Bothers You about Vaccines?

1. Andrew Wakefield et al., "Retracted: Ileal-Lymphoid-Nodular Hyperplasia, Non-Specific Colitis, and Pervasive Developmental Disorder in Children," *Lancet* 351, no. 9103 (February 1998): 637–41, https://doi.org/10.1016/S0140-6736(97)11096-0. This article was coauthored but is generally referred to as the "Wakefield article," and I follow that practice in this book. It was formally retracted by *The Lancet* in 2010.

2. Vaccinology is the science of vaccine development and testing.

3. James Colgrove, "Immunity for the People: The Challenge of Achieving High Vaccine Coverage in American History," *Public Health Reports* 122, no. 2 (March–April 2007): 248–57, https://doi.org/10.1177/003335490712200215. See also Colgrove, *State of Immunity: The Politics of Vaccination in Twentieth-Century America* (Berkeley: University of California Press, 2006).

4. David M. Oshinsky, *Polio: An American Story* (Oxford: Oxford University Press, 2006).

5. Elena Conis, *Vaccine Nation: America's Changing Relationship with Immunization* (Chicago: University of Chicago Press, 2014).

6. Lea Thompson, prod., *DPT: Vaccine Roulette* (Washington, DC: WRC-TV, 1982).

7. Seth Mnookin, *The Panic Virus: A True Story of Medicine, Science, and Fear* (New York: Simon & Schuster, 2011); Paul A. Offit, *Deadly Choices: How the Anti-vaccine Movement Threatens Us* (New York: Basic Books, 2012). Both Seth Mnookin and Paul Offit see *DPT: Vaccine Roulette* as a harbinger of irresponsible news reporting on vaccination that continues to the present day.

8. Holly A. Hill et al., "Vaccination Coverage among Children Aged 19–35 Months—United States, 2015," *Morbidity and Mortality Weekly Report* 65, no. 39 (October 7, 2016): 1065–71.

9. DTP was an acronym for the diphtheria, tetanus, and pertussis combination vaccine. Later it became known as DPT. Most recently, formulations were designated DTaP and Tdap to designate the acellular pertussis component. DTaP is the children's vaccine, and Tdap is the adult version.

10. Mark A. Largent, *Vaccine: The Debate in Modern America* (Baltimore: Johns Hopkins University Press, 2012).

11. Conis, *Vaccine Nation*, 162; Largent, *Vaccine*.

12. Kennedy, Robert F. Jr., "Deadly Immunity," *Rolling Stone*, July 14, 2005, 57–66.

13. Wakefield et al., "Retracted: Ileal-Lymphoid-Nodular Hyperplasia."

14. See Largent, *Vaccine*; Melissa Leach and James Fairhead, *Vaccine Anxieties: Global Science, Child Health, and Society* (Sterling, VA: Earthscan, 2007).

15. Edward Hooper, *The River* (New York: Little Brown, 1999).

16. Meredith Wadman's *The Vaccine Race: Science, Politics, and the Human Costs of Defeating Disease* (New York: Viking, 2017) includes an extended discussion of this controversy and the attendant scientific consequences of vaccines grown using animal or human tissue.

17. John Iliffe, *The African AIDS Epidemic: A History* (Athens: Ohio University Press, 2006); Bernice L. Hausman, *Viral Mothers* (Ann Arbor: University of Michigan Press, 2010), 227n34.

18. Patrick Tierney, *Darkness in El Dorado: How Scientists and Journalists Devastated the Amazon* (New York: Norton, 2002); Tierney, "The Fierce Anthropologist," *New Yorker*, October 9, 2000, https://www.newyorker.com/magazine/2000/10/09/the-fierce-anthropologist-2.

19. Alice Dreger, *Galileo's Middle Finger: Heretics, Activists, and One Scholar's Research* (London: Penguin, 2015); Conis, *Vaccine Nation.*

20. Bernice Hausman et al., "'Poisonous, Filthy, Loathsome, Dangerous Stuff': The Rhetorical Ecology of Vaccination Concern," *YJBM* 87, no. 4 (December 2014): 403–16.

21. "Timeline: The Rise and Fall of Vioxx," *NPR*, November 10, 2007, http://www.npr.org/templates/story/story.php?storyId=5470430. Vioxx was a prescription nonsteroidal anti-inflammatory medication made by Merck Pharmaceuticals. After being approved by the FDA in 1999, it was pulled in 2004 because of concerns that it could cause serious cardiovascular complications in some patients. At this writing, Gardasil has been modified to prevent an increased number of HPV strains.

22. "Docket of Omnibus Autism Proceeding," *United States Court of Federal Claims*, updated January 12, 2011, http://www.uscfc.uscourts.gov/docket-omnibus-autism-proceeding.

23. Jennifer Zipprich et al., "Measles Outbreak—California, December 2014–February 2015," *Morbidity and Mortality Weekly Report* 64, no. 6 (February 20, 2015): 153–54, https://www.cdc.gov/mmwr/preview/mmwrhtml/mm6406a5.htm; Nakia S. Clemmons et al., "Measles—United States, January 4–April 2, 2015," *Morbidity and Mortality Weekly Report* 64, no. 14 (April 17, 2015): 373–76, https://www.cdc.gov/MMWR./preview/mmwrhtml/mm6414a1.htm. The actual number of cases is variously reported as between 111 and 125, depending on the timing of the report.

24. Centers for Disease Control and Prevention, "U.S. Infant Vaccination Rates High," CDC.gov, accessed August 28, 2014, https://www.cdc.gov/media/releases/2014/p0828-infant-vaccination.html. See also note 8 above.

25. Conis, *Vaccine Nation*, 223.

26. Brendan Nyhan et al., "Effective Messages in Vaccine Promotion: A Randomized Trial," *Pediatrics* 133, no. 4 (April 2014): 1–9.

27. There are things that I left out of this history—attacks on Nigerian vaccination workers in 2013, for example, or the fact that the CIA sent spies pretending to be vaccinators into Pakistan in the hunt for Osama bin Laden, thereby damaging trust in vaccination workers in that country and slowing its control of polio and other endemic diseases. The global politics of vaccination and infectious disease are tremendously complex; I only brought to attention those international stories that significantly animated US public debates about vaccination and contagion.

28. Pew Research Center, "83% Say Measles Vaccine Is Safe for Healthy Children," *Pew Research Center*, February 9, 2015, http://www.people-press.org/2015/02/09/83-percent-say-measles-vaccine-is-safe-for-healthy-children/.

2. Immune to Reason

1. Ginia Bellafante, "Refuse to Vaccinate? Little Religious Ground to Stand On," *New York Times*, February 13, 2015, https://www.nytimes.com/2015/02/15/nyregion/refuse-to-vaccinate-little-religious-ground-to-stand-on.html?mcubz=0.

2. Paloma Esquivel and Sandra Poindexter, "Plunge in Kindergartners' Vaccination Rate Worries Health Officials," *Los Angeles Times*, September 2, 2014, http://www.latimes.com/local/education/la-me-school-vaccines-20140903-story.html#page=1. The run started in the *LA Times* with this article, which opens with "California parents are deciding against vaccinating their kindergarten-age children at twice the rate they did seven years ago, a fact public health experts said is contributing to the reemergence of measles across the state and may lead to outbreaks of other serious diseases." It includes this quote about risks: "'It's only ethical for a person to decide what risk they are willing to take with their body,' said Dawn Richardson of the National Vaccine Information Center, which argues for the right of parents

to decide. The American Academy of Pediatrics, however, has said the group promotes unscientific approaches to vaccines. 'No one group should demand that another group take a risk to benefit them, that's where it crosses the line,' Richardson said." The following day brought an article entitled "Rich, Educated, and Stupid Parents Are Driving the Vaccination Crisis." It opens with this: "The most shocking and disheartening story you'll read in the *Los Angeles Times* today may be our piece on the stunning decline in vaccination rates among California's kindergarten-age children." See Michael Hiltzik, "Rich, Educated, and Stupid Parents Are Driving the Vaccination Crisis," *Los Angeles Times*, September 3, 2014, http://www.latimes.com/business/hiltzik/la-fi-mh-vaccination-crisis-20140903-column.html. See also Paloma Esquivel, "Vaccination Controversy Swirls around O.C.'s 'Dr. Bob,'" *Los Angeles Times*, September 6, 2014, http://www.latimes.com/local/orangecounty/la-me-adv-vaccines-doctor-bob-20140907-story.html.

3. The *Atlantic* ran with the title "Wealthy L.A. Schools' Vaccination Rates Are as Low as South Sudan's." See Olga Khazan, "Wealthy L.A. Schools' Vaccination Rates Are as Low as South Sudan's," *Atlantic*, September 26, 2014, https://www.theatlantic.com/health/archive/2014/09/wealthy-la-schools-vaccination-rates-are-as-low-as-south-sudans/380252/. *Slate* ran an article somewhat late in the news cycle, referring to the *LA Times* and the *Hollywood Reporter* coverage in a December article about a whooping cough outbreak. See Filipa Ioannou, "California's Whooping Cough Epidemic Hits Latino Babies Disproportionately Hard," *Slate*, December 18, 2014, http://www.slate.com/blogs/the_slatest/2014/12/18/california_whooping_cough_latino_babies_hit_hard_by_epidemic_newborns_can.html.

4. Their original research papers can be found at http://www.vaccination.english.vt.edu under Research Outcomes: Media Analysis Reports.

5. Articles surveyed from *Salon* include Lesli Mitchell, "Secrets and Lies," *Salon*, August 2, 2000, http://www.salon.com/2000/08/02/autism/; Lindsay Abrams and Arthur Allen, "The Scramble for the Smallpox Vaccine," *Salon*, November 21, 2001, http://www.salon.com/2001/11/12/smallpox_2/; Julia Scott, "'The World Just Fell out from under Me,'" *Salon*, June 16, 2005, http://www.salon.com/2005/06/16/clark/; Sarah Goldstein, "HPV Vaccine Recommended for Preteen Girls," *Salon*, June 29, 2006, http://www.salon.com/2006/06/29/hpv_shots/; Page Rockwell, "Vaccinating Boys against HPV," *Salon*, July 31, 2006, https://www.salon.com/2006/07/31/boys_and_hpv_vaccine/; Tracy Clark-Flory, "Texas Governor Orders Mandatory HPV Vaccination," *Salon*, February 3, 2007, https://www.salon.com/2007/02/03/hpv_4/; Lynn Harris, "Why Not Vaccinate Boys for HPV?," *Salon*, February 14, 2007, https://www.salon.com/2007/02/14/boys_and_hpv_shot/; Carol Lloyd, "How Safe Is the HPV Vaccine?," *Salon,* April 20, 2007, http://www.salon.com/2007/04/20/hpv/; Tracy Clark-Flory, "Guarding Boys with Gardasil?," *Salon,* May 18, 2007, http://www.salon.com/2007/05/18/hpv_vaccine/; Tracy Clark-Flory, "Texas House Attacks HPV Order," *Salon,* March 14, 2007, http://www.salon.com/2007/03/14/hpv/; Carol Lloyd, "Autism Debate, Take 5,832," *Salon,* September 27, 2007, http://www.salon.com/2007/09/27/autism/; Katharine Mieszkowski, "Amanda Peet Gets Her Shot On," *Salon,* July 15, 2008, http://www.salon.com/2008/07/15/amanda_peet/; Rahul K. Parikh, "Inside the Vaccine-and-Autism Scare," *Salon,* September 22, 2008, http://www.salon.com/2008/09/22/autism_2/; Kate Harding, "Why Are Parents Skipping Swine Flu Vaccines?" *Salon,* September 25, 2009, http://www.salon.com/2009/09/25/swine_flu_vaccine/; Mary Elizabeth Williams, "A 'Sex Jab' Didn't Kill Natalie Morton," *Salon,* October 1, 2009, http://www.salon.com/2009/10/01/hpv_vaccine/; Alex Koppelman, "Glenn Beck Flirts with Sanity," *Salon,* October 8, 2009, http://www.salon.com/2009/10/08/beck/; Mary Elizabeth Williams, "Jenny McCarthy's Autism Fight Grows More Misguided," *Salon,* January 6, 2011, http://www.salon.com/2011/01/06/jenny_mccarthy_autism_debate/; Mary Elizabeth Williams, "My Twitter Battle over Vaccination," *Salon,* July 21, 2011, http://www.salon.com/2011/07/21/vaccination_twitter_battle/; Mary Elizabeth Williams, "A Sexually

Transmitted Virus That's Nothing to Be Ashamed About," *Salon,* September 16, 2011, http://www.salon.com/2011/09/16/hpv_ayelet_waldman_michele_bachmann/; Lindsay Abrams, "Study: Trying to Convince Parents to Vaccinate Their Kids Just Makes the Problem Worse," *Salon,* March 3, 2014, http://www.salon.com/2014/03/03/study_trying_to_convince_parents_to_vaccinate_their_kids_just_makes_the_problem_worse/; Daniel D'Addario, "Andy Cohen to Anti-vaccine Nut Kristin Cavallari: 'Personal Decision, Very Good,'" *Salon,* March 19, 2014, http://www.salon.com/2014/03/19/andy_cohen_to_anti_vaccine_nut_kristin_cavallari_personal_decision_very_good/; Lindsay Abrams, "'The Daily Show': Anti-Vaxxers Are the Climate-Denying 'Nutjobs' of the Left," *Salon,* June 3, 2014, http://www.salon.com/2014/06/03/the_daily_show_anti_vaxxers_are_the_climate_denying_nutjobs_of_the_left/.

Articles surveyed from *Slate* include Atul Gawande, "Gulf War Syndrome," *Slate,* October 26, 1996, http://www.slate.com/articles/news_and_politics/the_gist/1996/10/gulf_war_syndrome.html; Scott Shuger, "Vaccine but Not Heard," *Slate,* March 11, 1999, LexisNexis Academic; John Tooby, "Jungle Fever," *Slate,* October 25, 2000, http://www.slate.com/articles/news_and_politics/hey_wait_a_minute/2000/10/jungle_fever.html; "The *New Yorker* Replies," *Slate,* October 28, 2000, http://www.slate.com/articles/briefing/articles/2000/10/the_new_yorker_replies.html; John Armstrong, "Delusion in El Dorado," *Slate,* November 2, 2000, http://www.slate.com/articles/news_and_politics/best_of_the_fray/2000/11/delusion_in_el_dorado.html; Judith Shulevitz, "Is Anthropology Evil?," *Slate,* December 8, 2000, http://www.slate.com/articles/news_and_politics/culturebox/2000/12/is_anthropology_evil.html; Jon Cohen, "Vax Populi," *Slate,* September 25, 2001, http://www.slate.com/authors.jon_cohen.html; Jon Cohen, "And Now, the Good News about Smallpox," *Slate,* October 26, 2001, http://www.slate.com/articles/news_and_politics/politics/2001/10/and_now_the_good_news_about_smallpox.html; Caroline Benner, "Drop the Anthrax or I'll Shoot," *Slate,* December 16, 2001, http://www.slate.com/articles/news_and_politics/todays_papers/2001/12/drop_the_anthrax_or_ill_shoot.html; Brendan Koerner, "Horses Have a West Nile Vaccine; So Why Don't We?," *Slate,* August 14, 2002, http://www.slate.com/articles/news_and_politics/explainer/2002/08/horses_have_a_west_nile_vaccine_so_why_dont_we.html; Jon Cohen, "There's a Safer Smallpox Vaccine," *Slate,* October 10, 2002, http://www.slate.com/articles/health_and_science/medical_examiner/2002/10/theres_a_safer_smallpox_vaccine_.html; Timothy Noah, "Voulez Vous le Smallpox?," *Slate,* November 5, 2002, http://www.slate.com/articles/news_and_politics/chatterbox/2002/11/voulez_vous_le_smallpox.html; Jon Cohen, "Outbreak," *Slate,* March 21, 2003, http://www.slate.com/articles/health_and_science/medical_examiner/2003/03/outbreak.html; Robert Bazell, "Big Shot," *Slate,* December 2, 2003, http://www.slate.com/articles/health_and_science/medical_examiner/2003/12/big_shot.html; Robert Bazell, "No Immunity," *Slate,* December 9, 2003, http://www.slate.com/articles/health_and_science/medical_examiner/2003/12/no_immunity.htm; Ed Finn, "Why No More Flu Vaccine?," *Slate,* December 12, 2003, http://www.slate.com/articles/news_and_politics/explainer/2003/12/whyno_more_flu_vaccine.html; Eric Umansky, "Doc Block," *Slate,* April 2, 2004; "Flu Shot Shortage," *Slate,* October 6 2004, http://www.slate.com/articles/news_and_politics/recycled/2004/10/flushot_shortage.html; Brendan Koerner, "I Want a Flu Shot," *Slate,* October 8, 2004, http://www.slate.com/articles/news_and_politics/explainer/2004/10/i_want_a_flu_shot.html; Brendan Koerner, "Why Develop Vaccines in Space?," *Slate,* October 15, 2004, http://www.slate.com/articles/news_and_politics/explainer/2004/10/why_develop_vaccines_in_space.html; Emily Biuso, "Vaccination Frustration," *Slate,* October 17, 2004, http://www.slate.com/articles/news_and_politics/todays_papers/2004/10/vaccination_frustration.html; Timothy Noah, "Vaccine Hogs, Part 3," *Slate,* October 23, 2004, http://www.slate.com/articles/news_and_politics/chatterbox/2004/10/vaccine_hogs_part_3.html; Timothy Noah, "Vaccine Hogs, Part 4," *Slate,* October 25, 2004, http://www.slate.com/articles/news_and_politics/chatterbox/2004/10/vaccine_hogs_part_4.html; Jon Cohen, "Anthrax Scare," *Slate,*

November 16, 2004, http://www.slate.com/articles/health_and_science/medical_examiner/ 2004/11/anthrax_scare.html; Sydney Spiesel, "A Shot in the Dark," *Slate*, March 15, 2005, http://www.slate.com/articles/health_and_science/medical_examiner/2005/03/a_shot_in_the_ dark.html; Arthur Allen, "The Unsung Vaccinologist," *Slate*, April 13, 2005, http://www. slate.com/articles/health_and_science/medical_examiner/2005/04/the_unsung_vaccinologist. html; David Sarno, "Running Out of Shots," *Slate*, April 17, 2005, http://www.slate.com/ar ticles/news_and_politics/todays_papers/2005/04/running_out_of_shots.html; Sydney Spiesel, "The Doctor Is In," *Slate*, June 3, 2005; Arthur Allen, "Sticking Up for Thimerosal," *Slate*, August 2, 2005, http://www.slate.com/articles/health_and_science/medical_examiner/ 2005/08/sticking_up_for_thimerosal.html; Jesse Stanchak, "Entangled Sub-Plots," *Slate*, August 7, 2005, http://www.slate.com/articles/news_and_politics/todays_papers/2005/08/ entangled_subplots.html; Keelin McDonell, "How to Make an Avian-Flu Vaccine," *Slate*, Au gust 10, 2005, http://www.slate.com/articles/news_and_politics/explainer/2005/08/how_to_ make_an_avianflu_vaccine.html; David Dobbs, "Where's My Avian Flu Shot?," October 20, 2005, http://www.slate.com/articles/health_and_science/medical_examiner/2005/10/wheres_ my_avian_flu_shot.html; Arthur Allen, "The Last Big Virus," *Slate*, November 22, 2005, http://www.slate.com/articles/health_and_science/medical_examiner/2005/11/the_last_big_ virus.html; Arthur Allen, "The Vaccine Fairy," *Slate*, December 27, 2005, http://www.slate. com/articles/health_and_science/medical_examiner/2005/12/the_vaccine_fairy.html; Marc Siegel, "Forget the Chicken and the Egg," *Slate*, February 7, 2006, http://www.slate. com/articles/health_and_science/medical_examiner/2006/02/forget_the_chicken_and_the_ egg.html; Amanda Schaffer, "Chastity, M.D.," *Slate*, April 11, 2006, http://www.slate.com/ar ticles/health_and_science/medical_examiner/2006/04/chastity_md.html; Arthur Allen, "The Microbes Are Back," *Slate*, April 20, 2006, http://www.slate.com/articles/health_and_science/ medical_examiner/2006/04/the_microbes_are_back.html; Arthur Allen, "And Now, the HPV Vaccine," *Slate*, June 8, 2006, http://www.slate.com/articles/health_and_science/medical_ex aminer/2006/06/and_now_the_hpv_vaccine.html; Amanda Schaffer, "Viral Effect," *Slate*, July 3, 2006, http://www.slate.com/articles/health_and_science/medical_examiner/2006/07/ viral_effect.html; Gregg Easterbrook, "In Search of the Cause of Autism," *Slate*, September 5, 2006, http://www.slate.com/articles/health_and_science/science/2006/09/in_search_of_the_ cause_of_autism.html; Arthur Allen, "The Autism Numbers," *Slate*, January 15, 2007, http:// www.slate.com/articles/health_and_science/medical_examiner/2007/01/the_autism_numbers. html; Ann Hulbert, "Inside Autism," *Slate*, March 28, 2007, http://www.slate.com/articles/ news_and_politics/memoir_week/2007/03/inside_autism.html; Arthur Allen, "Thimerosal on Trial," *Slate*, May 28, 2007, http://www.slate.com/articles/health_and_science/medical_ex aminer/2007/05/thimerosal_on_trial.html; Arthur Allen, "True Believers," *Slate*, June 29, 2007, http://www.slate.com/articles/health_and_science/medical_examiner/2007/06/true_be lievers.html; Meghan O'Rourke, "Cancer Sluts," *Slate*, September 27, 2007, http://www. slate.com/articles/life/the_sex_issue/2007/09/cancer_sluts.html; Dana Stevens, "I Am Leg end," *Slate*, December 13, 2007, http://www.slate.com/articles/arts/movies/2007/12/i_am_ legend.html; Arthur Allen, "Can Vaccines Cause Autism?," *Slate*, January 30, 2008, http:// www.slate.com/articles/news_and_politics/recycled/2008/01/can_vaccines_cause_autism. html; Michelle Tsai, "Fix the Flu Shot," *Slate*, February 22, 2008, http://www.slate.com/arti cles/news_and_politics/explainer/2008/02/fix_the_flu_shot.html; Juliet Lapidos, "The AIDS Conspiracy Handbook," *Slate*, March 19, 2008, http://www.slate.com/articles/news_and_ politics/explainer/2008/03/the_aids_conspiracy_handbook.html; Daniel Engber, "The Para noid Style in American Science," *Slate*, April 15, 2008, http://www.slate.com/articles/ health_and_science/science/features/2008/the_paranoid_style_in_american_science/contrary_ imaginations.html; Juliet Lapidos, "How Do You Diagnose Autism?," *Slate*, July 22, 2008, http://www.slate.com/articles/news_and_politics/explainer/2008/07/how_do_you_diagnose_

autism.html; Sydney Spiesel, "The Good News and Bad News about MS," *Slate*, October 31, 2008, http://www.slate.com/articles/health_and_science/whats_up_doc/2008/10/the_good_news_and_bad_news_about_ms.html; Sydney Spiesel, "Shots All Around!," *Slate*, November 19, 2008, http://www.slate.com/articles/health_and_science/whats_up_doc/2008/11/shots_all_around.html; Arthur Allen, "In Your Eye, Jenny McCarthy," *Slate*, February 12, 2009, http://www.slate.com/articles/health_and_science/medical_examiner/2009/02/in_your_eye_jenny_mccarthy.html; Arthur Allen, "Treating Autism as If Vaccines Caused It," *Slate*, April 1, 2009, http://www.slate.com/articles/health_and_science/medical_examiner/2009/04/treating_autism_as_if_vaccines_caused_it.html; Christopher Beam, "Flu Fighters," *Slate*, April 27, 2009, http://www.slate.com/articles/news_and_politics/politics/2009/04/flu_fighters.html; "Swine Flu," *Slate*, April 27, 2009, http://www.slate.com/articles/health_and_science/science/2009/04/swine_flu.html; Michelle Tsai, "Why Isn't There a Cure-All Influenza Vaccine?," *Slate*, April 27, 2009, http://www.slate.com/articles/news_and_politics/recycled/2009/04/why_isnt_there_a_cureall_influenza_vaccine.html; Chris Wilson, "How Does a Pandemic Ever End?" *Slate*, April 27, 2009, http://www.slate.com/articles/news_and_politics/explainer/2009/04/how_does_a_pandemic_ever_end.html; Timothy Noah, "The Swine Last Time," *Slate*, April 28, 2009, http://www.slate.com/articles/news_and_politics/chatterbox/2009/04/the_swine_last_time.html; Daniel Politi, "To Panic or Not to Panic," April 28, 2009, http://www.slate.com/articles/news_and_politics/todays_papers/2009/04/to_panic_or_not_to_panic.html; Sydney Spiesel, "What Happened to Avian Flu?," *Slate*, April 28, 2009, http://www.slate.com/articles/health_and_science/medical_examiner/2009/04/what_happened_to_avian_flu.html; Christopher Beam, "Swine Flu FAQ," *Slate*, May 1, 2009, http://www.slate.com/articles/news_and_politics/explainer/2009/05/swine_flu_faq.html; John Dickerson, "Prudence or Panic?," *Slate*, May 1, 2009; Arthur Allen, "Say It Ain't So, O," *Slate*, May 6, 2009, http://www.slate.com/articles/health_and_science/medical_examiner/2009/05/say_it_aint_so_o.html; Anne Applebaum, "The Talking Cure," *Slate*, May 12, 2009, http://www.slate.com/articles/news_and_politics/foreigners/2009/05/the_talking_cure.html; Marc Siegel, "WHO and the Flu," *Slate*, May 14, 2009, http://www.slate.com/articles/health_and_science/medical_examiner/2009/05/who_and_the_flu.html; Marc Siegel, "Cabin Fever," *Slate*, July 10, 2009, http://www.slate.com/articles/health_and_science/medical_examiner/2009/07/cabin_fever.html; Jack Shafer, "Burying the Swine Flu Lede," *Slate*, September 12, 2009, http://www.slate.com/articles/news_and_politics/press_box/2009/09/burying_the_swine_flu_lede.html; David Dobbs, "To Boost or Not to Boost," *Slate*, September 17, 2009, http://www.slate.com/articles/health_and_science/medical_examiner/2009/09/to_boost_or_not_to_boost.html; Christopher Beam, "Up Your Nose or Down Your Throat?" *Slate*, October 2, 2009, http://www.slate.com/articles/news_and_politics/explainer/2009/10/up_your_nose_or_down_your_throat.html; Amanda Schaffer, "Sniffing Out Swine Flu," *Slate*, October 7, 2009, http://www.slate.com/articles/health_and_science/medical_examiner/2009/10/sniffing_out_swine_flu.html; Stephanie Tatel, "A Pox on You," *Slate*, October 20, 2009, http://www.slate.com/articles/health_and_science/medical_examiner/2009/10/a_pox_on_you.html; William Saletan, "Sexually Transmitted Injection," *Slate*, October 15, 2009, http://www.slate.com/articles/health_and_science/human_nature/2009/10/sexually_transmitted_injection.html; Marc Siegel, "Blowing the Shot," *Slate*, November 2, 2009, http://www.slate.com/articles/health_and_science/medical_examiner/2009/11/blowing_the_shot.html; Chris Mooney and Michael Specter, "Denialism," *Slate*, November 5, 2009, http://www.slate.com/articles/arts/the_book_club/features/2009/denialism/are_we_antiscience_or_are_we_inconsistent.html; Anne Applebaum, "Coughing, Sneezing, and Spreading Rumors," *Slate*, November 17, 2009, http://www.slate.com/articles/news_and_politics/foreigners/2009/11/coughing_sneezing_and_spreading_rumors.html; Rahul Parikh, "Doc Hollywood," *Slate*, December 9, 2009, http://www.slate.com/articles/health_and_science/medical_examiner/2009/12/doc_hollywood.html; Nayanah

Siva, "Wakefield's First Try," *Slate*, June 2, 2010, http://www.slate.com/articles/health_and_science/medical_examiner/2010/06/wakefields_first_try.html; Arthur Allen, "The Real Problem with Vaccines," *Slate*, February 23, 2011, http://www.slate.com/articles/health_and_science/medical_examiner/2011/02/the_real_problem_with_vaccines.html; Andrew Jack, "Reclaiming Skepticism," *Slate*, June 26, 2011, http://www.slate.com/articles/life/ft/2011/06/reclaiming_skepticism.html; Tom Scocca, "No One Is Immune," *Slate*, July 25, 2011, http://www.slate.com/articles/life/scocca/2011/07/no_one_is_immune.html; Kent Sepkowitz, "Finally, a Selfish Reason to Get Boys Vaccinated for HPV," *Slate*, June 15, 2011, http://www.slate.com/articles/double_x/doublex/2011/06/finally_a_selfish_reason_to_get_boys_vaccinated_for_hpv.html; Arthur Allen and Carl Zimmer, "Contagion: A Dialogue," *Slate*, September 8, 2011, http://www.slate.com/articles/health_and_science/science/features/2011/contagion_a_dialogue/could_they_really_makea_vaccine_so_quickly.html; Forrest Wickman, "Steven Soderbergh's Contagion," *Slate*, September 9, 2011, http://www.slate.com/articles/arts/movies/2011/09/steven_soderberghs_contagion.html; David Weigel, "Political Inoculation," *Slate*, September 13, 2011, http://www.slate.com/articles/news_and_politics/politics/2011/09/political_inoculation.html; Fiona Fox, "What If There Were Rules for Science Journalism?" *Slate*, December 11, 2011, http://www.slate.com/articles/health_and_science/new_scientist/2011/12/science_journalism_guidelines_might_be_a_good_idea.html; Evgeny Morozov, "Warning: This Site Contains Conspiracy Theories," *Slate*, January 23, 2012, http://www.slate.com/articles/technology/future_tense/2012/01/anti_vaccine_activists_9_11_deniers_and_google_s_social_search_.html; Elon Green, "The Longform Guide to Autism," *Slate*, April 28, 2012, http://www.slate.com/articles/life/longform/2012/04/longform_s_guide_to_autism_the_best_stories_ever_written_about_people_on_the_spectrum_.html; Amanda Schaffer, "Why Are Babies Dying of Old-Fashioned Whooping Cough?," *Slate*, September 5, 2012, http://www.slate.com/articles/double_x/doublex/2012/09/why_babies_are_dying_of_whooping_cough_.html; Amanda Schaffer, "Should You Go to the Drugstore for Your Flu Shots?," *Slate*, October 17, 2012, http://www.slate.com/articles/double_x/doublex/2012/10/vaccines_at_the_pharmacy_states_should_let_drugstores_give_shots.html; Darshak Sanghavi, "The Flu Vaccine Controversy," *Slate*, December 18, 2012, http://www.slate.com/articles/health_and_science/pandemics/2012/12/flu_vaccine_safety_tamiflu_and_vaccines_save_lives_and_show_public_health.html; Mark Joseph Stern, "The Worst Pandemic in History," *Slate*, December 26, 2012, http://www.slate.com/articles/health_and_science/pandemics/2012/12/spanish_flu_mystery_why_don_t_scientists_understand_the_1918_flu_even_after.html; Andrea Pitzer, "Why Is It So Tough to Get a Flu Vaccine?" *Slate*, January 10, 2013, http://www.slate.com/articles/health_and_science/medical_examiner/2013/01/flu_vaccine_shortage_cdc_and_fda_have_plans_for_a_crisis_but_in_january.html; Heidi Larson, "Some Mercury Is Good for You," *Slate*, January 18, 2013, http://www.slate.com/articles/health_and_science/new_scientist/2013/01/mercury_treaty_debate_should_thimerosal_be_banned_as_a_vaccine_preservative.html; Jake Blumgart, "Should You Get the HPV Vaccine?," *Slate*, January 25, 2013, http://www.slate.com/articles/health_and_science/medical_examiner/2013/01/who_should_get_the_hpv_vaccine_more_men_and_women_could_be_protected_from.html; Helena Rho, "What's the Matter with Vermont?," *Slate*, February 21, 2013, http://www.slate.com/articles/health_and_science/medical_examiner/2013/02/pertussis_epidemic_how_vermont_s_anti_vaxxer_activists_stopped_a_vaccine.html; Amanda Schaffer, "How to Superpower the Immune System," *Slate*, May 16, 2013, http://www.slate.com/articles/health_and_science/superman/2013/05/new_vaccines_and_immune_boosters_for_flu_cancer_newborns_the_elderly.html; Melinda Wenner Moyer, "Does My Toddler Have Autism?," *Slate*, May 23, 2013, http://www.slate.com/articles/double_x/the_kids/2013/05/does_my_child_have_autism_how_to_identify_the_disorder_s_early_signs.html; Laura Helmuth, "So Robert F. Kennedy Jr. Called Us to Complain," *Slate*, June 11, 2013, http://www.slate.com/articles/health_and_

science/medical_examiner/2013/06/robert_f_kennedy_jr_vaccine_conspiracy_theory_scien tists_and_journalists.html; Robert Stone, "Orthodox Environmentalists Don't Want You to See My Environmental Film," *Slate*, June 20, 2013, http://www.slate.com/articles/health_ and_science/science/2013/06/pandora_s_promise_producer_nuclear_energy_is_necessary_ to_fight_climate.html; Ray Fisman, "Why Aren't There More Cancer Vaccines?," *Slate*, August 26, 2013, http://www.slate.com/articles/health_and_science/the_dismal_science/2013/ 08/cancer_treatment_is_american_patent_law_hindering_the_discovery_of_more.html; Carey Goldberg and Rachel Zimmerman, "Vaccine Facts and Fictions," *Slate*, September 23, 2013, http://www.slate.com/articles/podcasts/the_checkup/2013/09/the_checkup_vaccina tion_flu_hpv_myths_and_truths.html; Melinda Wenner Moyer, "What to Do if You Get In- vited to a Chickenpox Party," *Slate*, November 15, 2013, http://www.slate.com/articles/ double_x/the_kids/2013/11/chickenpox_vaccine_is_it_really_necessary.html; Amy Parker, "Growing Up Unvaccinated," *Slate*, January 6, 2014, http://www.slate.com/articles/life/fam ily/2014/01/growing_up_unvaccinated_a_healthy_lifestyle_couldn_t_prevent_many_child hood.html; Jessica Martin, "The Flu Vaccine Is Safer than We Knew," *Slate*, January 22, 2014, http://www.slate.com/articles/health_and_science/medical_examiner/2014/01/flu_vac cine_is_safe_for_people_with_egg_allergies_why_i_vaccinated_my_child.html; Phil Plait, "Should Public Schools Have Mandatory Vaccinations for Students?," *Slate*, February 26, 2014, http://www.slate.com/blogs/bad_astronomy/2014/02/26/colorado_vaccinations_mak ing_it_harder_for_parents_to_opt_out.html; Phil Plait, "Jenny McCarthy Asks; the Internet Slam Dunks," *Slate*, March 17, 2014, http://www.slate.com/blogs/bad_astronomy/2014/03/17/ jenny_mccarthy_antivaxxer_gets_remedied_on_twitter.html; Sydney Spiesel, "I'm a Pediatri- cian. Should I Treat All Kids, or Just the Vaccinated Ones?," *Slate*, March 18, 2014, http:// www.slate.com/articles/life/family/2014/03/measles_outbreak_in_new_york_city_should_pe diatricians_treat_unvaccinated.html; Phil Plait, "Chili's Reception: Restaurant Cancels Event with Anti-Vax Group," *Slate*, April, 9, 2014, http://www.slate.com/articles/life/family/ 2014/03/measles_outbreak_in_new_york_city_should_pediatricians_treat_unvaccinated. html; Phil Plait, "Unvaccinated People Cause a 20-Year High in U.S. Measles Cases," *Slate*, May 31, 2014, http://www.slate.com/blogs/bad_astronomy/2014/05/31/measles_2014_infec tion_rate_at_highest_levels_in_20_years.html; Phil Plait, "*The Daily Show* and the Anti- Vaxxers," *Slate*, June 4, 2014, http://www.slate.com/blogs/bad_astronomy/2014/06/04/ anti_vaxxers_the_daily_show_mocks_anti_science.html; Mark O'Connell, "Vaccine as Meta- phor," *Slate*, October 9, 2014, http://www.slate.com/articles/arts/books/2014/10/on_immu nity_an_inoculation_reviewed_eula_biss_book_explores_fear_of_vaccines.html; Emily Yoffe, "Gut Shot," *Slate*, November 13, 2014, http://www.slate.com/articles/life/dear_prudence/ 2014/11/dear_prudence_our_midwives_are_anti_vaccination_activists_should_we_fire.html; Betsy Woodruff, "The Danger of Reading the Comments," *Slate*, January 27, 2015, http:// www.slate.com/articles/health_and_science/medical_examiner/2015/01/internet_comment_ credibility_study_vaccine_decisions_influenced_by_online.html; Ann Bauer, "My Life with Anti-Vaxxers," *Slate*, February 2, 2015, http://www.slate.com/articles/life/family/2015/02/ anti_vaxxers_and_the_measles_outbreak_understanding_why_parents_don_t_vaccinate. html; Jed Lipinski, "Endangering the Herd," *Slate*, February 2, 2015, http://www.slate.com/ articles/news_and_politics/jurisprudence/2013/08/anti_vaxxers_why_parents_who_don_t_ vaccinate_their_kids_should_be_sued_or.html; Brian Plamer, "What Do Pediatricians *Really* Think about Anti-Vaxxers?," *Slate*, February 5, 2015, http://www.slate.com/articles/health_ and_science/medical_examiner/2015/02/how_do_pediatricians_work_with_anti_vaccine_ parents_mds_frustrations_failures.html; Jamelle Bouie, "How to Deal with Anti-Vaxxers," *Slate*, February 3, 2015, http://www.slate.com/articles/news_and_politics/politics/2015/02/ anti_vaxxers_resist_persuasion_if_they_refuse_we_have_to_force_them_to_vaccinate.html; Melinda Wenner Moyer, "Does Breast-Feeding Protect My Baby from Measles?," *Slate*,

February 10, 2015, http://www.slate.com/articles/double_x/the_kids/2015/02/measles_and_infants_advice_for_parents_of_unvaccinated_babies.html; Padmananda Rama, "Joining the Herd," *Slate*, February 19, 2015, http://www.slate.com/articles/health_and_science/medical_examiner/2015/02/adult_measles_vaccination_child_of_california_new_age_parents_joins_the.html; Theresa Macphail, "WebMD Knows Best?," *Slate*, March 3, 2015, http://www.slate.com/articles/technology/future_tense/2015/03/webmd_and_self_diagnosis_how_the_internet_is_changing_medical_decisions.html; Emily Yoffe, "Deserves a Shot," *Slate*, March 10, 2015, http://www.slate.com/articles/life/dear_prudence/2015/03/dear_prudence_should_i_secretly_vaccinate_my_grandson.html; Jerry A. Coyne, "Faith Healing Kills Children," *Slate*, May 21, 2015, http://www.slate.com/articles/health_and_science/medical_examiner/2015/05/religious_exemptions_from_medical_care_faith_healing_kills_children.html; William Saletan, "Unhealthy Fixation," *Slate*, July 15, 2015, http://www.slate.com/articles/health_and_science/science/2015/07/are_gmos_safe_yes_the_case_against_them_is_full_of_fraud_lies_and_errors.html; Laura Miller, "What Are the Odds?," *Slate*, August 31, 2015, http://www.slate.com/articles/life/classes/2015/08/take_a_statistics_and_probability_class_in_college_to_improve_critical_thinking.html; Eric Posner, "Why Are People So Scared of Syrian Refugees?," *Slate*, November 20, 2015, http://www.slate.com/articles/news_and_politics/view_from_chicago/2015/11/why_american_people_are_scared_of_syrian_refugees.html.

6. Gawande, "Gulf War Syndrome."

7. Shuger, "Vaccine but Not Heard."

8. See note 5 for the list of titles surveyed.

9. Christine Gorman, "Hope Meets Hype," *Time*, July 19, 1999, 88. This article provides an example concerning a potential Alzheimer's vaccine and includes a discussion of the risks of vaccines in general seldom seen in reporting these days: "Then there's the possibility that a vaccine will do more harm than good. Every time you stimulate the immune system, you run the risk of triggering an inflammatory reaction, marked by fever, swelling and tissue destruction. In fact, many researchers believe the real destructive power of Alzheimer's comes not from the plaques but from the immune system's overreaction to them. The vaccine might also cross react with other proteins, triggering an autoimmune reaction in which the body attacked its own brain cells."

10. Tooby, "Jungle Fever"; "The *New Yorker* Replies"; Armstrong, "Delusion in El Dorado"; and Shulevitz, "Is Anthropology Evil?" See also Daniel Zalewski, "Ideas & Trends; Anthropology Enters the Age of Cannibalism," *New York Times*, October 8, 2000, http://www.nytimes.com/2000/10/08/weekinreview/ideas-trends-anthropology-enters-the-age-of-cannibalism.html?mcubz=0; John Horgan, "Hearts of Darkness," *New York Times*, November 12, 2000, http://www.nytimes.com/books/00/11/12/reviews/001112.12horgant.html?mcubz=0; and John Noble Wilford, "Book Leads Anthropologists to Look Inward," *New York Times*, November 18, 2000, http://www.nytimes.com/2000/11/18/us/book-leads-anthropologists-to-look-inward.html?mcubz=0.

11. While not reported on in *Slate* at the time, *The River* is mentioned by Elena Conis in her book *Vaccine Nation: America's Changing Relationship with Immunization* (Chicago: University of Chicago Press, 2014) as being influential: "The book's reception gave credence to the notion that vaccines were not just fallible in minor, insignificant ways, but could very well be implicated in the nation's most devastating epidemic in decades" (206; see also 310nn9–12).

12. Charles Krauthammer, "Smallpox Shots: Make Them Mandatory," *Time*, December 23, 2002, 84.

13. Spiesel, "Shot in the Dark." See also Harris L. Coulter and Barbara Loe Fisher, *DPT: A Shot in the Dark* (San Diego: Harcourt Brace Jovanovich, 1985). This book claiming vaccine injury, cowritten by Barbara Loe Fisher, the founder of the National Vaccine Information

Center (NVIC), demonstrates the popularity of the title in vaccine-skeptical publications as well. The NVIC hosts a website promoting vaccine safety and vaccine skepticism.

14. See Leon Jaroff, "This Will Only Hurt for a Minute," *Time*, October 2, 2000, 80. An example of the unevenness of tone in reporting can be found in Jaroff's article, which is highly inflammatory and refers to people who don't vaccinate as "quacks" and "fanatics," and uses phrases such as "preposterous medical illiteracy" and "appalling ignorance of history." This article's tone is unusual for its publication date.

15. Christine Gorman, "The Chicken Pox Conundrum," *Time*, July 19, 1993, 53. This article is from the period before the vaccine was licensed, and refers to chicken pox as a "mild disease," an "itchy nuisance of childhood for most kids rather than a real danger." While the article mentions that 100 people die on average per year from chicken pox, some attention is given to potential risks of the vaccine and the cost. In comparison, an article from the 2000s, "Preventing the Pox," *Time*, March 1, 2004, 78, states: "As unpleasant as its itchy rash can be, getting chicken pox may still be the best way to protect against catching it again, especially in the youngest children. Doctors from Yale and Columbia found that the chicken-pox vaccine's ability to protect against the varicella virus weakens after the first year and is particularly ineffective in infants who were immunized before the age of 15 months." In 2015 *Time* published Jeffrey Kluger's "Why 'Tolerating' Anti-Vaxxers Is a Losing Strategy," *Time*, December 10, 2015, http://time.com/4144359/vaccines-tolerance-anti-vaxxers-melbourne-aus tralia/. This article on varicella included the following, in reference to a chicken-pox outbreak: "Tolerance is one of the greatest of human impulses—the social and intellectual flexibility that allows a society to function at all—but there are limits. There is no reason to tolerate a virus in our midst that could have been kept out. *And there's no reason to tolerate the kind of thinking that allowed it to get there.*"

16. See, for example, Abrams, "Study: Trying to Convince Parents to Vaccinate Their Kids," and Abrams, "'The Daily Show,'" both of which feature prominent pictures of Jenny McCarthy.

17. Allen, "Sticking Up for Thimerosal."

18. Gardiner Harris and Anahad O'Connor, "On Autism's Cause, It's Parents vs. Research," *New York Times*, June 25, 2005, http://www.nytimes.com/2005/06/25/science/on-autisms-cause-its-parents-vs-research.html?_r=0. Melinda Wharton, the director of the Immunization Services Division at the CDC, told me that she thought Harris and O'Connor's article was a signal reporting event, after which reputable news sources tended to write disparagingly of parents who resisted vaccination. The article focused on thimerosal and pitted science researchers who trusted the studies exonerating thimerosal as a cause of autism against parents and their preferred researchers, who believed that thimerosal had a role in autism's increasing incidence among children.

19. Travertine Orndorff, "Vaccination Reporting in *Mother Jones*," *Vaccination Research Group*, Spring 2015, http://www.vaccination.english.vt.edu/wp-content/uploads/2015/06/Or ndorff_Mother-Jones.pdf.

20. Robert F. Kennedy, Jr., "Deadly Immunity," *Rolling Stone*, July 14, 2005, 57–66; Scott, "The World Just Fell out from under Me." *Salon* has since taken down the Kennedy article, although in 2016 it was still available on the *Rolling Stone* website. In fall 2017, *Rolling Stone* online claimed that the article was available, but the link did not work. The article was available for a time on Robert F. Kennedy Jr.'s, own website, but that entire website is unavailable in August 2018.

21. Kennedy, "Deadly Immunity," 57.

22. Seth Mnookin, *The Panic Virus: A True Story of Medicine, Science, and Fear* (New York: Simon & Schuster, 2011); Paul A. Offit, *Deadly Choices: How the Anti-vaccine Movement Threatens Us All* (New York: Basic Books, 2012).

23. The Omnibus Autism Proceeding was an action taken by the vaccine court to consolidate the thousands of claims being made that thimerosal or the MMR vaccine cause autism. The court allowed the plaintiffs to choose three emblematic cases to prove their allegations. Three theories were presented: (1) MMR vaccine and thimerosal-containing vaccines cause autism, (2) thimerosal-containing vaccines cause autism, or (3) MMR vaccine causes autism. In February 2009 the vaccine court ruled that there was no evidence to prove theory 1. In March 2010 the court ruled that theory 2 was also not supported by the evidence. Given that theory 1 was not supported by the evidence, the plaintiffs declined to continue to press theory 3 in vaccine court. The major source for this information was Health Resources and Services Administration, "About the Omnibus Autism Proceeding," http://www.hrsa.gov/vaccinecom pensation/omnibusautism.html. After the writing of this book, however, the URL now returns a page not found error, and a search of the site reveals no replacement page.

24. Harris and O'Connor, "On Autism's Cause." Harris and O'Connor's article heralded this change, although the article itself is not inflammatory in its tone and does not portray vaccine-skeptical parents in a derogatory way. It does, however, suggest that their concerns are misguided, given the research. Melinda Wharton, the director of the Immunization Services Division of the CDC, pointed me toward this article.

25. See John F. Burns, "British Medical Council Bars Doctor Who Linked Vaccine with Autism," *New York Times*, May 24, 2010, http://www.nytimes.com/2010/05/25/health/policy/25autism.html. Even so, there was publishing in *Time* up through 2008 still questioning vaccination: Alice Park, "How Safe Are Vaccines?," *Time*, June 2, 2008, 36–41. The article suggests that there may be a need for more targeted guidance for inoculations, based on personal genetic history and possible adverse reactions linked to personal genomics:

> Whether tests like these, combined with detailed family histories, will make a difference in the rates of developmental disorders like autism isn't yet clear. But such a strategy could reveal new avenues of research and lead to safer inoculations overall. Parents concerned about vaccine safety would then have stronger answers to their questions about how their child might be affected by the shots. Vaccines may be a medical marvel, but they are only one salvo in our fight against disease-causing bugs. It's worth remembering that viruses and bacteria have had millions of years to perfect their host-finding skills; our abilities to rebuff them are only two centuries old. And in that journey, both parents and public health officials want the same thing: to protect future generations from harm. (41)

26. Orndorff, "Vaccination Reporting in *Mother Jones*."

27. B. A. Slade et al., "Postlicensure Safety Surveillance for Quadrivalent Human Papillomavirus Recombinant Vaccine," *JAMA* 302, no. 7 (August 19, 2009): 750–57, https://www.ncbi.nlm.nih.gov/pubmed/19690307.

28. Saletan, "Unhealthy Fixation."

29. Conis, *Vaccine Nation*, 212.

30. Tetanus, of course, is an illness that is included in a required vaccine but is not communicable at all. Thus, one could argue that it sets the standard for a mandated vaccine that is not communicable in a school setting.

31. Virginia allows an easy exemption from HPV vaccination, unlike its religious and medical exemption processes.

3. Whom Do You Trust?

1. Frank Bruni, "The Vaccine Lunacy: Disneyland, Measles, and Madness," *New York Times*, January 31, 2015, https://www.nytimes.com/2015/02/01/opinion/sunday/frank-

bruni-disneyland-measles-and-madness.html?mcubz=0; Ginia Bellafante, "Refuse to Vaccinate? Little Religious Ground to Stand On," *New York Times*, February 13, 2015, https://www.nytimes.com/2015/02/15/nyregion/refuse-to-vaccinate-little-religious-ground-to-stand-on.html?mcubz=0.

2. "Anti-vaccine Moms Speak Out amid Fierce Backlash," CBSNews.com, February 22, 2015, https://www.cbsnews.com/news/anti-vaccine-moms-speak-out-amid-fierce-backlash/. This article has an AP byline. I first read it in the *Roanoke Times* and have notes from that, but I currently cannot locate that version. It appears that the piece was broadly circulated, as it also turns up in the United Kingdom's *Daily Mail*.

3. Abigail Zuger, "Defending Vaccination Once Again, with Feeling," *New York Times*, March 29, 2011, D5.

4. Paul Offit, interviewed by Stephen Colbert, *The Colbert Report*, January 31, 2011, https://www.youtube.com/watch?v=KXntMFfrbjc.

5. Paul A. Offit, *Deadly Choices: How the Anti-vaccine Movement Threatens Us* (New York: Basic Books, 2012), 56.

6. It's interesting in the context of this argument that Offit doesn't discuss Gulf War Syndrome, which is understood by many to be an imaginary illness. See Elaine Showalter, *Hystories: Hysterical Epidemics and Modern Media* (New York: Columbia University Press, 1998).

7. Offit, *Deadly Choices*, 80–82, 163, 88–91.

8. Saad B. Omer et al., "Nonmedical Exemptions to School Immunization Requirements," *JAMA* 296, no. 14 (October 11, 2006): 1757–63, doi:10.1001/jama.296.14.1757.

9. Offit, *Deadly Choices*, 92.

10. Michael J. Smith et al., "Media Coverage of the Measles-Mumps-Rubella Vaccine and Autism Controversy and Its Relationship to MMR Immunization Rates in the United States," *Pediatrics* 121, no. 4 (2008): e836–e843, doi:10.1542/peds.2007-1760.

11. Offit, *Deadly Choices*, 143; Omer et al., "Nonmedical Exemptions."

12. Offit, *Deadly Choices*, 92, 143; Smith et al., "Media Coverage of the Measles-Mumps-Rubella Vaccine and Autism Controversy"; Omer et al., "Nonmedical Exemptions."

13. Seth Mnookin, *The Panic Virus: A True Story of Medicine, Science, and Fear* (New York: Simon & Schuster, 2011), 199–200.

14. There were actually two large studies to test the Salk injected polio vaccine, which included a killed virus. One study included a control group of children who received placebo shots. The other study simply included a large number of children as "observed controls," that is, subjects whose disease status was followed but who received no shots. Parsing the numbers from the Salk polio vaccine trials is quite difficult. The 1,800,000 number for the total number of children involved in the trials is cited in a number of sources and appears to be an accurate number for the total number of first, second, and third graders in the study population. See, for example, Marcia Meldrum, "'A Calculated Risk': The Salk Polio Vaccine Trials," *BMJ* 317 (1998): 1233–36. Meldrum writes, "Across the United States, 623,972 schoolchildren were injected with vaccine or placebo, and more than a million others participated as 'observed' controls" (1233), clearly indicating the 1,800,000+ figure.

David Oshinsky, a very reliable historian, uses the figure 1,349,135 in his book *Polio: An American Story* (Oxford: Oxford University Press, 2006), 200. It appears that he gets this figure by adding together the number of children receiving all three vaccine injections and the children receiving placebos in the controlled study, the children receiving all three injections in the observation study, and the total number of first- and third-grade observed controls in the latter study (204). It is true that in the observation study, the second graders receiving vaccine were to be compared to first and third graders who did not receive the vaccine or a placebo. Yet most other accounts use the 1,800,000+ figure for the entire population of first through third graders in the study population overall, as it appears that the incidence of disease was tracked for all of these children to compare to those injected with vaccine. For example, Liza Dawson, "The Salk Polio Vaccine Trial of 1954: Risks, Randomization, and Public Involvement in Research," *Clinical Trials* 1, no. 1 (2004): 122–30, doi. org/10.1191/1740774504cn010xx, mentions "this enormous clinical trial, involving 1.8 million children," in the abstract of her article. Yet it is very clear from all sources that in no way did almost two million children receive polio vaccine in the trials.

Thomas Francis's articles about the study design of the 1954 trials were published in the *American Journal of Public Health* in May 1955, part 2. See the following articles, which are listed without author but are usually credited to Thomas Francis: "Introduction," *American Journal of Public Health* 45, no. 5, pt. 2 (May 1, 1955): xii–xiv, doi:10.2105/ AJPH.45.5_Pt_2.xii; "I. Plan of Study," ibid., 1–14, doi:10.2105/AJPH.45.5_Pt_2.1; "II. Results," ibid., 15–48, doi:10.2105/AJPH.45.5_Pt_2.15; "III. Summary of Effectiveness of Vaccine," ibid., 49–51, doi:10.2105/AJPH.45.5_Pt_2.49. A full table appears on p. 25 of the study results. Jonas Salk's article about vaccine effectiveness was published in the same journal, part 1. See Jonas E. Salk, "Vaccination against Paralytic Poliomyelitis Performance and Prospects," *American Journal of Public Health* 45, no. 5, pt. 1 (May 1, 1955): 575–96, doi. org/10.2105/AJPH.45.5_Pt_1.575, for the scientific account of vaccine effectiveness and his recommendation for the 1955 vaccination schedule.

15. Mnookin, *The Panic Virus*, 277–78, 305.

16. Ibid., 56. See also Offit, *Deadly Choices*, 208.

17. Robert M. Jacobson, Paul V. Targonski, and Gregory A. Poland, "Taxonomy of Reasoning Flaws," *Vaccine* 25, no. 15 (2007): 3146–52, doi:10.1016/j.vaccine.2007.01.046.

18. Elena Conis, *Vaccine Nation: America's Changing Relationship with Immunization* (Chicago: University of Chicago Press, 2014), 223–24.

4. Being a Responsible Parent

1. Ginia Bellafante, "Refuse to Vaccinate? Little Religious Ground to Stand On," *New York Times*, February 13, 2015, https://www.nytimes.com/2015/02/15/nyregion/refuse-to-vaccinate-little-religious-ground-to-stand-on.html?mcubz=0.

2. Mark A. Largent, *Vaccine: The Debate in Modern America* (Baltimore: Johns Hopkins University Press, 2012); Eula Biss, *On Immunity: An Inoculation* (Minneapolis: Graywolf Press, 2014).

3. According to the publisher's website, *On Immunity* was one of the *New York Times Book Review*'s Ten Best Books of 2014, a *Publishers Weekly* Most Anticipated Book of fall 2014, a finalist for the 2015 Midwest Booksellers Choice Award, and an Indies Choice Awards Honoree. See https://www.graywolfpress.org/books/immunity.

4. Jennifer Reich, *Calling the Shots: Why Parents Reject Vaccines* (New York: New York University Press, 2016).

5. Largent, *Vaccine*, 25.

6. In 2014, Michigan instituted an education requirement for any parent requesting a nonmedical waiver of vaccination for a school-aged child. See Michigan Department of Health and Human Services, "Immunization Waiver Information," http://www.michigan.gov/ mdhhs/0,5885,7-339-73971_4911_4914_68361-344843—,00.html.

7. Biss, *On Immunity*, 23–24.

8. Reich, *Calling the Shots*, 248.

9. See Pru Hobson-West, "'Trusting Blindly Can Be the Biggest Risk of All': Organized Resistance to Childhood Vaccination in the UK," *Sociology of Health and Illness* 29, no. 2

(2007): 195–215. See esp. pp. 206–7, where she discusses the use of individualist discourses in interviews with people associated with vaccine-skeptical groups in the United Kingdom. She finds that "the data do not support accusations of 'rampant individualism' that have been levied at vaccination critics and the groups do not present themselves as the defenders of the individual. Rather, their critique is articulated through stressing the complex, multifaceted nature of both risk and health."

10. Heidi Y. Lawrence, Bernice L. Hausman, and Clare J. Dannenburg, "Reframing Medicine's Publics: The Local as a Public of Vaccine Refusal," *Journal of Medical Humanities* 35, no. 2 (2014): 111–29, doi:10.1007/s10912-014-9278-4. See also Rachel Conrad Bracken, "Social (Ir)Responsibility: Vaccine Exemption and the Ethics of Immunity," in *Transforming Contagion: Risky Contacts among Bodies, Disciplines, and Nations*, ed. Breanne Fahs et al. (New Brunswick: Rutgers University Press, 2018), 56–70.

11. See Susan Marmagas et al., "Cumberland Plateau Health District 2009–2010 Flu Season Vaccine Study Final Report," *Vaccination Research Group*, 2011, www.vaccination. english.vt.edu/publications.html, for extended demographic information about this community.

12. Pew Research Center, "83% Say Measles Vaccine Is Safe for Healthy Children," *Pew Research Center*, February 9, 2015, http://www.people-press.org/2015/02/09/83-percent-say-measles-vaccine-is-safe-for-healthy-children/.

13. Reich, *Calling the Shots*, 95.

14. See Nikolas Rose, *The Politics of Life Itself: Biomedicine, Power, and Subjectivity in the Twenty-First Century* (Princeton, NJ: Princeton University Press, 2007).

15. Largent, *Vaccine*, 166.

16. Melissa Leach and James Fairhead, *Vaccine Anxieties: Global Science, Child Health, and Society* (Sterling, VA: Earthscan, 2007), 98.

17. Nadja Durbach, *Bodily Matters: The Anti-vaccination Movement in England, 1853–1907* (Durham, NC: Duke University Press, 2005); Bernice Hausman et al., "'Poisonous, Filthy, Loathsome, Dangerous Stuff': The Rhetorical Ecology of Vaccination Concern," *YJBM* 87, no. 4 (December 2014): 403–16; Michael Willrich, *Pox: An American History* (New York: Penguin, 2011).

5. Is Vaccine Refusal a Form of Science Denial?

1. Emma Bloomfield, "Rhetorical Patterns of History and Science Denial," *Papers of the Strassler Center for Holocaust and Genocide Studies*, 2014, http://commons.clarku.edu/chgspapers/5/?utm_source=commons.clarku.edu%2Fchgspapers%2F5&utm_medium=PDF&utm_campaign=PDFCoverPages.

2. Bernice L. Hausman, *Viral Mothers* (Ann Arbor: University of Michigan Press, 2010), 166.

3. Bloomfield, "Rhetorical Patterns," 3.

4. Deborah E. Lipstadt, *Denying the Holocaust: The Growing Assault on Truth and Memory* (New York: Plume, 1994), 65.

5. Ibid., 18–19; see also Michael Shermer and Alex Grobman, *Denying History: Who Says the Holocaust Never Happened and Why Do They Say It?* (Berkeley: University of California Press, 2000), 29.

6. Lipstadt, *Denying the Holocaust*, 18.

7. Shermer and Grobman, *Denying History*, 241.

8. Ibid., 75.

9. Anna Kata, "A Postmodern Pandora's Box: Anti-vaccination Misinformation on the Internet," *Vaccine* 28, no. 7 (2010): 1709–16.

10. Nicoli Nattrass, *The AIDS Conspiracy: Science Fights Back* (New York: Columbia University Press, 2012), articulates a similar concern: "But it is also likely that the 'postmodern turn' in the social sciences encouraged scholars to concentrate on the rhetorical strategies employed by those making truth claims, rather than take a stance on those truth claims themselves" (64–65). She believes that postmodern sensibilities allow scholars to give themselves too much leeway, to be too relative in their approaches to truth; her discussion of some poststructuralist responses to one attempt to refute AIDS denialism accuses those scholars of moral relativity by engaging in "a rhetorical move that excuses the analyst from having to confront the very issue of weighing the credibility of rival claims and coming to reasoned judgments of them" (66).

11. Bloomfield, "Rhetorical Patterns," 2.

12. Dan Kahan, "A Risky Science Communication Environment for Vaccines," *Science* 342 (October 4, 2013): 53–54, doi:10.1126/science.1245724.

13. Mark Hoofnagle, "About," *Denialism Blog*, April 30, 2007, http://scienceblogs.com/denialism/about/.

14. Hausman, *Viral Mothers*, 168.

15. John Cook, "Inoculating against Science Denial," *The Conversation*, April 26, 2015, http://theconversation.com/inoculating-against-science-denial-40465.

16. Michael Specter, *Denialism: How Irrational Thinking Hinders Scientific Progress, Harms the Planet, and Threatens Our Lives* (New York: Penguin, 2009).

17. Sara E. Gorman and Jack M. Gorman, *Denying to the Grave: Why We Ignore the Facts That Will Save Us* (New York: Oxford University Press, 2017).

18. Andrew Shtulman, *scienceblind: Why Our Intuitive Theories about the World Are So Often Wrong* (New York: Basic Books, 2017).

19. Specter, *Denialism*, 11–12.

20. Gorman and Gorman, *Denying to the Grave*, 5–6; emphasis in original.

21. Shtulman, *scienceblind*, 10.

22. Melissa Leach and James Fairhead, *Vaccine Anxieties: Global Science, Child Health, and Society* (Sterling, VA: Earthscan, 2007), 83–99. Leach and Fairhead provide an excellent discussion of parental research into autism and vaccines as a form of citizen science. The assumption made in most books on so-called science denial is that only experts can evaluate scientific data, which, as I will show, contradicts the notion that people who believe in mainstream science do so because they trust in scientific facts.

23. It's important to note that Specter himself uses "the Great Denial" ironically, as that is a term used by Barbara Loe Fisher, a prominent vaccine skeptic and founder of the National Vaccine Information Center, to refer to establishment denial of vaccine risks. See Specter, *Denialism*, 80.

24. Shtulman, *scienceblind*, 255.

25. Ibid., 254.

26. Mary Douglas and Aaron Wildavsky, *Risk and Culture: An Essay on the Selection of Technological and Environmental Dangers* (Berkeley: University of California Press, 1983).

27. Melissa Leach and James Fairhead, in *Vaccine Anxieties*, explicitly compare British and West African concerns about vaccines, linking them to broader trends and political ideas in each society.

28. Fine 1992, quoted in Nattrass, *The AIDS Conspiracy*, 16.

29. "Cultropreneurs" are defined as "those who both promote conspiracy theories about Western medicine while offering seemingly safer (more 'natural' or 'holistic') alternatives in its place." Nattrass, *The AIDS Conspiracy*, 4.

30. Gorman and Gorman, *Denying to the Grave*, 260.

31. Mary Poovey, *A History of the Modern Fact* (Chicago: University of Chicago Press, 1998).

32. Hausman, *Viral Mothers*, 168, 179.

6. What Are Facts, and How Do We Trust Them?

1. Eric Bradner, "Conway: Trump White House Offered 'Alternative Facts' on Crowd Size," *CNN*, modified January 23, 2017, http://www.cnn.com/2017/01/22/politics/kellyanne-conway-alternative-facts/index.html.

2. Andrew Shtulman, "In Public Understanding of Science, Alternative Facts Are the Norm," *NPR*, May 29, 2017, http://www.npr.org/sections/13.7/2017/05/29/527892222/in-public-understanding-of-science-alternative-facts-are-the-norm.

3. Mary C. Politi, Katherine M. Jones, and Sydney E. Philpott, "The Role of Patient Engagement in Addressing Parents' Perceptions about Immunization," *JAMA* 318, no. 3 (July 18, 2017): 237–38, doi:10.1001/jama.2017.7168. Politi, Jones, and Philpott use the phrase *alternative facts* similarly, in their viewpoint article in *JAMA*. They link *alternative facts* to "pseudoscientific articles, fake news stories generating an artificial controversy, or anecdotes from personal connections" (237).

4. See, for example, Anthony Giddens, *The Consequences of Modernity* (Redwood City, CA: Stanford University Press, 1991).

5. Paula Treichler, *How to Have Theory in an Epidemic: Cultural Chronicles of AIDS* (Durham, NC: Duke University Press, 1999).

6. For a discussion of the controversy over naming HIV and determining what type of virus it is, see Elizabeth Ohneck, "The Discovery of HIV: A Tale of Two Scientists," *Scizzle*, June 6, 2014, http://www.myscizzle.com/blog/hiv-discovery-controversy/.

7. Steve Epstein, *Impure Science: AIDS, Activism, and the Politics of Knowledge* (Berkeley: University of California Press, 1996).

8. Treichler, *How to Have Theory*, 175; emphasis in original.

9. *A History of the Modern Fact* is not without its detractors. The book has been criticized for misunderstanding some basic historical facts that distort Poovey's conclusions about how numerical facts—statistics—come to support the emerging administrative state of the nineteenth century; see, for example, Margaret C. Jacob, "Factoring Mary Poovey's *A History of the Modern Fact*," *History and Theory* 40, no. 2 (2001): 280–89. My use of Poovey's findings, however, relies less on the accuracy of her historical interpretation than on the theoretical implications of her discussion. However, I would be remiss not to note the critical reception of the book, as the question of accuracy and correctness is at the heart of controversies over facts.

10. Poovey, *A History*, 2.

11. Nicoli Nattrass, *The AIDS Conspiracy: Science Fights Back* (New York: Columbia University Press, 2012), 163.

12. See the winter 2016 issue of *Narrative Inquiry in Bioethics* for examples.

13. Heidi Y. Lawrence, Bernice L. Hausman, and Clare J. Dannenburg, "Reframing Medicine's Publics: The Local as a Public of Vaccine Refusal," *Journal of Medical Humanities* 35, no. 2 (2014): 111–29, doi:10.1007/s10912-014-9278-4. See also Rachel Conrad Bracken, "Social (Ir)Responsibility: Vaccine Exemption and the Ethics of Immunity," in *Transforming Contagion: Risky Contacts among Bodies, Disciplines, and Nations*, ed. Breanne Fahs et al. (New Brunswick: Rutgers University Press, 2018), 56–70.

14. Nattrass, *AIDS Conspiracy*, 163.

15. Naomi Oreskes and Erik Conway, *Merchants of Doubt: How a Handful of Scientists Obscured the Truth on Issues from Tobacco Smoke to Global Warming* (London: Bloomsbury Press, 2010).

16. Interestingly, this claim against Rachel Carson shows up in Eula Biss's *On Immunity*, where she cites one of the *New York Times* articles about DDT and Carson that Oreskes and Conway claim uses fraudulent evidence. See pp. 42–46.

17. Treichler, *How to Have Theory*, 273.

18. Carl Elliott, "Pharmaceutical Propaganda," in *Against Health: How Health Became the New Morality*, ed. Jonathan M. Metzl and Anna Kirkland (New York: New York University Press, 2010), 93–104.

19. Pru Hobson-West, "'Trusting Blindly Can Be the Biggest Risk of All': Organized Resistance to Childhood Vaccination in the UK," *Sociology of Health & Illness* 29, no. 2 (2007): 209, doi:10.1111/j.1467-9566.2007.00544.x.

7. Medicalization and Biomedicalization

1. Adele E. Clarke et al., eds., *Biomedicalization: Technoscience, Health, and Illness* (Durham, NC: Duke University Press, 2010); and Adele E. Clarke et al., "Biomedicalization: Technoscientific Transformations of Health, Illness, and U.S. Biomedicine," *American Sociological Review* 68, no. 2 (April 2003): 161–94.

2. Nikolas Rose, *The Politics of Life Itself: Biomedicine, Power, and Subjectivity in the Twenty-First Century* (Princeton, NJ: Princeton University Press, 2007).

3. I am indebted to conversations and emails with my father, David H. Hausman, MD, to clarify this history.

4. Lester S. King and Marjorie C. Meehan, "A History of the Autopsy: A Review," *American Journal of Pathology* 73, no. 2 (Nov. 1973): 514–44, esp. 538.

5. Indeed, he once told me a darkly amusing story about a surgical resident who had been recommended to pathology because of questions about his mental stability. My father was offended that pathology was seen as a "less stressful" specialization than surgery, more appropriate to a doctor with a history of mental illness.

6. King and Meehan, "A History of the Autopsy," esp. 519–20. See also Sanjib Kumar Ghosh, "Human Cadaveric Dissection: A Historical Account from Ancient Greece to the Modern Era," *Anatomy and Cell Biology* 48, no. 3 (2015): 153–69.

7. In an interesting link to vaccination history, I learned in fall 2014, while attending a symposium at New York University on Jonas Salk's 100th birthday, that both Salk and Sabin attended NYU's medical school in the 1920s and 1930s because at the time it was the only medical school in New York City without a quota for Jews.

8. John Ehrenreich, "Introduction: The Cultural Crisis of Modern Medicine," in *The Cultural Crisis of Modern Medicine* (New York: Monthly Review Press, 1978), 5.

9. R. D. Laing, *The Divided Self: A Study of Sanity and Madness* (London: Tavistock, 1960); Thomas Szasz, *The Myth of Mental Illness* (New York: Harper and Row, 1974).

10. Ken Kesey, *One Flew Over the Cuckoo's Nest* (New York; Viking Press, 1962); Miloš Forman, dir., *One Flew Over the Cuckoo's Nest* (Fantasy Films, 1975).

11. Susanna Kaysen, *Girl, Interrupted* (New York: Turtle Bay Books, 1993); James Mangold, dir., *Girl, Interrupted* (Columbia Pictures, 2000).

12. Irving Kenneth Zola, "Medicine as an Institution of Social Control," in *The Cultural Crisis of Modern Medicine*, ed. John Ehrenreich (New York: Monthly Review Press, 1978), 80; emphasis in original.

13. Peter Conrad, *The Medicalization of Society: On the Transformation of Human Conditions into Treatable Disorders* (Baltimore: Johns Hopkins University Press, 2007), 7–8.

14. Zola, "Medicine as an Institution," 86–91.

15. John Ehrenreich, "Introduction," 1–35.

16. Michel Foucault, "The Politics of Health in the Eighteenth Century," in *Power/Knowledge: Selected Interviews and Other Writings, 1972–1977*, ed. Colin Gordon (New

York: Vintage, 1980), 166–82; Michel Foucault, "The Politics of Health in the Eighteenth Century," *Foucault Studies* 1, no. 18 (2014): 113–27, https://rauli.cbs.dk/index.php/foucault-studies/article/view/4654/5087. There are two versions of this essay available in English. The most popular was originally published in French in 1976 and then included in English in a popular collection called *Power/Knowledge* that came out in 1980. The second version was first published in 1979 in French and was not translated into English until 2014, when it appeared in an issue of *Foucault Studies*, which is an online open-access journal. The first third of the essay differs considerably in the two versions, but the final two-thirds are almost exactly the same. Readers can easily access both versions to compare. I refer to both versions of the essay in this chapter.

17. Foucault, "The Politics of Health in the Eighteenth Century," *Foucault Studies*, 114.

18. Ibid., 118.

19. Michel Foucault, *The History of Sexuality, Volume 1: An Introduction*, trans. Robert Hurley (New York: Vintage, 1990).

20. This passage has always bedeviled me and my students when we talk about it in class. Does Foucault think that the reader will be sympathetic to the "village halfwit," as he refers to him later? He writes on p. 32, "So it was that our society—and it was doubtless the first in history to take such measures—assembled around these timeless gestures, these barely furtive pleasures between simple-minded adults and alert children, a whole machinery for speechifying, analyzing, and investigating." Clearly, Foucault *does* think the reader will be sympathetic, if not to the "halfwit" himself, at least to his predicament. But why? Most of my students are not sympathetic; they identify the little girl, not the farm hand, as the victim. They think she is being sexually molested. (I did have one student, years ago, who stood up for the little girl's independent desire and agency in seeking out sexual adventure, but in my experience that is an anomalous interpretation of the passage.) It certainly appears to be so, based on the description. In spring 2015, however, I had an extraordinary group of graduate students who, in my view, cracked this passage and made me understand *how* Foucault understood it to solicit sympathy for the farm hand. My rendering here is based on the interpretation we developed in class, one that relies on the medicalization thesis to be convincing. The students who forwarded this interpretation included Tarryn Abrahams, Andrew Kulak, Kari Putterman, Jessica Beckett, and Hung-Yin Tsai.

21. Clarke et al., "Biomedicalization: Technoscientific Transformations," 164.

22. Clarke et al., *Biomedicalization*, 22.

23. Ibid., 2.

24. Clarke et al., "Biomedicalization: Technoscientific Transformations," 163, 169; Clarke et al., *Biomedicalization*, 2.

25. Carl Elliott, *Better than Well: American Medicine Meets the American Dream* (New York: Norton, 2003).

26. Elliott, *Better than Well*, 128.

27. Elliott, *Better than Well*; Allan V. Horwitz, review of *Happy Pills in America: From Miltown to Prozac*, by David Herzberg, *The Age of Anxiety: A History of America's Turbulent Affair with Tranquilizers*, by Andrea Tone, and *Before Prozac: The Troubled History of Mood Disorders in Psychiatry*, by Edward Shorter, *New England Journal of Medicine* 360, no. 8 (February 19, 2009): 841–44, http://www.nejm.org/doi/full/10.1056/NEJMbkrev0809177. Many of the current antidepressant drugs that are popular have fewer side effects than previously prescribed psychiatric medications, making them easier to tolerate as everyday adjuncts to a normal life.

28. Elena Conis, *Vaccine Nation: America's Changing Relationship with Immunization* (Chicago: University of Chicago Press, 2014), 81–84.

29. Rima Apple, *Perfect Motherhood: Science and Childrearing in America* (New Brunswick, NJ: Rutgers University Press, 2006).

30. An antigen is a substance that produces an immune reaction. Some examples include proteins in foods, red blood cells from other organisms, and parts of viruses or bacteria.

31. Stephen R. Preblud, Walter A. Orenstein, and Kenneth J. Bart, "Varicella: Clinical Manifestations, Epidemiology, and Health Impact on Children," *Pediatric Infectious Disease* 3, no. 6 (1984): 506. In comparison to measles, chicken pox caused one-quarter to one-fifth the number of deaths per year, while mumps-related deaths were half those of chicken pox, prior to vaccines.

32. Centers for Disease Control and Prevention, *Epidemiology and Prevention of Vaccine-Preventable Diseases* (Atlanta: Centers for Disease Control and Prevention, 2015), 356; "Prevention of Varicella: Recommendations of the Advisory Committee on Immunization Practices (ACIP)," *MMWR Recommendations and Reports* 45, no. RR-11 (July 12, 1996): 1–36, https://www.cdc.gov/mmwr/preview/mmwrhtml/00042990.htm, indicates on p. 2 that between 1972 and 1976, the mean annual number of persons dying from varicella was 106, decreasing to 57 during 1982–1986. Between 1987 and 1992, that number increased to 94 for unknown reasons.

33. Lawrence K. Altman, "After Long Debate, Vaccine for Chicken Pox Is Approved," *New York Times*, March 18, 1995, http://www.nytimes.com/1995/03/18/us/after-long-debate-vaccine-for-chicken-pox-is-approved.html?pagewanted=all&mcubz=0.

34. Tracy A. Lieu et al., "Cost-Effectiveness of a Routine Varicella Vaccination Program for US Children," *JAMA* 271, no. 5 (1994): 381. See also M. Elizabeth Halloran et al., "Theoretical Epidemiologic and Morbidity Effects of Routine Varicella Immunization of Preschool Children in the United States," *American Journal of Epidemiology* 140, no. 2 (1994): 81–104.

35. See "State Information," *Immunization Action Coalition*, updated February 17, 2017, http://www.immunize.org/laws/varicella.asp, which is the Immunization Action Coalition's web page of state mandates for varicella vaccination, including dates of implementation. A few states were holdouts beyond ten years out from recommendation. The varicella vaccine is now required in all states, although requirements differ.

36. Rose, *The Politics of Life Itself*, 22–23.

37. Jonathan M. Metzl and Anna Kirkland, eds., *Against Health: How Health Became the New Morality* (New York: New York University Press, 2010).

38. Anna Kirkland, "Conclusion: What's Next?," in Metzl and Kirkland, *Against Health*, 199–200.

39. Carl Elliott, "Pharmaceutical Propaganda," in Metzl and Kirkland, *Against Health*, 93–104.

40. See, for example, Ariana Eungjung Cha, "New Statin Guidelines: Everyone 40 and Older Should Be Considered for the Drug Therapy," *Washington Post*, November 13, 2016, https://www.washingtonpost.com/news/to-your-health/wp/2016/11/13/new-statin-guidelines-everyone-age-40-should-be-considered-for-the-drug-therapy/?utm_term=.a1839e4e1ea5, and linked materials. The article was published after the conversation related here occurred, but refers to the pertinent debate.

41. Kirkland, "Conclusion," 202.

42. Simon Williams and Michael Calnan, "The 'Limits' of Medicalization? Modern Medicine and the Lay Populace in 'Late' Modernity," *Social Science & Medicine* 42, no. 12 (June 1996): 1609–20.

8. Antimedicine in Theory and Practice

1. Ivan Illich, *Medical Nemesis: The Expropriation of Health* (New York: Pantheon, 1982).

2. See Francine du Plessix Gray, *Divine Disobedience* (London: Hamish Hamilton, 1971), for an extended discussion of his radical career in the church.

3. Carl Mitcham, "The Challenges of This Collection," in *The Challenges of Ivan Illich*, ed. Lee Hoinacki and Carl Mitcham (Albany: State University of New York Press, 2002), 9–10; Ivan Illich, *Deschooling Society* (London: Marion Boyars, 1971); Ivan Illich, *Tools for Conviviality* (London: Marion Boyars, 2001).

4. Illich, *Medical Nemesis*, 32.

5. His example is the United Kingdom, which established the National Health Service (NHS) in the 1940s.

6. Ivan Illich, *Limits to Medicine: Medical Nemesis, the Expropriation of Health* (London: Marion Boyars, 2000), iii.

7. Michel Foucault, "The Crisis of Medicine or the Crisis of Antimedicine?," trans. Edgar C. Knowlton Jr. and Clare O'Farrell, *Foucault Studies* 1 (December 2004): 5–19, https://rauli.cbs.dk/index.php/foucault-studies/article/view/562.

8. Robert S. Mendelsohn, *Confessions of a Medical Heretic* (Chicago: Contemporary Books, 1979); Mendelsohn, *Male Practice: How Doctors Manipulate Women* (Chicago: Contemporary Books, 1982); Mendelsohn, *How to Raise a Healthy Child in Spite of Your Doctor* (New York: Ballantine Books, 1987).

9. La Leche League is an international breastfeeding support organization that was started by seven mothers in the Chicago area in the mid-1950s.

10. Mendelsohn, *Confessions*, 141–42; emphasis in original.

11. Mendelsohn, *How to Raise a Healthy Child*, 19–22.

12. His comments about polio vaccine are interesting. In *Confessions of a Medical Heretic*, he commented on Jonas Salk's testimony in the late 1970s that the Sabin oral polio vaccine was by that time the primary cause of the few remaining polio cases in the United States. Mendelsohn writes, "Today, when the man credited with stamping out polio points to the vaccine as the source of the handful of cases which exist, it's high time to question what we are gaining by using the vaccine on an entire population" (145). This statement suggests that he was not against vaccination per se, but against its use without an understanding of the costs in relation to the benefits. Polio is indeed here a "frightening spectre raised in our minds" (145)—Mendelsohn does not diminish the effects of illness or the importance of the vaccine in eliminating the disease. Rather, his attention was focused on the situation at the time (the early 1980s), when the disease was largely eradicated in the United States. Is any risk from the vaccine valid in a context in which the natural disease no longer appears? ACIP agreed almost two decades later when, in 2000, it ended use of the oral polio vaccine in favor of the injected vaccine, which uses an inactivated virus rather than an attenuated virus.

13. Ivan Illich and Robert Mendelsohn, "Medical Ethics: A Call to De-bunk Bio-ethics," in *Ivan Illich: In the Mirror of the Past; Lectures and Addresses, 1978–1990* (New York: Marion Boyars, 1992), 233.

14. Ivan Illich, "The Institutional Construction of a New Fetish," in *Ivan Illich: In the Mirror of the Past*, 220; emphasis in original. It is fascinating to consider how much Illich's ideas resonate with concerns about a risk society, the elaboration of theories of modernity, and criticisms of the instrumental morality and sensibility that appear to emerge in tandem with modern medicalization and neoliberal conceptions of the individual and the state.

15. See Rima Apple, *Mothers and Medicine* (Madison: University of Wisconsin Press, 1987), for a historical discussion of this point.

16. Peter Gøtzsche, *Deadly Medicines and Organized Crime: How Big Pharma Has Corrupted Healthcare* (Boca Raton, FL: CRC Press, 2013); John Abramson, *Overdo$ed America: The Broken Promise of American Medicine* (New York: Harper Perennial, 2004); Marcia Angell, *The Truth about Drug Companies: How They Deceive Us and What to Do about It* (New York: Random House, 2004); Jeremy A. Greene, *Prescribing by Numbers: Drugs and the Definition of Disease* (Baltimore: Johns Hopkins University Press, 2008); Joseph

Dumit, *Drugs for Life: How Pharmaceutical Companies Define Our Health* (Durham, NC: Duke University Press, 2012); H. Gilbert Welch et al., *Overdiagnosed: Making People Sick in the Pursuit of Health* (Boston: Beacon Press, 2012); Carl Elliott, *Better than Well: American Medicine Meets the American Dream* (New York: Norton, 2003). Though I don't specifically refer to all of these books in this section of the chapter, I did consult each during the research phase of writing.

17. "Creating new patients and making more diagnoses benefits an entire medical-industrial complex that includes Pharma but also manufacturers of medical devices and diagnostic technologies, freestanding diagnostic centers, surgical centers, hospitals, and even academic medical centers"; Welch et al., *Overdiagnosed*, 156.

18. Greene, *Prescribing by Numbers*, 4.

19. Dumit, *Drugs for Life*, 208; emphasis added.

20. Dumit's chapter 2 in *Drugs for Life*, "Responding to Facts," contains a more extended discussion on the construction of facts in medical research than I can portray here.

21. Interestingly, and disturbingly, while my mother was in the hospital during her last illness, her heart went into an abnormal rhythm for about six hours, then reverted to normal. Upon discharge, she was given a prescription for statins, in addition to the other medications she was prescribed for her gastric bleeding and stomach ulcer (later found to be caused by cancer). The resident I questioned about the statin prescription didn't have a very good answer as to why she was being prescribed a medication to lower her cholesterol for a problem with her cardiac rhythm. The resident implied it was prescribed for all cardiac abnormalities as a precaution. I was shocked at the routine prescription of a statin, especially because her medication regimen upon discharge was so complicated that we had to create a schedule to make sure that she could take her meds throughout the day without adverse interactions between the drugs or with food. A documented side effect of statins is muscle pain or weakness, and my mother was extremely weak anyway from almost a week in the hospital with little food. I pressed my father to discuss this issue with my mother's primary care doctor, who suggested she not take the statin at that time. This was one time that my parents took my concerns about too much medication seriously.

22. Angell, *The Truth about Drug Companies*, 261.

23. Ivan Illich, "Preface to the 1995 Edition," in *Limits to Medicine*, x.

24. Dumit, *Drugs for Life*, 34.

9. Viral Imaginations

1. Hausman et al., "Urban Legends and the Flu: A Survey of College Students' Perceptions," *Vaccination Research Group*, 2011, http://www.vaccination.english.vt.edu/?page_id=96.

2. Francis Lawrence, dir., *I Am Legend* (Burbank, CA: Warner Bros. Pictures, 2007).

3. Stephen King, *Danse Macabre* (New York: Gallery Books, 2010). And vampires sometimes appear as animals, or "familiars." In King's pandemic apocalypse narrative, *The Stand*, the archetypal evil character, sometimes called Randall Flagg, uses wolves as his familiars and sometimes takes the shape of crows. In Bram Stoker's *Dracula*, the count appears at times as a wolf. Stephen King, *The Stand* (New York: Doubleday, 1978); Bram Stoker, *Dracula* (London: Archibald Constable and Company, 1897).

4. Roger Luckhurst, *Zombies: A Cultural History* (London: Reaktion Books, 2015).

5. The reference to "other-directed society" is to David Reisman, Reuel Denney, and Nathan Glazer, *The Lonely Crowd: A Study of Changing American Character* (New Haven, CT: Yale University Press, 1950).

6. "A Definition of Irreversible Coma: Report of the Ad Hoc Committee of the Harvard Medical School to Examine the Definition of Brain Death," *JAMA* 205, no. 6 (August 1968): 337–40.

7. An epidemic of encephalitis lethargica, or "sleepy-sickness," affected over a million people worldwide in the 1920s. See "Mystery of the Forgotten Plague," *BBC News*, July 27, 2004, http://news.bbc.co.uk/2/hi/health/3930727.stm.

8. George Romero, dir., *Dawn of the Dead* (United Film Distribution Company, 1979).

9. George Romero, dir., *Night of the Living Dead* (Walter Reade Organization and Continental Distributing, 1968).

10. Sarah J. Lauro, *Transatlantic Zombie: Slavery, Rebellion, and Living Death* (New Brunswick, NJ: Rutgers University Press, 2015), 94.

11. King, *Danse Macabre*, 374.

12. Jonathan Maberry, *Dead of Night* (New York: St. Martin's Griffin, 2014).

13. Wolfgang Peterson, dir., *Outbreak* (Burbank, CA: Warner Bros. Pictures, 1995).

14. Max Brooks, *World War Z* (New York: Crown, 2006).

15. Justin Cronin, *The Passage* (New York: Ballantine Books, 2010).

16. The thymus gland creates a type of immune cell and undergoes involution as the person approaches puberty. The notion here is that if the thymus gland is restored, people retain youthful vigor and live longer, perhaps forever.

17. Details about Jonas Lear's emotional situation, which is due in part to his wife's untimely death from lymphoma, are related more fully in the third volume of the trilogy. See Justin Cronin, *The City of Mirrors* (New York: Ballantine Books, 2016).

18. Justin Cronin, *The Twelve* (New York: Ballantine Books, 2012).

19. James F. Thompson, "The Rise of the Zombie in Popular Culture," in . . . *But If a Zombie Apocalypse* Did *Occur: Essays on Medical, Military, Governmental, Ethical, Economic, and Other Implications*, ed. Amy L. Thompson and Antonio S. Thompson (Jefferson, NC: McFarland, 2015), 21.

20. Emily St. John Mandel, *Station Eleven* (New York: Vintage, 2014); King, *The Stand*; Margaret Atwood, *Oryx and Crake* (New York: Doubleday, 2003).

21. Richard Matheson, *I Am Legend* (New York: Gold Medal Books, 1954).

22. Marc Forster, dir., *World War Z* (Hollywood: Paramount Pictures, 2013).

23. Steven Soderbergh, dir., *Contagion* (Burbank, CA: Warner Bros. Pictures, 2011).

24. Kim Sung-su, dir., *Flu* (Seoul: CJ Entertainment, 2013).

10. Anti/Vax

1. Members of the research group change semester to semester, as undergraduates usually enroll for only one semester at a time for research credits. But the main researchers on these studies are Heidi Lawrence, currently an assistant professor of English at George Mason University, and Tarryn Abrahams, a doctoral candidate in science and technology studies at Virginia Tech, as well as Kari Campeau, a doctoral candidate in rhetoric at the University of Minnesota Twin Cities. Erica Palladino and Shelby Turner were also involved in the collection of data for these studies.

2. All three studies have been approved by the Virginia Tech Institutional Review Board for research involving human subjects, and the pertussis study also involved a Virginia Department of Health IRB protocol, because of the involvement of health department personnel, not reported on here: VT-IRB-11-429 (H1N1), VT-IRB-14-903 with VDH-40203 (pertussis), and VT-IRB-15-905 (health beliefs). Susan West Marmagas was principal investigator on the H1N1 study, and I am principal investigator on the rest. Citations of these studies will indicate the interview number, the study, and the lines of the transcript quoted.

3. Health Beliefs and Vaccination, Interview 13, lines 59–66.

4. Health Beliefs and Vaccination, Interview 13, lines 75–84. See Jill Nienhiser, "Dietary Guidelines," *The Weston A. Price Foundation*, January 1, 2000, https://www.westonaprice.

org/health-topics/abcs-of-nutrition/dietary-guidelines/, for information about the Weston Price Foundation and its recommended "Wise Traditions."

5. Health Beliefs and Vaccination, Interview 14, lines 75–76, 94–105.

6. Health Beliefs and Vaccination, Interview 15, lines 801–4.

7. Health Beliefs and Vaccination, Interview 6, lines 218–22.

8. Health Beliefs and Vaccination, Interview 4, lines 845–48.

9. Health Beliefs and Vaccination, Interview 1, lines 314–18.

10. Pertussis and Health Beliefs, Interview 9, lines 669–80.

11. Pertussis and Health Beliefs, Interview 9, line 533.

12. World Health Organization, "About WHO," WHO.int, http://www.who.int/about/mission/en.

13. Health Beliefs and Vaccination, Interview 15, lines 750–76.

14. Health Beliefs and Vaccination, Interview 12, lines 453–55.

15. Health Beliefs and Vaccination, Interview 10, lines 782–87.

16. Pertussis and Health Beliefs, Interview 9, lines 488–515.

17. Pertussis and Health Beliefs, Interview 5, lines 391–97.

18. Pertussis and Health Beliefs, Interview 5, lines 344–51.

19. Pertussis and Health Beliefs, Interview 9, lines 391–93.

20. Pertussis and Health Beliefs, Interview 7, lines 765–72.

21. Health Beliefs and Vaccination, Interview 1, lines 420–27.

22. Health Beliefs and Vaccination, Interview 7, lines 2912–33.

23. Health Beliefs and Vaccination, Interview 7, lines 748–71.

24. Health Beliefs and Vaccination, Interview 15, lines 1559–63.

25. I thought about this criticism of Jell-O a lot when my mother was hospitalized for a gastrointestinal bleed. She was put on a clear diet for almost a week, and I watched her slurp up a pretty disgusting looking broth and eat Jell-O each noon and night. It was hard not to think that the entire experience could have been different, and she wouldn't have become so debilitated, if the hospital had been willing to feed her more nourishing foods while she was there.

Conclusion

1. See Jacob Heller, *The Vaccine Narrative* (Nashville: Vanderbilt University Press, 2008).

2. Julie Steenhuysen, "U.S. Vaccination Rates High, but Pockets of Unvaccinated Pose Risk," *Reuters*, August 27, 2015, http://www.reuters.com/article/us-usa-vaccine-exemptions/u-s-vaccination-rates-high-but-pockets-of-unvaccinated-pose-risk-idUSKCN0QW2JY20150827. In 2016, according to the National Immunization Survey, only 0.8 percent of children under 36 months of age had received no vaccinations. Holly A. Hill et al., "Vaccination Coverage Among Children Aged 19–35 Months—United States, 2016," *Morbidity and Mortality Weekly Report* 66, no. 43 (November 3, 2017): 1171–77.

3. Virginia Woolf, *On Being Ill* (Ashfield, MA: Paris Press, 2002), 13–14.

4. Virginia Woolf, *A Room of One's Own* (New York: Harcourt, Brace, 1929), 15.

5. See Emily Martin, "The Pharmaceutical Person," *Biosocieties* 1, no. 3 (September 2006): 273–87.

6. Virginia Woolf, *Three Guineas* (New York: Harcourt, Brace, 1938).

BIBLIOGRAPHY

Abrams, Lindsay. "'The Daily Show': Anti-vaxxers Are the Climate-Denying 'Nutjobs' of the Left." *Salon*, June 3, 2014. http://www.salon.com/2014/06/03/the_daily_show_anti_vaxxers_are_the_climate_denying_nutjobs_of_the_left/.

——. "Study: Trying to Convince Parents to Vaccinate Their Kids Just Makes the Problem Worse." *Salon*, March 3, 2014. http://www.salon.com/2014/03/03/study_trying_to_convince_parents_to_vaccinate_their_kids_just_makes_the_problem_worse/.

Abrams, Lindsay, and Arthur Allen. "The Scramble for the Smallpox Vaccine." *Salon*, November 21, 2001. http://www.salon.com/2001/11/12/smallpox_2/.

Abramson, John. *Overdo$ed America: The Broken Promise of American Medicine.* New York: Harper Perennial, 2004.

Allen, Arthur. "And Now, the HPV Vaccine." *Slate*, June 8, 2006. http://www.slate.com/articles/health_and_science/medical_examiner/2006/06/and_now_the_hpv_vaccine.html.

——. "The Autism Numbers." *Slate*, January 15, 2007. http://www.slate.com/articles/health_and_science/medical_examiner/2007/01/the_autism_numbers.html.

——. "Can Vaccines Cause Autism?" *Slate*, January 30, 2008. http://www.slate.com/articles/news_and_politics/recycled/2008/01/can_vaccines_cause_autism.html.

——. "In Your Eye, Jenny McCarthy." *Slate*, February 12, 2009. http://www.slate.com/articles/health_and_science/medical_examiner/2009/02/in_your_eye_jenny_mccarthy.html.

———. "The Last Big Virus." *Slate,* November 22, 2005. http://www.slate.com/articles/health_and_science/medical_examiner/2005/11/the_last_big_virus.html.

———. "The Microbes Are Back." *Slate,* April 20, 2006. http://www.slate.com/articles/health_and_science/medical_examiner/2006/04/the_microbes_are_back.html.

———. "The Real Problem with Vaccines." *Slate,* February 23, 2011. http://www.slate.com/articles/health_and_science/medical_examiner/2011/02/the_real_problem_with_vaccines.html.

———. "Say It Ain't So, O." *Slate,* May 6, 2009. http://www.slate.com/articles/health_and_science/medical_examiner/2009/05/say_it_aint_so_o.html.

———. "Sticking Up for Thimerosal." *Slate,* August 2, 2005. http://www.slate.com/articles/health_and_science/medical_examiner/2005/08/sticking_up_for_thimerosal.html.

———. "Thimerosal on Trial." *Slate,* May 28, 2007. http://www.slate.com/articles/health_and_science/medical_examiner/2007/05/thimerosal_on_trial.html.

———. "Treating Autism as If Vaccines Caused It." *Slate,* April 1, 2009. http://www.slate.com/articles/health_and_science/medical_examiner/2009/04/treating_autism_as_if_vaccines_caused_it.html.

———. "True Believers." *Slate,* June 29, 2007. http://www.slate.com/articles/health_and_science/medical_examiner/2007/06/true_believers.html.

———. "The Unsung Vaccinologist." *Slate,* April 13, 2005. http://www.slate.com/articles/health_and_science/medical_examiner/2005/04/the_unsung_vaccinologist.html.

———. "The Vaccine Fairy." *Slate,* December 27, 2005. http://www.slate.com/articles/health_and_science/medical_examiner/2005/12/the_vaccine_fairy.html.

———. *Vaccine: The Controversial Story of Medicine's Greatest Lifesaver.* New York: W. W. Norton, 2007.

Allen, Arthur, and Carl Zimmer. "Contagion: A Dialogue." *Slate,* September 8, 2011. http://www.slate.com/articles/health_and_science/science/features/2011/contagion_a_dialogue/could_they_really_makea_vaccine_so_quickly.html.

Altman, Lawrence K. "After Long Debate, Vaccine for Chicken Pox Is Approved." *New York Times,* March 18, 1995. http://www.nytimes.com/1995/03/18/us/after-long-debate-vaccine-for-chicken-pox-is-approved.html?pagewanted=all&mcubz=0.

Angell, Marcia. *The Truth about Drug Companies: How They Deceive Us and What to Do about It.* New York: Random House, 2004.

"Anti-vaccine Moms Speak Out amid Fierce Backlash." CBSNews.com, February 22, 2015. https://www.cbsnews.com/news/anti-vaccine-moms-speak-out-amid-fierce-backlash/.

Apple, Rima. *Mothers and Medicine.* Madison: University of Wisconsin Press, 1987.

———. *Perfect Motherhood: Science and Childrearing in America.* New Brunswick, NJ: Rutgers University Press, 2006.

Applebaum, Anne. "Coughing, Sneezing, and Spreading Rumors." *Slate,* November 17, 2009. http://www.slate.com/articles/news_and_politics/foreigners/2009/11/coughing_sneezing_and_spreading_rumors.html.

———. "The Talking Cure." *Slate,* May 12, 2009. http://www.slate.com/articles/news_and_politics/foreigners/2009/05/the_talking_cure.html.

Armstrong, John. "Delusion in El Dorado." *Slate,* November 2, 2000. http://www.slate.com/articles/news_and_politics/best_of_the_fray/2000/11/delusion_in_el_dorado.html.

Atwood, Margaret. *Oryx and Crake*. New York: Doubleday, 2003.

Bauer, Ann. "My Life with Anti-Vaxxers." *Slate*, February 2, 2015. http://www.slate.com/articles/life/family/2015/02/anti_vaxxers_and_the_measles_outbreak_under standing_why_parents_don_t_vaccinate.html.

Bazell, Robert. "Big Shot." *Slate*, December 2, 2003. http://www.slate.com/articles/health_and_science/medical_examiner/2003/12/big_shot.html.

——. "No Immunity." *Slate*, December 9, 2003. http://www.slate.com/articles/health_and_science/medical_examiner/2003/12/no_immunity.html.

Beam, Christopher. "Flu Fighters." *Slate*, April 27, 2009. http://www.slate.com/articles/news_and_politics/politics/2009/04/flu_fighters.html.

——. "Swine Flu FAQ." *Slate*, May 1, 2009. http://www.slate.com/articles/news_and_politics/explainer/2009/05/swine_flu_faq.html.

——. "Up Your Nose or down Your Throat?" *Slate*, October 2, 2009. http://www.slate.com/articles/news_and_politics/explainer/2009/10/up_your_nose_or_down_your_throat.html.

Bellafante, Ginia. "Refuse to Vaccinate? Little Religious Ground to Stand On." *New York Times*, February 13, 2015. https://www.nytimes.com/2015/02/15/nyregion/refuse-to-vaccinate-little-religious-ground-to-stand-on.html?mcubz=0.

Benner, Caroline. "Drop the Anthrax or I'll Shoot." *Slate*, December 16, 2001. Lexis-Nexis Academic.

Biss, Eula. *On Immunity: An Inoculation*. Minneapolis: Graywolf Press, 2014.

Bitzer, Lloyd. "The Rhetorical Situation." *Philosophy & Rhetoric* 1, no. 1 (January 1968): 1–14.

Biuso, Emily. "Vaccination Frustration." *Slate*, October 17, 2004. http://www.slate.com/articles/news_and_politics/todays_papers/2004/10/vaccination_frustration.html.

Bloomfield, Emma. "Rhetorical Patterns of History and Science Denial." *Papers of the Strassler Center for Holocaust and Genocide Studies*, 2014. http://commons.clarku.edu/chgspapers/5/?utm_source=commons.clarku.edu%2Fchgspapers%2F5&utm_medium=PDF&utm_campaign=PDFCoverPages.

Blumgart, Jake. "Should You Get the HPV Vaccine?" *Slate*, January 25, 2013. http://www.slate.com/articles/health_and_science/medical_examiner/2013/01/who_should_get_the_hpv_vaccine_more_men_and_women_could_be_protected_from.html.

Bouie, Jamelle, "How to Deal with Anti-Vaxxers." *Slate*, February 3, 2015. http://www.slate.com/articles/news_and_politics/politics/2015/02/anti_vaxxers_resist_persuasion_if_they_refuse_we_have_to_force_them_to_vaccinate.html.

Bracken, Rachel Conrad. "Social (Ir)Responsibility: Vaccine Exemption and the Ethics of Immunity." In *Transforming Contagion: Risky Contacts among Bodies, Disciplines, and Nations*, edited by Breanne Fahs, Annika Mann, Eric Swank, and Sarah Stage, 56–70. New Brunswick: Rutgers University Press, 2018.

Bradner, Eric. "Conway: Trump White House Offered 'Alternative Facts' on Crowd Size." *CNN*, modified January 23, 2017. http://www.cnn.com/2017/01/22/politics/kellyanne-conway-alternative-facts/index.html.

Brooks, Max. *World War Z*. New York: Crown, 2006.

Bruni, Frank. "The Vaccine Lunacy: Disneyland, Measles, and Madness." *New York Times*, January 31, 2015. https://www.nytimes.com/2015/02/01/opinion/sunday/frank-bruni-disneyland-measles-and-madness.html?mcubz=0.

Burns, John F. "British Medical Council Bars Doctor Who Linked Vaccine with Autism." *New York Times*, May 24, 2010. http://www.nytimes.com/2010/05/25/health/policy/25autism.html.

Centers for Disease Control and Prevention. *Epidemiology and Prevention of Vaccine-Preventable Diseases*. Atlanta: Centers for Disease Control and Prevention, 2015.

——. "U.S. Infant Vaccination Rates High: Unvaccinated Still Vulnerable." CDC.gov, August 28, 2014. https://www.cdc.gov/media/releases/2014/p0828-infant-vaccination.html.

Cha, Ariana Eungjung. "New Statin Guidelines: Everyone 40 and Older Should Be Considered for the Drug Therapy." *Washington Post*, November 13, 2016. https://www.washingtonpost.com/news/to-your-health/wp/2016/11/13/new-statin-guidelines-everyone-age-40-should-be-considered-for-the-drug-therapy/?utm_term=.a1839e4e1ea5.

Clarke, Adele E., Laura Mamo, Jennifer Ruth Fosket, Jennifer R. Fishman, and Janet K. Shim, eds. *Biomedicalization: Technoscience, Health, and Illness*. Durham, NC: Duke University Press, 2010.

Clarke, Adele E., Janet K. Shim, Laura Mamo, Jennifer Ruth Fosket, and Jennifer R. Fishman. "Biomedicalization: Technoscientific Transformations of Health, Illness, and U.S. Biomedicine." *American Sociological Review* 68, no. 2 (April 2003): 161–94.

Clark-Flory, Tracy. "Guarding Boys with Gardasil?" *Salon*, May 18, 2007. http://www.salon.com/2007/05/18/hpv_vaccine/.

——. "Texas Governor Orders Mandatory HPV Vaccination." *Salon*, February 3, 2007. https://www.salon.com/2007/02/03/hpv_4/.

——. "Texas House Attacks HPV Order." *Salon*, March 14, 2007. http://www.salon.com/2007/03/14/hpv/.

Clemmons, Nakia S., Paul A Gastanaduy, Amy Parker Fiebelkorn, Susan B. Redd, and Gregory S. Wallace. "Measles—United States, January 4–April 2, 2015." *Morbidity and Mortality Weekly Report* 64, no. 14 (April 17, 2015): 373–76. https://www.cdc.gov/MMWR/preview/mmwrhtml/mm6414a1.htm.

Cohen, Jon. "And Now, the Good News about Smallpox." *Slate*, October 26, 2001. http://www.slate.com/articles/news_and_politics/politics/2001/10/and_now_the_good_news_about_smallpox.html.

——. "Anthrax Scare." *Slate*, November 16, 2004. http://www.slate.com/articles/health_and_science/medical_examiner/2004/11/anthrax_scare.html.

——. "Outbreak." *Slate*, March 21, 2003. http://www.slate.com/articles/health_and_science/medical_examiner/2003/03/outbreak.html.

——. "There's a Safer Smallpox Vaccine." *Slate*, October 10, 2002. http://www.slate.com/articles/health_and_science/medical_examiner/2002/10/theres_a_safer_smallpox_vaccine_.html.

——. "Vax Populi." *Slate*, September 25, 2001. http://www.slate.com/authors.jon_cohen.html.

Colgrove, James. "Immunity for the People: The Challenge of Achieving High Vaccine Coverage in American History." *Public Health Reports* 122, no. 2 (March–April 2007): 248–57. https://doi.org/10.1177/003335490712200215.

——. *State of Immunity: The Politics of Vaccination in Twentieth-Century America.* Berkeley: University of California Press, 2006.

Conis, Elena. *Vaccine Nation: America's Changing Relationship with Immunization.* Chicago: University of Chicago Press, 2014.

Conrad, Peter. *The Medicalization of Society: On the Transformation of Human Conditions into Treatable Disorders.* Baltimore: Johns Hopkins University Press, 2007.

Cook, John. "Inoculating against Science Denial." *The Conversation*, April 26, 2015. http://theconversation.com/inoculating-against-science-denial-40465.

Coulter, Harris L., and Barbara Loe Fisher. *DPT: A Shot in the Dark.* San Diego: Harcourt Brace Jovanovich, 1985.

Coyne, Jerry A. "Faith Healing Kills Children." *Slate*, May 21, 2015. http://www.slate.com/articles/health_and_science/medical_examiner/2015/05/religious_exemptions_from_medical_care_faith_healing_kills_children.html.

Cronin, Justin. *The City of Mirrors.* New York: Ballantine Books, 2016.

——. *The Passage.* New York: Ballantine Books, 2010.

——. *The Twelve.* New York: Ballantine Books, 2012.

D'Addario, Daniel. "Andy Cohen to Anti-vaccine Nut Kristin Cavallari: 'Personal Decision, Very Good.'" *Salon*, March 19, 2014. http://www.salon.com/2014/03/19/andy_cohen_toanti_vaccine_nut_kristin_cavallari_personal_decision_very_good/.

Dawson, Liza. "The Salk Polio Vaccine Trial of 1954: Risks, Randomization, and Public Involvement in Research." *Clinical Trials* 1, no. 1 (2004): 122–30. doi.org/10.1191/1740774504cn010xx.

"A Definition of Irreversible Coma: Report of the Ad Hoc Committee of the Harvard Medical School to Examine the Definition of Brain Death." *JAMA* 205, no. 6 (August 1968): 337–40.

Dickerson, John. "Prudence or Panic?" *Slate*, May 1, 2009. LexisNexis Academic.

Dobbs, David. "To Boost or Not to Boost." *Slate*, September 17, 2009. http://www.slate.com/articles/health_and_science/medical_examiner/2009/09/to_boost_or_not_to_boost.html.

——. "Where's My Avian Flu Shot." October 20, 2005. http://www.slate.com/articles/health_and_science/medical_examiner/2005/10/wheres_my_avian_flu_shot.html.

"Docket of Omnibus Autism Proceeding." *United States Court of Federal Claims.* Updated January 12, 2011. http://www.uscfc.uscourts.gov/docket-omnibus-autism-proceeding.

Douglas, Mary, and Aaron Wildavsky. *Risk and Culture: An Essay on the Selection of Technological and Environmental Dangers.* Berkeley: University of California Press, 1983.

Dreger, Alice. *Galileo's Middle Finger: Heretics, Activists, and One Scholar's Research.* London: Penguin, 2015.

Dumit, Joseph. *Drugs for Life: How Pharmaceutical Companies Define Our Health.* Durham, NC: Duke University Press, 2012.

Durbach, Nadja. *Bodily Matters: The Anti-vaccination Movement in England, 1853–1907.* Durham, NC: Duke University Press, 2005.

Easterbrook, Gregg. "In Search of the Cause of Autism." *Slate,* September 5, 2006. http://www.slate.com/articles/health_and_science/science/2006/09/in_search_of_the_ cause_of_autism.html.

——. "TV Might Really Cause Autism." *Slate,* October 16, 2006. http://www.slate.com/ articles/health_and_science/science/2006/10/tv_really_might_cause_autism.html.

Ehrenreich, John, ed. *The Cultural Crisis of Modern Medicine.* New York: Monthly Review Press, 1978.

——. "Introduction: The Cultural Crisis of Modern Medicine." In *The Cultural Crisis of Modern Medicine,* edited by John Ehrenreich, 1–35. New York: Monthly Review Press, 1978.

Elliott, Carl. *Better than Well: American Medicine Meets the American Dream.* New York: Norton, 2003.

——. "Pharmaceutical Propaganda." In *Against Health: How Health Became the New Morality,* edited by Jonathan M. Metzl and Anna Kirkland, 93–104. New York: New York University Press, 2010.

Engber, Daniel. "The Paranoid Style in American Science." *Slate,* April 15, 2008. http:// www.slate.com/articles/health_and_science/science/features/2008/the_paranoid_ style_in_american_science/contrary_imaginations.html.

Epstein, Steve. *Impure Science: AIDS, Activism, and the Politics of Knowledge.* Berkeley: University of California Press, 1996.

Esquivel, Paloma. "Vaccination Controversy Swirls around O.C.'s 'Dr. Bob.'" *Los Angeles Times,* September 6, 2014. http://www.latimes.com/local/orangecounty/ la-me-adv-vaccines-doctor-bob-20140907-story.html.

Esquivel, Paloma, and Sandra Poindexter. "Plunge in Kindergartners' Vaccination Rate Worries Health Officials." *Los Angeles Times,* September 2, 2014. http://www.latimes. com/local/education/la-me-school-vaccines-20140903-story.html#page=1.

Finn, Ed. "Why No More Flu Vaccine?" *Slate,* December 12, 2003. http://www.slate. com/articles/news_and_politics/explainer/2003/12/whyno_more_flu_vaccine.html.

Fisman, Ray. "Why Aren't There More Cancer Vaccines?" *Slate,* August 26, 2013. http://www.slate.com/articles/health_and_science/the_dismal_science/2013/08/ cancer_treatment_is_american_patent_law_hindering_the_discovery_of_more.html.

"Flu Shot Shortage." *Slate,* October 6 2004. http://www.slate.com/articles/news_and_ politics/recycled/2004/10/flushot_shortage.html.

Forman, Miloš, dir. *One Flew Over the Cuckoo's Nest.* Film. Fantasy Films, 1975.

Forster, Marc, dir. *World War Z.* Paramount Pictures, 2013.

Foucault, Michel. "The Crisis of Medicine or the Crisis of Antimedicine?" Translated by Edgar C. Knowlton Jr. and Clare O'Farrell. *Foucault Studies* 1 (December 2004): 5–19. https://rauli.cbs.dk/index.php/foucault-studies/article/view/562.

——. *The History of Sexuality, Volume 1: An Introduction.* Translated by Robert Hurley. New York: Vintage, 1990.

——. "The Politics of Health in the Eighteenth Century." In *Power/Knowledge: Selected Interviews and Other Writings, 1972–1977,* edited by Colin Gordon, 166–82. New York: Vintage, 1980.

——. "The Politics of Health in the Eighteenth Century." *Foucault Studies* 1, no. 18 (2014): 113–27. https://rauli.cbs.dk/index.php/foucault-studies/article/view/4654/5087.

Fox, Fiona. "What If There Were Rules for Science Journalism?" *Slate,* December 11, 2011. http://www.slate.com/articles/health_and_science/new_scientist/2011/12/science_journalism_guidelines_might_be_a_good_idea.html.

Francis, Thomas. "Introduction." *American Journal of Public Health* 45, no. 5, pt. 2 (May 1, 1955): xii–xiv. doi:10.2105/AJPH.45.5_Pt_2.xii.

——. "I. Plan of Study." *American Journal of Public Health* 45, no. 5, pt. 2 (May 1, 1955): 1–14. doi:10.2105/AJPH.45.5_Pt_2.1.

——. "II. Results." *American Journal of Public Health* 45, no. 5, pt. 2 (May 1, 1955): 15–48. doi:10.2105/AJPH.45.5_Pt_2.15.

——. "III. Summary of Effectiveness of Vaccine." *American Journal of Public Health* 45, no. 5, pt. 2 (May 1, 1955): 49–51. doi:10.2105/AJPH.45.5_Pt_2.49.

Gawande, Atul. "Gulf War Syndrome." *Slate,* October 26, 1996. http://www.slate.com/articles/news_and_politics/the_gist/1996/10/gulf_war_syndrome.html.

Ghosh, Sanjib Kumar. "Human Cadaveric Dissection: A Historical Account from Ancient Greece to the Modern Era." *Anatomy and Cell Biology* 48, no. 3 (2015): 153–69.

Giddens, Anthony. *The Consequences of Modernity.* Redwood City, CA: Stanford University Press, 1991.

Goldberg, Carey, and Rachel Zimmerman. "Vaccine Facts and Fictions." *Slate,* September 23, 2013. http://www.slate.com/articles/podcasts/the_checkup/2013/09/the_checkup_vaccination_flu_hpv_myths_and_truths.html.

Goldstein, Sarah. "HPV Vaccine Recommended for Preteen Girls." *Salon,* June 29, 2006. http://www.salon.com/2006/06/29/hpv_shots/.

Gorman, Christine. "The Chicken Pox Conundrum." *Time,* July 19, 1993, 53.

——. "Hope Meets Hype." *Time,* July 19, 1999, 88.

Gorman, Sara E., and Jack M. Gorman. *Denying to the Grave: Why We Ignore the Facts That Will Save Us.* New York: Oxford University Press, 2017.

Gøtzsche, Peter. *Deadly Medicines and Organized Crime: How Big Pharma Has Corrupted Healthcare.* Boca Raton, FL: CRC Press, 2013.

Gray, Francine du Plessix. *Divine Disobedience.* London: Hamish Hamilton, 1971.

Green, Elon. "The Longform Guide to Autism." *Slate,* April 28, 2012. http://www.slate.com/articles/life/longform/2012/04/longform_s_guide_to_autism_the_best_stories_ever_written_about_people_on_the_spectrum_.html.

Greene, Jeremy A. *Prescribing by Numbers: Drugs and the Definition of Disease.* Baltimore: Johns Hopkins University Press, 2008.

Halloran, M. Elizabeth, Stephen L. Cochi, Tracy A. Lieu, Melinda Wharton, and Lara Fehrs. "Theoretical Epidemiologic and Morbidity Effects of Routine Varicella Immunization of Preschool Children in the United States." *American Journal of Epidemiology* 140, no. 2 (1994): 81–104.

Harding, Kate. "Why Are Parents Skipping Swine Flu Vaccines?" *Salon,* September 25, 2009. http://www.salon.com/2009/09/25/swine_flu_vaccine/.

Harris, Gardiner, and Anahad O'Connor. "On Autism's Cause, It's Parents vs. Research." *New York Times,* June 25, 2005. http://www.nytimes.com/2005/06/25/science/on-autisms-cause-its-parents-vs-research.html?_r=0.

Harris, Lynn. "Why Not Vaccinate Boys for HPV?" *Salon*, February 14, 2007, https://www.salon.com/2007/02/14/boys_and_hpv_shot/.

Hausman, Bernice L. *Viral Mothers*. Ann Arbor: University of Michigan Press, 2010.

Hausman, Bernice L., Mecal Ghebremich, Phillip Hayek, and Erin Mack. "'Poisonous, Filthy, Loathsome, Dangerous Stuff': The Rhetorical Ecology of Vaccination Concern." *YJBM* 87, no. 4 (December 2014): 403–16.

Hausman, Bernice L., Heidi Y. Lawrence, Megan Casady, Jessica Fuller, Leanne Shelley, and Andria Wallen. "Urban Legends and the Flu: A Survey of College Students' Perceptions." *Vaccination Research Group*. 2011. http://www.vaccination.english.vt.edu/?page_id=96.

Hausman, Bernice L., Heidi Y. Lawrence, Susan West Marmagas, Lauren F. Fortenberry, and Clare J. Dannenberg. "H1N1 Vaccination and Health Beliefs in a Rural Community in the Southeastern United States: Lessons Learned." Forthcoming.

Heller, Jacob. *The Vaccine Narrative*. Nashville: Vanderbilt University Press, 2008.

Helmuth, Laura. "So Robert F. Kennedy Jr. Called Us to Complain." *Slate*, June 11, 2013. http://www.slate.com/articles/health_and_science/medical_examiner/2013/06/robert_f_kennedy_jr_vaccine_conspiracy_theory_scientists_and_journalists.html.

Hill, Holly A., Laurie D. Elam-Evans, David Yankey, James Singleton, and Vance Dietz. "Vaccination Coverage among Children Aged 19–35 Months—United States, 2015." *Morbidity and Mortality Weekly Report* 65, no. 39 (October 7, 2016): 1065–71.

Hill, Holly A., Laurie D. Elam-Evans, David Yankey, James Singleton, and Yoonjae Kang. "Vaccination Coverage Among Children Aged 19–35 Months—United States, 2016." *Morbidity and Mortality Weekly Report* 66, no. 43 (November 3, 2017): 1171–77.

Hiltzik, Michael. "Rich, Educated, and Stupid Parents Are Driving the Vaccination Crisis," *Los Angeles Times*, September 3, 2014. http://www.latimes.com/business/hiltzik/la-fi-mh-vaccination-crisis-20140903-column.html.

Hobson-West, Pru. "'Trusting Blindly Can Be the Biggest Risk Of All': Organized Resistance to Childhood Vaccination in the UK." *Sociology of Health and Illness* 29, no. 2 (2007): 198–215. doi:10.1111/j.1467–9566.2007.00544.x.

Hoofnagle, Mark. "About." *Denialism Blog*, April 30, 2007. http://scienceblogs.com/denialism/about/.

Hooper, Edward. *The River*. New York: Little Brown, 1999.

Horgan, John. "Hearts of Darkness." *New York Times*, November 12, 2000. http://www.nytimes.com/books/00/11/12/reviews/001112.12horgant.html?mcubz=0.

Horwitz, Allan V. Review of *Happy Pills in America: From Miltown to Prozac*, by David Herzberg, *The Age of Anxiety: A History of America's Turbulent Affair with Tranquilizers*, by Andrea Tone, and *Before Prozac: The Troubled History of Mood Disorders in Psychiatry*, by Edward Shorter. *New England Journal of Medicine* 360, no. 8 (February 19, 2009): 841–44. http://www.nejm.org/doi/full/10.1056/NEJMbkrev0809177.

Hulbert, Ann. "Inside Autism." *Slate,* March 28, 2007. http://www.slate.com/articles/news_and_politics/memoir_week/2007/03/inside_autism.html.

Illich, Ivan. *Deschooling Society*. London: Marion Boyars, 1971.

———. "The Institutional Construction of a New Fetish." In *Ivan Illich: In the Mirror of the Past; Lectures and Addresses, 1978–1990*, 218–31. New York: Marion Boyars, 1992.

———. *Limits to Medicine: Medical Nemesis, the Expropriation of Health.* London: Marion Boyars, 2000.

———. *Medical Nemesis: The Expropriation of Health.* New York: Pantheon, 1982.

———. *Tools for Conviviality.* London: Marion Boyars, 2001.

Illich, Ivan, and Robert Mendelsohn. "Medical Ethics: A Call to De-bunk Bio-ethics." In *Ivan Illich: In the Mirror of the Past; Lectures and Addresses, 1978–1990*, 233. New York: Marion Boyars, 1992.

Iliffe, John. *The African AIDS Epidemic: A History.* Athens: Ohio University Press, 2006.

Institute of Medicine. *Immunization Safety Review: Vaccines and Autism.* Washington, DC: National Academic Press, 2004. doi.org/10.17226/10997.

Ioannou, Filipa. "California's Whooping Cough Epidemic Hits Latino Babies Disproportionately Hard." *Slate*, December 18, 2014. http://www.slate.com/blogs/the_slatest/2014/12/18/california_whooping_cough_latino_babies_hit_hard_by_epidemic_newborns_can.html.

Jack, Andrew. "Reclaiming Skepticism." *Slate*, June 26, 2011. http://www.slate.com/articles/life/ft/2011/06/reclaiming_skepticism.html.

Jacob, Margaret C. "Factoring Mary Poovey's *A History of the Modern Fact*." *History and Theory* 40, no. 2 (2001): 280–89.

Jacobson, Robert M., Paul V. Targonski, and Gregory A. Poland. "A Taxonomy of Reasoning Flaws." *Vaccine* 25, no. 15 (2007): 3146–52. doi:10.1016/j.vaccine.2007.01.046.

Jaroff, Leon. "This Will Only Hurt for a Minute." *Time*, October 2, 2000, 80.

Kahan, Dan. "A Risky Science Communication Environment for Vaccines." *Science* 342 (October 4, 2013): 53–54. doi:10.1126/science.1245724.

Kata, Anna. "A Postmodern Pandora's Box: Anti-vaccination Misinformation on the Internet." *Vaccine* 28, no. 7 (2010): 1709–16.

Kaysen, Susanna. *Girl, Interrupted.* New York: Turtle Bay Books, 1993.

Kennedy, Robert F., Jr. "Deadly Immunity." *Rolling Stone*, July 14, 2005, 57–66.

Kesey, Ken. *One Flew Over the Cuckoo's Nest.* New York: Viking Press, 1962.

Khazan, Olga. "Wealthy L.A. Schools' Vaccination Rates Are as Low as South Sudan's." *Atlantic*, September 26, 2014. https://www.theatlantic.com/health/archive/2014/09/wealthy-la-schools-vaccination-rates-are-as-low-as-south-sudans/380252/.

King, Lester S., and Marjorie C. Meehan. "A History of the Autopsy: A Review." *American Journal of Pathology* 73, no. 2 (Nov. 1973): 514–44.

King, Stephen. *Danse Macabre.* New York: Gallery Books, 2010.

———. *The Stand.* New York: Doubleday, 1978.

Kirby, David. *Evidence of Harm: Mercury in Vaccines and the Autism Epidemic: A Medical Controversy.* Boston: St. Martin's Griffin, 2006.

Kirkland, Anna. "Conclusion: What's Next?" In *Against Health*, edited by Jonathan Metzl and Anna Kirkland, 199–200. New York: New York University Press, 2010.

Kluger, Jeffrey. "Why 'Tolerating' Anti-Vaxxers Is a Losing Strategy." *Time*, December 10, 2015. http://time.com/4144359/vaccines-tolerance-anti-vaxxers-melbourne-australia/.

Koerner, Brendan. "Horses Have a West Nile Vaccine; So Why Don't We?" *Slate*, August 14, 2002. http://www.slate.com/articles/news_and_politics/explainer/2002/08/horses_have_a_west_nile_vaccine_so_why_dont_we.html.

——. "I Want a Flu Shot." *Slate*, October 8, 2004. http://www.slate.com/articles/news_and_politics/explainer/2004/10/i_want_a_flu_shot.html.

——. "Why Develop Vaccines in Space?" *Slate*, October 15, 2004. http://www.slate.com/articles/news_and_politics/explainer/2004/10/why_develop_vaccines_in_space.html.

Koppelman, Alex. "Glenn Beck Flirts with Sanity." *Salon*, October 8, 2009. http://www.salon.com/2009/10/08/beck/

Krauthammer, Charles. "Smallpox Shots: Make Them Mandatory." *Time*, December 23, 2002, 84.

Laing, R. D. *The Divided Self: A Study of Sanity and Madness*. London: Tavistock, 1960.

Lapidos, Juliet. "The AIDS Conspiracy Handbook." *Slate*, March 19, 2008. http://www.slate.com/articles/news_and_politics/explainer/2008/03/the_aids_conspiracy_handbook.html.

——. "How Do You Diagnose Autism?" *Slate*, July 22, 2008. http://www.slate.com/articles/news_and_politics/explainer/2008/07/how_do_you_diagnose_autism.html.

Largent, Mark A. *Vaccine: The Debate in Modern America*. Baltimore: Johns Hopkins University Press, 2012.

Larson, Heidi. "Some Mercury Is Good for You." *Slate*, January 18, 2013. http://www.slate.com/articles/health_and_science/new_scientist/2013/01/mercury_treaty_debate_should_thimerosal_be_banned_as_a_vaccine_preservative.html.

Lauro, Sarah J. *Transatlantic Zombie: Slavery, Rebellion, and Living Death*. New Brunswick, NJ: Rutgers University Press, 2015.

Lawrence, Francis, dir. *I Am Legend*. Burbank, CA: Warner Bros. Pictures, 2007.

Lawrence, Heidi Y., Bernice L. Hausman, and Clare J. Dannenburg. "Reframing Medicine's Publics: The Local as a Public of Vaccine Refusal." *Journal of Medical Humanities* 35, no. 2 (2014): 111–29. doi:10.1007/s10912-014-9278-4.

Leach, Melissa, and James Fairhead. *Vaccine Anxieties: Global Science, Child Health, and Society*. Sterling, VA: Earthscan, 2007.

Lieu, Tracey A., Stephen L. Cochi, Steven B. Black, M. Elizabeth Halloran, Henry R. Shinefield, Sandra J. Holmes, Melinda Wharton, and A. Eugene Washington. "Cost-Effectiveness of a Routine Varicella Vaccination Program for US Children." *JAMA* 271, no. 5 (1994): 375–81.

Lipinski, Jed. "Endangering the Herd." *Slate*, February 2, 2015. http://www.slate.com/articles/news_and_politics/jurisprudence/2013/08/anti_vaxxers_why_parents_who_don_t_vaccinate_their_kids_should_be_sued_or.html.

Lipstadt, Deborah E. *Denying the Holocaust: The Growing Assault on Truth and Memory*. New York: Plume, 1994.

Lloyd, Carol. "Autism Debate, Take 5,832." *Salon*, September 27, 2007. http://www.salon.com/2007/09/27/autism/.

———. "How Safe Is the HPV Vaccine?" *Salon*, April 20, 2007. http://www.salon. com/2007/04/20/hpv/.

Luckhurst, Roger. *Zombies: A Cultural History*. London: Reaktion Books, 2015.

Maberry, Jonathan. *Dead of Night*. New York: St. Martin's Griffin, 2014.

Macphail, Theresa. "WebMD Knows Best?" *Slate*, March 3, 2015. http://www.slate. com/articles/technology/future_tense/2015/03/webmd_and_self_diagnosis_how_the_ internet_is_changing_medical_decisions.html.

Mandel, Emily St. John. *Station Eleven*. New York: Vintage, 2014.

Mangold, James, dir. *Girl, Interrupted*. Columbia Pictures, 2000.

Marmagas, Susan, Clare Dannenberg, Francois Elvinger, Bernice L. Hausman, Elizabeth Anthony, Stacy Boyer, Lauren Fortenberry, and Heidi Y. Lawrence. "Cumberland Plateau Health District 2009–2010 Flu Season Vaccine Study Final Report." *Vaccination Research Group*, 2011. www.vaccination.english.vt.edu/publications.html.

Martin, Emily. "The Pharmaceutical Person." *Biosocieties* 1, no. 3 (September 2006): 273–87.

Martin, Jessica. "The Flu Vaccine Is Safer than We Knew." *Slate*, January 22, 2014. http://www.slate.com/articles/health_and_science/medical_examiner/2014/01/flu_ vaccine_is_safe_for_people_with_egg_allergies_why_i_vaccinated_my_child.html.

Matheson, Richard. *I Am Legend*. New York: Gold Medal Books, 1954.

McDonell, Keelin. "How to Make an Avian-Flu Vaccine." *Slate*, August 10, 2005. http://www.slate.com/articles/news_and_politics/todays_papers/2005/08/entangled_ subplots.html.

Meldrum, Marcia. "'A Calculated Risk': The Salk Polio Vaccine Trials." *BMJ* 317 (1998): 1233–36.

Mendelsohn, Robert S. *Confessions of a Medical Heretic*. Chicago: Contemporary Books, 1979.

———. *How to Raise a Healthy Child in Spite of Your Doctor*. New York: Ballantine, 1987.

———. *Male Practice: How Doctors Manipulate Women*. Chicago: Contemporary Books, 1982.

Metzl, Jonathan M., and Anna Kirkland, eds. *Against Health: How Health Became the New Morality*. New York: New York University Press, 2010.

Michigan Department of Health and Human Services. "Immunization Waiver Information." http://www.michigan.gov/mdhhs/0,5885,7-339-73971_4911_4914_68361- 344843—,00.html.

Mieszkowski, Katharine. "Amanda Peet Gets Her Shot On." *Salon*, July 15, 2008. http://www.salon.com/2008/07/15/amanda_peet/.

Miller, Laura. "What Are the Odds?" *Slate*, August 31, 2015. http://www.slate.com/ articles/life/classes/2015/08/take_a_statistics_and_probability_class_in_college_to_ improve_critical_thinking.html.

Mitcham, Carl. "The Challenges of This Collection." In *The Challenges of Ivan Illich*, edited by Lee Hoinacki and Carl Mitcham, 9–32. Albany: State University of New York Press, 2002.

Mitchell, Lesli. "Secrets and Lies." *Salon*, August 2, 2000. http://www.salon.com/ 2000/08/02/autism/.

Mnookin, Seth. *The Panic Virus: A True Story of Medicine, Science, and Fear*. New York: Simon & Schuster, 2011.

Mooney, Chris, and Michael Specter. "Denialism." *Slate*, November 5, 2009. http://www.slate.com/articles/arts/the_book_club/features/2009/denialism/are_we_anti science_or_are_we_inconsistent.html.

Morozov, Evgeny. "Warning: This Site Contains Conspiracy Theories." *Slate*, January 23, 2012. http://www.slate.com/articles/technology/future_tense/2012/01/anti_vaccine_ activists_9_11_deniers_and_google_s_social_search_.html.

Moyer, Melinda Wenner. "Does Breast-Feeding Protect My Baby from Measles?" *Slate*, February 10, 2015. http://www.slate.com/articles/double_x/the_kids/2015/02/measles_ and_infants_advice_for_parents_of_unvaccinated_babies.html.

——. "Does My Toddler Have Autism?" *Slate*, May 23, 2013. http://www.slate.com/articles/double_x/the_kids/2013/05/does_my_child_have_autism_how_to_identify_ the_disorder_s_early_signs.html.

——. "What to Do If You Get Invited to a Chickenpox Party." *Slate*, November 15, 2013. http://www.slate.com/articles/double_x/the_kids/2013/11/chickenpox_vaccine_ is_it_really_necessary.html.

"Mystery of the Forgotten Plague." *BBC News*, July 27, 2004. http://news.bbc.co.uk/2/ hi/health/3930727.stm.

National Immunization Survey (NIS)—Children (19–35 months), Centers for Disease Control and Prevention. CDC.gov. https://www.cdc.gov/vaccines/imz-managers/ coverage/nis/child/index.html.

National Vaccine Information Center. "Is the Childhood Vaccine Schedule Safe?" NVIC.org. http://www.nvic.org/NVIC-Vaccine-News/October-2017/is-the-childhood-vaccine-schedule-safe.aspx.

Nattrass, Nicoli. *The AIDS Conspiracy: Science Fights Back*. New York: Columbia University Press, 2012.

"The *New Yorker* Replies." *Slate*, October 28, 2000. http://www.slate.com/articles/ briefing/articles/2000/10/the_new_yorker_replies.html.

Nienhiser, Jill. "Dietary Guidelines." *The Weston A. Price Foundation*, January 1, 2000. https://www.westonaprice.org/health-topics/abcs-of-nutrition/dietary-guidelines/.

Noah, Timothy. "The Swine Last Time." *Slate*, April 28, 2009. http://www.slate.com/ articles/news_and_politics/chatterbox/2009/04/the_swine_last_time.html.

——. "Vaccine Hogs, Part 3." *Slate*, October 23, 2004. http://www.slate.com/articles/ news_and_politics/chatterbox/2004/10/vaccine_hogs_part_3.html.

——. "Vaccine Hogs, Part 4." *Slate*, October 25, 2004. http://www.slate.com/articles/ news_and_politics/chatterbox/2004/10/vaccine_hogs_part_4.html.

——. "Voulez Vous le Smallpox?" *Slate*, November 5, 2002. http://www.slate.com/ articles/news_and_politics/chatterbox/2002/11/voulez_vous_le_smallpox.html.

Nyhan, Brendan, Jason Reifler, Sean Richey, and Gay L. Freed. "Effective Messages in Vaccine Promotion: A Randomized Trial." *Pediatrics* 133, no. 4 (April 2014): 1–9.

O'Connell, Mark. "Vaccine as Metaphor." *Slate*, October 9, 2014. http://www.slate. com/articles/arts/books/2014/10/on_immunity_an_inoculation_reviewed_eula_biss_ book_explores_fear_of_vaccines.html.

Offit, Paul A. *Bad Faith: When Religious Belief Undermines Modern Medicine*. New York: Basic Books, 2015.

———. *Deadly Choices: How the Anti-vaccine Movement Threatens Us All.* New York: Basic Books, 2012.

Ohneck, Elizabeth. "The Discovery of HIV: A Tale of Two Scientists." *Scizzle,* June 6, 2014. http://www.myscizzle.com/blog/hiv-discovery-controversy/.

Omer, Saad B., William K. Y. Pan, Neal A. Halsey, Shannon Stokley, Lawrence H. Moulton, Ann Marie Navar, Mathew Pierce, and Daniel A. Salmon. "Nonmedical Exemptions to School Immunization Requirements." *JAMA* 296, no. 14 (October 11, 2006): 1757–63. doi:10.1001/jama.296.14.1757.

Oreskes, Naomi, and Erik M. Conway. *Merchants of Doubt: How a Handful of Scientists Obscured the Truth on Issues from Tobacco Smoke to Global Warming.* London: Bloomsbury Press, 2010.

Orndorff, Travertine. "Vaccination Reporting in *Mother Jones.*" *Vaccination Research Group,* Spring 2015. http://www.vaccination.english.vt.edu/wp-content/up loads/2015/06/Orndorff_Mother-Jones.pdf.

O'Rourke, Meghan. "Cancer Sluts." *Slate,* September 27, 2007. http://www.slate.com/articles/life/the_sex_issue/2007/09/cancer_sluts.html.

Oshinsky, David M. *Polio: An American Story.* Oxford: Oxford University Press, 2006.

Parikh, Rahul K. "Doc Hollywood." *Slate,* December 9, 2009. http://www.slate.com/articles/health_and_science/medical_examiner/2009/12/doc_hollywood.html.

———. "Inside the Vaccine-and-Autism Scare." *Salon,* September 22, 2008. http://www.salon.com/2008/09/22/autism_2/.

Park, Alice. "How Safe Are Vaccines?" *Time,* June 2, 2008, 36–41.

Parker, Amy. "Growing Up Unvaccinated." *Slate,* January 6, 2014. http://www.slate.com/articles/life/family/2014/01/growing_up_unvaccinated_a_healthy_lifestyle_couldn_t_prevent_many_childhood.html.

Peterson, Wolfgang, dir. *Outbreak.* Burbank, CA: Warner Bros. Pictures, 1995.

Pew Research Center. "83% Say Measles Vaccine Is Safe for Healthy Children." *Pew Research Center,* February 9, 2015. http://www.people-press.org/2015/02/09/83-percent-say-measles-vaccine-is-safe-for-healthy-children/.

Pitzer, Andrea. "Why Is It So Tough to Get a Flu Vaccine?" *Slate,* January 10, 2013. http://www.slate.com/articles/health_and_science/medical_examiner/2013/01/flu_vaccine_shortage_cdc_and_fda_have_plans_for_a_crisis_but_in_january.html.

Plait, Phil. "Chili's Reception: Restaurant Cancels Event with Anti-Vax Group." *Slate,* April 9, 2014. http://www.slate.com/articles/life/family/2014/03/measles_outbreak_in_new_york_city_should_pediatricians_treat_unvaccinated.html.

———. "*The Daily Show* and the Anti-Vaxxers." *Slate,* June 4, 2014. http://www.slate.com/blogs/bad_astronomy/2014/06/04/anti_vaxxers_the_daily_show_mocks_anti_science.html.

———. "Jenny McCarthy Asks; the Internet Slam Dunks." *Slate,* March 17, 2014. http://www.slate.com/blogs/bad_astronomy/2014/03/17/jenny_mccarthy_antivaxxer_gets_remedied_on_twitter.html.

———. "Should Public Schools Have Mandatory Vaccinations for Students?" *Slate,* February 26, 2014. http://www.slate.com/blogs/bad_astronomy/2014/02/26/Colorado_vaccinations_making_it_harder_for_parents_to_opt_out.html.

——. "Unvaccinated People Cause a 20-Year High in U.S. Measles Cases." *Slate,* May 31, 2014. http://www.slate.com/blogs/bad_astronomy/2014/05/31/measles_2014_infection_rate_at_highest_levels_in_20_years.html.

Plamer, Brian. "What Do Pediatricians *Really* Think about Anti-Vaxxers?" *Slate,* February 5, 2015. http://www.slate.com/articles/health_and_science/medical_examiner/2015/02/how_do_pediatricians_work_with_anti_vaccine_parents_mds_frustrations_failures.html.

Politi, Daniel. "To Panic or Not to Panic." *Slate,* April 28, 2009. http://www.slate.com/articles/news_and_politics/todays_papers/2009/04/to_panic_or_not_to_panic.html.

Politi, Mary C., Katherine M. Jones, and Sydney E. Philpott. "The Role of Patient Engagement in Addressing Parents' Perceptions about Immunization." *JAMA* 318, no. 3 (July 18, 2017): 237–38. doi:10.1001/jama.2017.7168.

Poovey, Mary. *A History of the Modern Fact.* Chicago: University of Chicago Press, 1998.

Posner, Eric. "Why Are People So Scared of Syrian Refugees?" *Slate,* November 20, 2015. http://www.slate.com/articles/news_and_politics/view_from_chicago/2015/11/why_american_people_are_scared_of_syrian_refugees.html.

Preblud, Stephen R., Walter A. Orenstein, and Kenneth J. Bart. "Varicella: Clinical Manifestations, Epidemiology, and Health Impact on Children." *Pediatric Infectious Disease* 3, no. 6 (1984): 506.

"Preventing the Pox." *Time,* March 1, 2004, 78.

"Prevention of Varicella: Recommendations of the Advisory Committee on Immunization Practices (ACIP)." *MMWR Recommendations and Reports* 45, no. RR-11 (July 12, 1996): 1–36. https://www.cdc.gov/mmwr/preview/mmwrhtml/00042990.htm.

Rama, Padmananda. "Joining the Herd." *Slate,* February 19, 2015. http://www.slate.com/articles/health_and_science/medical_examiner/2015/02/adult_measles_vaccination_child_of_california_new_age_parents_joins_the.html.

Reich, Jennifer. *Calling the Shots: Why Parents Reject Vaccines.* New York: New York University Press, 2016.

Reisman, David, Reuel Denney, and Nathan Glazer. *The Lonely Crowd: A Study of Changing American Character.* New Haven, CT: Yale University Press, 1950.

Rho, Helena. "What's the Matter with Vermont?" *Slate,* February 21, 2013. http://www.slate.com/articles/health_and_science/medical_examiner/2013/02/pertussis_epidemic_how_vermont_s_anti_vaxxer_activists_stopped_a_vaccine.html.

Rockwell, Page. "Vaccinating Boys against HPV." *Salon,* July 31, 2006. https://www.salon.com/2006/07/31/boys_and_hpv_vaccine/.

Romero, George, dir. *Dawn of the Dead.* United Film Distribution Company, 1979.

——. *Night of the Living Dead.* Walter Reade Organization and Continental Distributing, 1968.

Rose, Nikolas. *The Politics of Life Itself: Biomedicine, Power, and Subjectivity in the Twenty-First Century.* Princeton, NJ: Princeton University Press, 2007.

Saletan, William. "Sexually Transmitted Injection." *Slate,* October 15, 2009. http://www.slate.com/articles/health_and_science/human_nature/2009/10/sexually_transmitted_injection.html.

——. "Unhealthy Fixation." *Slate,* July 15, 2015. http://www.slate.com/articles/health_and_science/science/2015/07/are_gmos_safe_yes_the_case_against_them_is_full_of_fraud_lies_and_errors.html.

Salk, Jonas E. "Vaccination against Paralytic Poliomyelitis Performance and Prospects." *American Journal of Public Health* 45, no. 5, pt. 1 (May 1, 1955): 575–96. doi:10.2105/AJPH.45.5_Pt_1.575.

Sanghavi, Darshak. "The Flu Vaccine Controversy." *Slate,* December 18, 2012. http://www.slate.com/articles/health_and_science/pandemics/2012/12/flu_vaccine_safety_tamiflu_and_vaccines_save_lives_and_show_public_health.html.

Sarno, David. "Running Out of Shots." *Slate,* April 17, 2005. http://www.slate.com/articles/news_and_politics/todays_papers/2005/04/running_out_of_shots.html.

Schaffer, Amanda. "Chastity, M.D." *Slate,* April 11, 2006. http://www.slate.com/articles/health_and_science/medical_examiner/2006/04/chastity_md.html.

——. "How to Superpower the Immune System." *Slate,* May 16, 2013. http://www.slate.com/articles/health_and_science/superman/2013/05/new_vaccines_and_immune_boosters_for_flu_cancer_newborns_the_elderly.html.

——. "Should You Go to the Drugstore for Your Flu Shots?" *Slate,* October 17, 2012. http://www.slate.com/articles/double_x/doublex/2012/10/vaccines_at_the_pharmacy_states_should_let_drugstores_give_shots.html.

——. "Sniffing Out Swine Flu." *Slate,* October 7, 2009. http://www.slate.com/articles/health_and_science/medical_examiner/2009/10/sniffing_out_swine_flu.html.

——. "Viral Effect." *Slate,* July 3, 2006. http://www.slate.com/articles/health_and_science/medical_examiner/2006/07/viral_effect.html.

——. "Why Are Babies Dying of Old-Fashioned Whooping Cough?" *Slate,* September 5, 2012. http://www.slate.com/articles/double_x/doublex/2012/09/why_babies_are_dying_of_whooping_cough_.html.

Scocca, Tom. "No One Is Immune." *Slate,* July 25, 2011. http://www.slate.com/articles/life/scocca/2011/07/no_one_is_immune.html.

Scott, Julia. "'The World Just Fell out from under Me.'" *Salon,* June 16, 2005. http://www.salon.com/2005/06/16/clark/.

Sears, Robert W. *The Vaccine Book: Making the Right Decision for Your Child.* 2nd ed. New York: Little, Brown and Company, 2011.

Sepkowitz, Kent. "Finally, a Selfish Reason to Get Boys Vaccinated for HPV." *Slate,* June 15, 2011. http://www.slate.com/articles/double_x/doublex/2011/06/finally_a_selfish_reason_to_get_boys_vaccinated_for_hpv.html.

Shafer, Jack. "Burying the Swine Flu Lede." *Slate,* September 12, 2009. http://www.slate.com/articles/news_and_politics/press_box/2009/09/burying_the_swine_flu_lede.html.

Shermer, Michael, and Alex Grobman. *Denying History: Who Says the Holocaust Never Happened and Why Do They Say It?* Berkeley: University of California Press, 2000.

Showalter, Elaine. *Hystories: Hysterical Epidemics and Modern Media.* New York: Columbia University Press, 1998.

Shtulman, Andrew. "In Public Understanding of Science, Alternative Facts Are the Norm." *NPR,* May 29, 2017. http://www.npr.org/sections/13.7/2017/05/29/527892222/in-public-understanding-of-science-alternative-facts-are-the-norm.

——. *scienceblind: Why Our Intuitive Theories about the World Are So Often Wrong.* New York: Basic Books, 2017.

Shuger, Scott. "Vaccine but Not Heard." *Slate,* March 11, 1999. LexisNexis Academic.

Shulevitz, Judith. "Is Anthropology Evil?" *Slate,* December 8, 2000. http://www.slate. com/articles/news_and_politics/culturebox/2000/12/is_anthropology_evil.html.

Siegel, Marc. "Blowing the Shot." *Slate,* November 2, 2009. http://www.slate.com/articles/ health_and_science/medical_examiner/2009/11/blowing_the_shot.html.

——. "Cabin Fever." *Slate,* July 10, 2009. http://www.slate.com/articles/health_and_ science/medical_examiner/2009/07/cabin_fever.html.

——. "Forget the Chicken and the Egg." *Slate,* February 7, 2006. http://www.slate.com/ articles/health_and_science/medical_examiner/2006/02/forget_the_chicken_and_ the_egg.html.

——. "WHO and the Flu." *Slate,* May 14, 2009. http://www.slate.com/articles/health_ and_science/medical_examiner/2009/05/who_and_the_flu.html.

Siva, Nayanah. "Wakefield's First Try." *Slate,* June 2, 2010. http://www.slate.com/articles/ health_and_science/medical_examiner/2010/06/wakefields_first_try.html.

Slade, B. A., L. Liedel, C. Vellozzi, E. J. Wool, W. Hua, A. Sutherland, H. S. Izurieta, R. Ball, N. Miller, M. M. Braun, L. E. Markowitz, and J. Iskander. "Postlicensure Safety Surveillance for Quadrivalent Human Papillomavirus Recombinant Vaccine." *JAMA* 302, no. 7 (August 19, 2009): 750–57. https://www.ncbi.nlm.nih.gov/ pubmed/19690307.

Smith, Michael J., Susan S. Ellenberg, Louis M. Bell, and David M. Rubin. "Media Coverage of the Measles-Mumps-Rubella Vaccine and Autism Controversy and Its Relationship to MMR Immunization Rates in the United States." *Pediatrics* 121, no. 4 (2008): e836–e843. doi:10.1542/peds.2007–1760.

Soderbergh, Steven, dir. *Contagion.* Burbank, CA: Warner Bros. Pictures, 2011.

Specter, Michael. *Denialism: How Irrational Thinking Hinders Scientific Progress, Harms the Planet, and Threatens Our Lives.* New York: Penguin, 2009.

Spiesel, Sydney. "The Doctor Is In." *Slate,* June 3, 2005. LexisNexis Academic.

——. "The Good News and Bad News about MS." *Slate,* October 31, 2008. http://www.slate.com/articles/health_and_science/whats_up_doc/2008/10/the_ good_news_and_bad_news_about_ms.html.

——. "I'm a Pediatrician. Should I Treat All Kids, or Just the Vaccinated Ones?" *Slate,* March 18, 2014. http://www.slate.com/articles/life/family/2014/03/measles_outbreak_ in_new_york_city_should_pediatricians_treat_unvaccinated.html.

——. "A Shot in the Dark." *Slate,* March 15, 2005. http://www.slate.com/articles/ health_and_science/medical_examiner/2005/03/a_shot_in_the_dark.html.

——. "Shots All Around!" *Slate,* November 19, 2008. http://www.slate.com/articles/ health_and_science/whats_up_doc/2008/11/shots_all_around.html.

——. "What Happened to Avian Flu?" *Slate,* April 28, 2009. http://www.slate.com/articles/ health_and_science/medical_examiner/2009/04/what_happened_to_avian_flu.html.

Stanchak, Jesse. "Entangled Sub-Plots." *Slate,* August 7, 2005. http://www.slate.com/ articles/news_and_politics/todays_papers/2005/08/entangled_subplots.html.

"State Information." *Immunization Action Coalition.* Updated February 17, 2017. http://www.immunize.org/laws/varicella.asp.

Steenhuysen, Julie. "U.S. Vaccination Rates High, but Pockets of Unvaccinated Pose Risk." *Reuters,* August 27, 2015. http://www.reuters.com/article/us-usa-vaccine-exemptions/u-s-vaccination-rates-high-but-pockets-of-unvaccinated-pose-risk-idUSKCN0QW2JY20150827.

Stern, Mark Joseph. "The Worst Pandemic in History." *Slate,* December 26, 2012. http://www.slate.com/articles/health_and_science/pandemics/2012/12/spanish_flu_mystery_why_don_t_scientists_understand_the_1918_flu_even_after.html.

Stevens, Dana. "I Am Legend." *Slate,* December 13, 2007. http://www.slate.com/articles/arts/movies/2007/12/i_am_legend.html.

Stoker, Bram. *Dracula.* London: Archibald Constable and Company, 1897.

Stone, Robert. "Orthodox Environmentalists Don't Want You to See My Environmental Film." *Slate,* June 20, 2013. http://www.slate.com/articles/health_and_science/science/2013/06/pandora_s_promise_producer_nuclear_energy_is_necessary_to_fight_climate.html.

Sung-su, Kim, dir. *Flu.* Seoul: CJ Entertainment, 2013.

"Swine Flu." *Slate,* April 27, 2009. http://www.slate.com/articles/health_and_science/science/2009/04/swine_flu.html.

Szasz, Thomas. *The Myth of Mental Illness.* New York: Harper and Row, 1974.

Tatel, Stephanie. "A Pox on You." *Slate,* October 20, 2009. http://www.slate.com/articles/health_and_science/medical_examiner/2009/10/a_pox_on_you.html.

Thompson, James F. "The Rise of the Zombie in Popular Culture." In *. . . But If a Zombie Apocalypse* Did *Occur: Essays on Medical, Military, Governmental, Ethical, Economic, and Other Implications,* edited by Amy L. Thompson and Antonio S. Thompson, 11–25. Jefferson, NC: McFarland, 2015.

Thompson, Lea, prod. *DPT: Vaccine Roulette.* Washington, DC: WRC-TV, 1982.

Tierney, Patrick. *Darkness in El Dorado: How Scientists and Journalists Devastated the Amazon.* New York: Norton, 2002.

——. "The Fierce Anthropologist." *New Yorker,* October 9, 2000. https://www.newyorker.com/magazine/2000/10/09/the-fierce-anthropologist-2.

"Timeline: The Rise and Fall of Vioxx." *NPR,* November 10, 2007. http://www.npr.org/templates/story/story.php?storyId=5470430.

Tooby, John. "Jungle Fever." *Slate,* October 25, 2000. http://www.slate.com/articles/news_and_politics/hey_wait_a_minute/2000/10/jungle_fever.html.

Treichler, Paula. *How to Have Theory in an Epidemic: Cultural Chronicles of AIDS.* Durham, NC: Duke University Press, 1999.

Tsai, Michelle. "Fix the Flu Shot." *Slate,* February 22, 2008. http://www.slate.com/articles/news_and_politics/explainer/2008/02/fix_the_flu_shot.html.

——. "Why Isn't There a Cure-All Influenza Vaccine?" *Slate,* April 27, 2009. http://www.slate.com/articles/news_and_politics/recycled/2009/04/why_isnt_there_a_cureall_influenza_vaccine.html.

Umansky, Eric. "Doc Block." *Slate,* April 2, 2004. LexisNexis Academic.

Vaccination Education Center, Children's Hospital of Philadelphia. "A Look at Each Vaccine: Rotavirus Vaccine." CHOP.edu. Accessed October 1, 2017. http://www.chop.edu/centers-programs/vaccine-education-center/vaccine-details/rotavirus-vaccine.

——. "Vaccine Safety: Are Vaccines Safe?" CHOP.edu. Accessed February 1, 2018. http://www.chop.edu/centers-programs/vaccine-education-center/vaccine-safety/are-vaccines-safe.

Wadman, Meredith. *The Vaccine Race: Science, Politics, and the Human Costs of Defeating Disease.* New York: Viking, 2017.

Wakefield, Andrew, S. H. Murch, A. Anthony, J. Linell, D. M. Casson, M. Malik, M. Berelowitz, A. P. Dhillon, M. A. Thomson, P. Harvey, A. Valentine, S. E. Davies, and J. A. Walker Smith. "Retracted: Ileal-Lymphoid-Nodular Hyperplasia, Non-Specific Colitis, and Pervasive Developmental Disorder in Children." *Lancet* 351, no. 9103 (February 1998): 637–41. https://doi.org/10.1016/S0140-6736(97)11096-0.

Weigel, David. "Political Inoculation." *Slate,* September 13, 2011. http://www.slate.com/articles/news_and_politics/politics/2011/09/political_inoculation.html.

Welch, H. Gilbert, Lisa Schwartz, and Steve Woloshin. *Overdiagnosed: Making People Sick in the Pursuit of Health.* Boston: Beacon Press, 2012.

Wickman, Forrest. "Steven Soderbergh's Contagion." *Slate,* September 9, 2011. http://www.slate.com/articles/arts/movies/2011/09/steven_soderberghs_contagion.html.

Wilford, John Noble. "Book Leads Anthropologists to Look Inward." *New York Times,* November 18, 2000. http://www.nytimes.com/2000/11/18/us/book-leads-anthropologists-to-look-inward.html?mcubz=0.

Williams, Mary Elizabeth. "Jenny McCarthy's Autism Fight Grows More Misguided." *Salon,* January 6, 2011. http://www.salon.com/2011/01/06/jenny_mccarthy_autism_debate/.

——. "My Twitter Battle over Vaccination." *Salon,* July 21, 2011. http://www.salon.com/2011/07/21/vaccination_twitter_battle/.

——. "A 'Sex Jab' Didn't Kill Natalie Morton." *Salon,* October 1, 2009. http://www.salon.com/2009/10/01/hpv_vaccine/.

——. "A Sexually Transmitted Virus That's Nothing to Be Ashamed About." *Salon,* September 16, 2011. http://www.salon.com/2011/09/16/hpv_ayelet_waldman_michele_bachmann/.

Williams, Simon, and Michael Calnan. "The 'Limits' of Medicalization? Modern Medicine and the Lay Populace in 'Late' Modernity." *Social Science & Medicine* 42, no. 12 (June 1996): 1609–20.

Willrich, Michael. *Pox: An American History.* New York: Penguin, 2011.

Wilson, Chris. "How Does a Pandemic Ever End?" *Slate,* April 27, 2009. http://www.slate.com/articles/news_and_politics/explainer/2009/04/how_does_a_pandemic_ever_end.html.

Woodruff, Betsy. "The Danger of Reading the Comments." *Slate,* January 27, 2015. http://www.slate.com/articles/health_and_science/medical_examiner/2015/01/internet_comment_credibility_study_vaccine_decisions_influenced_by_online.html.

Woolf, Virginia. *On Being Ill.* Ashfield, MA: Paris Press, 2002.

——. *A Room of One's Own.* New York: Harcourt, Brace, 1929.

——. *Three Guineas.* San Diego: Harcourt, Brace, 1938.

World Health Organization. "About WHO." WHO.int. http://www.who.int/about/mission/en.

Yoffe, Emily. "Deserves a Shot." *Slate,* March 10, 2015. http://www.slate.com/articles/life/
dear_prudence/2015/03/dear_prudence_should_i_secretly_vaccinate_my_grandson.
html.

———. "Gut Shot." *Slate,* November 13, 2014. http://www.slate.com/articles/life/dear_
prudence/2014/11/dear_prudence_our_midwives_are_anti_vaccination_activists_
should_we_fire.html.

Zalewski, Daniel. "Ideas & Trends; Anthropology Enters the Age of Cannibalism."
New York Times, October 8, 2000. http://www.nytimes.com/2000/10/08/weekinre
view/ideas-trends-anthropology-enters-the-age-of-cannibalism.html?mcubz=0.

Zipprich, Jennifer, Kathleen Winter, Jill Hacker, Dongxiang Xia, James Watt, and Kathleen Harriman. "Measles Outbreak—California, December 2014–February 2015."
Morbidity and Mortality Weekly Report 64, no. 6 (February 20, 2015): 153–54.
https://www.cdc.gov/mmwr/preview/mmwrhtml/mm6406a5.htm.

Zola, Irving Kenneth. "Medicine as an Institution of Social Control." In *The Cultural
Crisis of Modern Medicine,* edited by John Ehrenreich, 80–100. New York: Monthly
Review Press, 1978.

Zuger, Abigail. "Defending Vaccination Once Again, with Feeling." *New York Times,*
March 29, 2011.

INDEX

Page numbers in *italics* indicate tabular material. Nonfiction works cited appear under the author's name; fictional texts are listed by title.